# DENTAL ADMISSION TEST

*by THE ARCO EDITORIAL BOARD*

arco  219 Park Avenue South
New York, N.Y. 10003

Sixth Edition, B-2082
Third Printing, 1976

Published by Arco Publishing Company, Inc.
219 Park Avenue South, New York, N. Y. 10003

Library of Congress Catalog Card Number  72-94812
ISBN  0-668-01065-7


Printed in the United States of America

# CONTENTS

HOW TO USE THIS INDEX
Slightly bend the right-hand edge
of the book. This will expose
the corresponding Parts
which match the index, below.

PART ONE

## THREE PREDICTIVE PRACTICE EXAMINATIONS

BIOMEDICAL SCIENCE      SENTENCE COMPLETIONS

INTERPRETATION OF SCIENCE READINGS      QUANTITATIVE ABILITY

VOCABULARY      PERCEPTUAL MOTOR ABILITY

VERBAL ANALOGIES

PART

1

2

3

4

...continued on next page

# CONTENTS continued

**PART**

**1**

**2**

**3**

**4**

## PART FOUR
### PERCEPTUAL MOTOR ABILITY
### FINAL MODEL EXAM AND SOME FINAL ADVICE

...continued on next page

# CONTENTS continued

# WHAT THIS BOOK WILL DO FOR YOU

*To get the greatest help from this book, please understand that it has been carefully organized. You must, therefore, plan to use it accordingly. Study this concise, readable book earnestly and your way will be clear. You will progress directly to your goal. You will not be led off into blind alleys and useless fields of study.*

Arco Publishing Company has followed testing trends and methods ever since the firm was founded in 1937. We have specialized in books that prepare people for tests. Based on this experience it is our modest boast that you probably have in your hands the best book that could be prepared to help *you* score high. Now, if you'll take a little advice on using it properly, we can assure you that you will do well.

To write this book we carefully analyzed every detail surrounding the forthcoming examination . . .

* the job itself

* official and unofficial announcements concerning the examination

* all the available previous examinations

* many related examinations

* technical literature that explains and forecasts the examination.

As a result of all this (which you, happily, have not had to do) we've been able to create the "climate" of your test, and to give you a fairly accurate picture of what's involved. Some of this material, digested and simplified, actually appears in print

here, if it was deemed useful and suitable in helping you score high.

But more important than any other benefit derived from this research is our certainty that the study material, the text and the practice questions are right for you.

The practice questions you will study have been judiciously selected from hundreds of thousands of previous test questions on file here at Arco. But they haven't just been thrown at you pell mell. They've been organized into the subjects that you can expect to find on your test. As you answer the questions, these subjects will take on greater meaning for you. At the same time you will be getting valuable practice in answering test questions. You will proceed with a sure step toward a worthwhile goal: high test marks.

Studying in this manner, you will get the feel of the entire examination. You will learn by "insight," by seeing through a problem as a result of experiencing *previous similar situations*. This is true learning according to many psychologists.

In short, what you get from this book will help you operate at top efficiency . . . make you give the best possible account of yourself on the actual examination.

## CAN YOU PREPARE YOURSELF FOR YOUR TEST?

We believe, most certainly, that you *can* with the aid of this "self-tutor!"

It's not a "pony." It's not a complete college education. It's not a "crib sheet," and it's no HOW TO SUCCEED ON TESTS WITHOUT REALLY TRYING. There's nothing in it that will give you a higher score than you really deserve.

It's just a top quality course which you can readily review in less than twenty hours . . . a digest of material which you might easily have written yourself after about five thousand hours of laborious digging.

To really prepare for your test you must motivate yourself . . . get into the right frame of mind for learning from your "self-tutor." You'll have to urge *yourself* to learn and that's the only way people ever learn. Your efforts to score high on the test will be greatly aided by the fact that you will have to do this job on your own . . . perhaps without a teacher. Psychologists have demonstrated that studies undertaken for a clear goal . . . which you initiate yourself and actively pursue . . . are the most successful. You, yourself, want to pass this test. That's why you bought this book and embarked on this program. Nobody forced you to do it, and there may be nobody to lead you through the course. Your self-activity is going to be the key to your success in the forthcoming weeks.

Used correctly, your "self-tutor" will show you what to expect and will give you a speedy brush-up on the subjects peculiar to your exam. Some of these are subjects not taught in schools at all. Even if your study time is very limited, you should:

- Become familiar with the type of examination you will meet.

- Improve your general examination-taking skill.

- Improve your skill in analyzing and answering questions involving reasoning, judgment, comparison, and evaluation.

- Improve your speed and skill in reading and understanding what you read—an important part of your ability to learn and an important part of most tests.

- Prepare yourself in the particular fields which measure your learning—
    Vocabulary
    Problem solving
    Mathematics
    Arithmetic

This book will tell you exactly what to study by presenting in full every type of question you will get on the actual test. You'll do better merely by familiarizing yourself with them.

This book will help you find your weaknesses and find them fast. Once you know where you're weak you can get right to work (before the test) and concentrate your efforts on those soft spots. This is the kind of selective study which yields maximum test results for every hour spent.

This book will give you the *feel* of the exam. Almost all our sample and practice questions are taken from actual previous exams. Since previous exams are not always available for inspection by the public, these sample test questions are quite important for you. The day you take your exam you'll see how closely this book follows the format of the real test.

This book will give you confidence *now*, while you are preparing for the test. It will build your self-confidence as you proceed. It will beat those dreaded before-test jitters that have hurt so many other test-takers.

This book stresses the modern, multiple-choice type of question because that's the kind you'll undoubtedly get on your test. In answering these questions you will add to your knowledge by learning the correct answers, naturally. However, you will not be satisfied with merely the correct choice for each question. You will want to find out why the other choices are incorrect. This will jog your memory . . . help you remember much you thought you had forgotten. You'll be preparing and enriching yourself for the exam to come.

Of course, the great advantage in all this lies in narrowing your study to just those fields in which you're most likely to be quizzed. Answer enough questions in those fields and the chances are very good that you'll meet a few of them again on the actual test. After all, the number of questions an examiner can draw upon in these fields is rather limited. Examiners frequently employ the same questions on different tests for this very reason.

Probably the most important element of tests which you can learn is vocabulary. Most testers consider your vocabulary range an important indication of what you have learned in your life, and therefore, an important measuring rod of your learning ability. With some concentration and systematic study, you can increase your vocabulary substantially and thus increase your score on most tests.

After testing yourself, you may find that your reading ability is poor. It may be wise to take the proper remedial measures now.

If you find that your reasoning ability or your ability to handle mathematical problems is weak, there are ways of improving your skill in these fields.

There are other things which you should know and which various sections of this book will help you learn. Most important, not only for this examination but for all the examinations to come in your life, is learning how to take a test and how to prepare for it.

# WHAT YOU SHOULD KNOW ABOUT THE DENTAL ADMISSION TEST

## THE PURPOSE OF THE DENTAL ADMISSION TEST

The Dental Aptitude Test is under the direction of the Council on Dental Education of the American Dental Association in cooperation with the American Association of Dental Schools. The test is given to applicants who are seeking admission to any dental school. The DAT predicts, with great accuracy, the probable success that students will experience in dental schools. Because of the success of the Dental Aptitude Testing Program, all dental schools are presently cooperating in this Program which is nationwide.

## HOW IMPORTANT IS THE DAT* FOR DENTAL SCHOOL ADMISSION?

You should be aware of the fact that the results of the DAT will not be the sole factor in determining whether you will be admitted to a dental school. Other considerations come into play . . . your undergraduate scholastic record, standing in your graduating class, grades in certain specific subjects, the personal interview, etc. It is obvious, however, that doing well in the DAT will increase your chances substantially of being accepted by the Dental School of your choice.

The Dental Aptitude Test is a world-wide test. The Council on Dental Education of the American Dental Association, which administers the test, will release scores only to authorized dental institutions. The scores are not available to applicants. One phase of the score is your percentile ranking. The latter tells how many test-takers did better than you and how many were inferior. It is reasonable, therefore, that the admissions officer will consider very seriously your standing on the DAT to determine how well you are likely to do in dental school.

With the steady increase of student enrollment in dental schools throughout the country, some of these institutions are now "bursting at the seams." These schools of advanced learning are, accordingly, becoming more and more selective in student admission. Since undergraduate schools have varying standards of grading, it is understandable that college marks alone will not suffice in the effort to appraise objectively the ability of an undergraduate to do graduate work. An "A" in a course of "Shakespeare's Tragedies" in College X may be worth a "C" in College Y. Moreover, it is an accepted fact that even the professors within a college may differ among themselves in grading techniques. The DAT is highly objective. Consequently, it has become sine qua non for many dental school admissions officers in order to predict success or lack of success for applicants.

## NATURE OF THE TEST

The Dental Aptitude Test is designed to give the dental schools information concerning your educational background and general scholastic ability. It is not an intelligence test nor is it, in the strict sense, an achievement test. Included in the test are questions in these categories:

MORNING SESSION
    CARVING DEXTERITY
    READING COMPREHENSION
    PERCEPTUAL MOTOR ABILITY

AFTERNOON SESSION
    SENTENCE COMPLETIONS
    ARITHMETIC (Computations & Problems)
    VOCABULARY
    SCIENCE (Biology & Chemistry)

The test allows a total working time of approximately five hours, plus time to collect and check test-books, to answer questions, and to allow for a rest period.

## HOW QUESTIONS ARE TO BE ANSWERED

The following will help you become familiar with the way in which answers are to be recorded.

30.  Chicago is a
    (A) state            (B) city
    (C) country          (D) town
            (E) village.

*Sample Answer Spaces:*

A B C D E

30 || ▉ || || ||

Note that the letters of the suggested answers appear on the answer sheet and that *you are to blacken the sphere beneath the letter of the answer you wish to give.* The multiple choice questions on the actual test may consist of 4 or 5 choices: A, B, C, D (E).

## HOW TO PREPARE FOR THE TEST

Let us sound a warning at the very start of this discussion of "How to Prepare for the Test." Do not wait till a week or even a month before the examination, in starting your preparation for it. Cramming will do little for you.

Be systematic. First, take the sample Dental Aptitude Test. Analyze the results. You should, thereby, get a fairly good idea of your areas of strength and your areas of weakness. Then concentrate on fortifying yourself where you are weak. Work hard with questions in those fields where the Sample Test has spotlighted initial "softness." Work, work, work in these areas. You will fare considerably better in the DAT by following this simple procedure.

## HOW TO TAKE THE TEST

There is no reason to become disturbed if you find that you are unable to answer a number of questions in a test or if you are unable to finish. No one is expected to get a perfect score, and there are no established "passing" or "failing" grades. Your score compares your performance with that of other candidates taking the test, and the report to the dental school shows the relation of your score to the scores obtained by other candidates.

Although the test stresses accuracy more than speed, it is important for you to use your time as economically as possible. Work steadily and as rapidly as you can without becoming careless. Take the questions in order, but do not waste time in pondering over questions which contain extremely difficult or unfamiliar material.

In each section of a test you should read the directions with care. If you read too hastily, you may miss an important direction and thus lose credit for an entire section.

### Should You Guess?

Many candidates wonder whether or not to mark the answers to questions about which they are not certain. Your score will be based on the number of questions you answer correctly. No deduction will be made for wrong answers. You are advised to use your time effectively and to mark the best answer you can to every question, regardless of how sure you are of the answer you mark. However, do not waste your time on questions that are too difficult for you. Go on to the other questions and come back to the difficult ones later if you have time.

## SAMPLE TEST QUESTIONS

You will find a complete treatment of the sections that make up the Morning and Afternoon Session Tests in Chapter Three of this book. In these pages you have many examples of each of the types of DAT questions which are given on the actual test. Answer keys are provided in every case.

Samples of some of the questions that customarily appear in the DAT are illustrated below.

### Verbal Analogies

Directions: Each of the CAPITALIZED words have a certain relationship to each other. Select the pair of words which are related in the same way.

1. CONDONE : OFFENSE ::
   (A) punish : criminal
   (B) mitigate : penitence
   (C) overlook : abberation
   (D) mistake : judgment

2. PROTOPLASM : CELL ::
   (A) chain : link
   (B) fibre : plastic
   (C) coin : money
   (D) chemistry : elements

3. OXYGEN : GASEOUS ::
   (A) feather : light
   (B) mercury : fluid
   (C) iron : heavy
   (D) sand : grainy

ANSWERS

1. C 2. A 3. B

## Sentence Completions

*Directions:* Each of the sentences below has one or more blank spaces, each blank indicating that a word has been omitted. You are to choose the one word or set of words which, when inserted in the sentence, *best fits* in with the meaning of the sentence as a whole.

1. The progressive yearly _____ of the land, caused by the depositing of mud from the river, makes it possible to estimate the age of excavated remains by noting the depth at which they are found below the present level of the valley.
   (A) erosion  (B) elevation
   (C) improvement  (D) irrigation
   (E) displacement

2. It is a mistake to _____ the beliefs of an entire people from the _____ of a few representatives.
   (A) deduce - actions
   (B) influence - appointment
   (C) question - success
   (D) glorify - failures
   (E) criticize - abilities

### Answers

1. B    2. A

## Vocabulary

*Directions:* Select the word (or words) in each group nearest in meaning to the word in capitals. Then, on the answer sheet, blacken the space beneath the letter corresponding to the letter of the answer you have chosen.

1. ABNEGATION
   (A) renunciation
   (B) failure to conform to rule
   (C) utter humiliation
   (D) sudden departure
   (E) confirmation

2. XENOPHOBIC
   (A) susceptible to disease
   (B) opposed to gambling
   (C) hating or fearing strangers
   (D) hating or fearful of dogs
   (E) philosophic

3. SPUME
   (A) flood  (B) froth
   (C) fountain  (D) spillway in a dam
   (E) fume

### Answers

1. A    2. C    3. B

## Reading Comprehension

*Directions:* At the right of the passage below, you will find three incomplete statements about the passage. Each statement is followed by five words or expressions. Select the word or expression that most satisfactorily completes each statement in accordance with the meaning of the passage. Then, on the answer sheet, blacken the space beneath the letter corresponding to the letter of the answer you have chosen.

The teacher lives in what has happened to the minds of his students, and in what they remember of things infinitely greater than themselves or than himself. They will remember, perhaps, that once in a way, in the midst of the routine of the classroom, it was something not himself that spoke, something not themselves that listened. The teacher may well be content to be otherwise forgotten, or to live in something grown to ripeness in his students that he, however minutely, helped bring to birth. There are many students thus come to fruition whom I should be proud to have say: "He was my teacher." There is no other immortality a teacher can have.

1. The title below that best expresses the ideas of this passage is:
   (A) moments of genius
   (B) the forgotten teacher
   (C) artist in the classroom
   (D) infinity in education
   (E) immortality for the teacher.

2. A teacher is best known by
   (A) his jokes
   (B) what he quotes
   (C) his absent-mindedness
   (D) what his pupils achieve
   (E) his ability to manage class routine.

3. The writer probably taught
   (A) first grade  (B) mature adults
   (C) nursery school  (D) in ancient times
   (E) high school or college students.

### Answers

1. E    2. D    3. E

## Mathematics

The Mathematics part tests your understanding of basic quantitative concepts such as the following:

You will be asked to demonstrate your understanding of the above concepts by applying your knowledge to such problems as you had in secondary school and, possibly, in elementary school. The Mathematics part is not a test of Advanced College Mathematics. There are no problems in Calculus, Analytic Geometry, and such fields of advanced mathematical study.

Pages 72 to 91 will give you considerable practice for the Mathematics part of the Dental Aptitude Test. The Supplementary Practice Section (Chapter Five) includes an explanation of each concept, problems illustrating each concept, and solutions to these problems. Samples of each type of mathematical concept are given below:

*Directions:* Each of the questions in this section is followed by five possible answers lettered A through E. Select the correct answer to each question and mark the corresponding space on the answer sheet.

## FRACTIONS

1. The fractional equivalent of .0625 is

    (A) 1/16  (B) 1/15
    (C) 1/14  (D) 1/13
    (E) 1/6.

## CONVERSION OF UNITS

2. A boy picked one bushel of huckleberries and sold 24 quarts. How many quarts were left?

    (A) 4  (B) 8
    (C) 12  (D) 16
    (E) 20.

## RATIO AND PROPORTION

3. In a certain city 12% of the elementary school teachers are men, 40% of the high school teachers are men, and 20% of all the teachers in the elementary and high schools combined are men. What is the ratio of the number of elementary school teachers to the number of high school teachers?

    (A) $\dfrac{13}{50}$  (B) $\dfrac{1}{2}$

    (C) $\dfrac{5}{2}$  (D) $\dfrac{13}{5}$

    (E) $\dfrac{10}{3}$

## AVERAGES

4. The salary for a group of executives was listed as follows: 18 at $5,000; 10 at $6,000; 8 at $7,500; 2 at $9,000; 2 at $10,000. The average salary was

    (A) $5,400  (B) $6,000
    (C) $6,200  (D) $6,400
    (E) $7,000.

## INTEREST AND PERCENT

5. A man's income is $25,000 per annum; his expenses per annum are $15,000. What per cent of his income does he save?

    (A) 30%  (B) 40%
    (C) 37½%  (D) 60%
    (E) None of these.

## TIME AND WORK

6. A laborer in Japan worked 30 days. He paid 2/5 of his earnings for board and room and had $81 left. What was his daily wage?

    (A) $4.50  (B) $5.75
    (C) $6.75  (D) $7.25
    (E) $8.00.

## RATE, TIME, AND DISTANCE

7. A man traveling 100 miles at r miles per hour arrived at his destination 2 hours late. How many miles an hour should he have traveled to arrive on time?

    (A) $\dfrac{50-r}{50r}$  (B) $\dfrac{50r}{50+r}$

    (C) $\dfrac{100-2r}{r}$  (D) $\dfrac{50r}{50-r}$

    (E) $\dfrac{50r+1}{50}$

## SERIES

8. In the series .04, .2, 1, 5 _____ the number that follows logically is

   (A) 10    (B) 20
   (C) 25    (D) 50
           (E) 100.

## GEOMETRY

9. In the figure below, the length of diagonal AC is

   (A) 10 inches    (B) 14 inches
   (C) 18 inches    (D) 48 inches
           (E) 96 inches

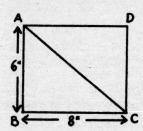

## GRAPHS, CHARTS, AND TABLES

Answer question 10 from the table below. Distribution of the Total Population of the United States by Age Group, 1940:

| Age Group | Per Cent |
|---|---|
| Under 15 | 25.00 |
| 15 to 34 | 34.50 |
| 35 to 54 | 25.62 |
| 55 to 74 | 12.90 |
| 74 and over | 1.98 |
| | 100.00 |

10. If, in the United States in 1940, 30 million persons were under 15 years of age, how many million persons (to the nearest 0.1 million) were in the 75 and over age group?

    (A) 1.7    (B) 2.0
    (C) 2.4    (D) 23.8
            (E) 37.9.

### ANSWERS

1. A    3. C    5. B    7. D    9. A
2. B    4. C    6. A    8. C    10. C

## Biology

*Directions:* Choose the correct answer from the choices given.

1. The term "amphibians of the plant world" is most applicable to

   (A) bryophytes    (B) pteridophytes
   (C) spermatophytes    (D) challophytes.

2. Damage to the cerebellum would interfere mainly with which one of the following?

   (A) memory    (B) voluntary acts
   (C) sensation    (D) equilibrium.

3. Blood coming from the lungs enters the heart by way of the

   (A) aorta    (B) pulmonary artery
   (C) vena cava    (D) pulmonary vein.

4. Which one of the following terms is not directly associated with the same sense organ as the three others?

   (A) stapes
   (B) cochlea
   (C) tympanic membrane
   (D) cornea

### ANSWERS

1. A    2. D    3. D    4. D

## Chemistry

*Directions:* Choose the correct answer from the choices given.

1. A sulfide which is insoluble in water and white in color is
   (A) $ZnS$    (B) $PbS$
   (C) $As_2S_3$    (D) $Na_2S$.

2. The compound which is used most frequently to melt snow is

   (A) $CaCl_2$    (B) $CaSO_4$
   (C) $CaCO_3$    (D) $Ca(OH)_2$

### ANSWERS

1. A    2. A

## PERCEPTUAL-MOTOR ABILITY

*These questions on matching parts and figures test your understanding of spatial relations.*

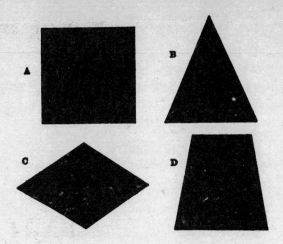

.   THE first two questions show, at the left side, two or more flat pieces. In each question select the arrangement lettered A, B, C, or D that shows how these pieces can be fitted together without gaps or overlapping. The pieces may be *turned around* or *turned over* in any way to make them fit together.

*From these pieces*

**1.**

*which one of these arrangements can you make?*

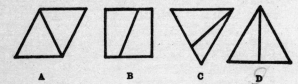

*From these pieces*

**2.**

*which one of these arrangements can you make?*

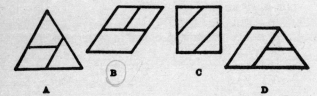

The next two questions are based on the four solid patterns shown.

Each of the questions shows *one* of these four patterns cut up into pieces. For each question, decide which one of the four patterns could be made by fitting *all of the pieces* together without having any edges overlap and without leaving any space between pieces. Some of the pieces may need to be *turned around* or *turned over* to make them fit. The pattern must be made in its exact size and shape.

Look at sample question 3. If the two pieces were fitted together they would make pattern D. The piece on the left fits at the bottom of pattern D, and the piece at the right is turned around and over to make the top of the pattern.

**3.**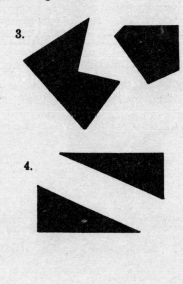

**4.**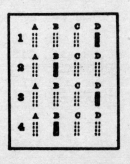

# PART ONE

# Three Predictive Practice Examinations

*DIRECTIONS: For each question read all the choices carefully. Then select that answer which you consider correct or most nearly correct. Write the letter preceding your best choice next to the question. Should you want to answer on the kind of answer sheet used on machine-scored examinations, we have provided several such facsimiles. On some machine-scored exams you are instructed to "place no marks whatever on the test booklet." In other examinations you may be instructed to mark your answers in the test booklet. In such cases you should be careful that no other marks interfere with the legibility of your answers. It is always best NOT to mark your booklet unless you are sure that it is permitted. It is most important that you learn to mark your answers clearly and in the right place.*

*FOR THE SAMPLE QUESTION that follows, select the appropriate letter preceding the word which is most nearly the same in meaning as the capitalized word:*

1. DISSENT:    (A) approve    (B) depart
              (C) disagree    (D) enjoy

*DISSENT is most nearly the same as (C), disagree, so that the acceptable answer is shown thus on your answer sheet:*

A  B  C  D

# Practice Using Answer Sheets

**Alter numbers to match the practice and drill questions in each part of the book.
Make only ONE mark for each answer. Additional and stray marks may be counted as mistakes.
In making corrections, erase errors COMPLETELY. Make glossy black marks.**

# I. PREDICTIVE PRACTICE EXAMINATION

*To begin your studies, test yourself now to see how you measure up. This examination is similar to the one you'll get, and is therefore a practical yardstick for charting your progress and planning your course. Adhere strictly to all test instructions. Mark yourself honestly and you'll find where your weaknesses are and where to concentrate your study.*

**TOTAL TIME: 4 hours 30 minutes.** In order to create the climate of the test to come, that's precisely what you should allow yourself . . . no more, no less. Use a watch and keep a record of your time, especially since you may find it convenient to take the test in several sittings.

In constructing this Examination we tried to visualize the questions you are *likely* to face on your actual exam. We included those subjects on which they are *probably* going to test you.

Although copies of past exams are not released, we were able to piece together a fairly complete picture of the forthcoming exam.

A principal source of information was our analysis of official announcements going back several years.

Critical comparison of these announcements, particularly the sample questions, revealed the testing trend; foretold the important subjects, and those that are likely to recur.

The various subjects expected on your exam are represented by separate Tests. Each Test has just about the number of questions you may find on the actual exam. And each Test is timed accordingly.

The questions on each Test are represented exactly on the special Answer Sheet provided. Mark your answers on this sheet. It's just about the way you'll have to do it on the real exam.

As a result you have an Examination which simulates the real one closely enough to provide you with important training.

Proceed through the entire exam without pausing after each Test.

Correct answers for all the questions in all the Tests of the Exam appear at the end of the Exam, after the suggestions for self diagnosis and further study.

Then you may convert your answers to a percentage score for each Test, using the score boxes we provide.

# PREDICTIVE PRACTICE EXAMINATION

| ANALYSIS AND TIMETABLE: PREDICTIVE PRACTICE EXAMINATION | |
|---|---|
| *Since the number of questions for each test may vary on different forms of the actual examination, the time allotments below are flexible.* | |
| **SUBJECT TESTED** | Time Allowed |
| TEST I. BIOMEDICAL SCIENCE | 65 Minutes |
| TEST II. INTERPRETATION OF SCIENCE READINGS | 75 Minutes |
| TEST III. VOCABULARY | 20 Minutes |
| TEST IV. VERBAL ANALOGIES | 15 Minutes |
| TEST V. SENTENCE COMPLETIONS | 15 Minutes |
| TEST VI. QUANTITATIVE ABILITY | 60 Minutes |
| TEST VII. PERCEPTUAL MOTOR ABILITY | 20 Minutes |

# ANSWER SHEET FOR PREDICTIVE EXAMINATION I.

## TEST I. BIOMEDICAL SCIENCE

| | | | | | | | |
|---|---|---|---|---|---|---|---|
| 1 A B C D E | 2 A B C D E | 3 A B C D E | 4 A B C D E | 5 A B C D E | 6 A B C D E | 7 A B C D E | 8 A B C D E |
| 9 A B C D E | 10 A B C D E | 11 A B C D E | 12 A B C D E | 13 A B C D E | 14 A B C D E | 15 A B C D E | 16 A B C D E |
| 17 A B C D E | 18 A B C D E | 19 A B C D E | 20 A B C D E | 21 A B C D E | 22 A B C D E | 23 A B C D E | 24 A B C D E |
| 25 A B C D E | 26 A B C D E | 27 A B C D E | 28 A B C D E | 29 A B C D E | 30 A B C D E | 31 A B C D E | 32 A B C D E |
| 33 A B C D E | 34 A B C D E | 35 A B C D E | 36 A B C D E | 37 A B C D E | 38 A B C D E | 39 A B C D E | 40 A B C D E |
| 41 A B C D E | 42 A B C D E | 43 A B C D E | 44 A B C D E | 45 A B C D E | 46 A B C D E | 47 A B C D E | 48 A B C D E |
| 49 A B C D E | 50 A B C D E | | | | | | |

## TEST II. INTERPRETATION OF SCIENCE READINGS

| | | | | | | | |
|---|---|---|---|---|---|---|---|
| 1 A B C D E | 2 A B C D E | 3 A B C D E | 4 A B C D E | 5 A B C D E | 6 A B C D E | 7 A B C D E | 8 A B C D E |
| 9 A B C D E | 10 A B C D E | 11 A B C D E | 12 A B C D E | 13 A B C D E | 14 A B C D E | 15 A B C D E | 16 A B C D E |
| 17 A B C D E | 18 A B C D E | 19 A B C D E | 20 A B C D E | 21 A B C D E | 22 A B C D E | 23 A B C D E | 24 A B C D E |
| 25 A B C D E | 26 A B C D E | 27 A B C D E | 28 A B C D E | 29 A B C D E | 30 A B C D E | 31 A B C D E | 32 A B C D E |

## TEST III. VOCABULARY

| | | | | | | | |
|---|---|---|---|---|---|---|---|
| 1 A B C D E | 2 A B C D E | 3 A B C D E | 4 A B C D E | 5 A B C D E | 6 A B C D E | 7 A B C D E | 8 A B C D E |
| 9 A B C D E | 10 A B C D E | 11 A B C D E | 12 A B C D E | 13 A B C D E | 14 A B C D E | 15 A B C D E | 16 A B C D E |
| 17 A B C D E | 18 A B C D E | 19 A B C D E | 20 A B C D E | 21 A B C D E | 22 A B C D E | 23 A B C D E | 24 A B C D E |
| 25 A B C D E | 26 A B C D E | | | | | | |

## TEST IV. VERBAL ANALOGIES

| | | | | | | | |
|---|---|---|---|---|---|---|---|
| 1 A B C D E | 2 A B C D E | 3 A B C D E | 4 A B C D E | 5 A B C D E | 6 A B C D E | 7 A B C D E | 8 A B C D E |
| 9 A B C D E | 10 A B C D E | 11 A B C D E | 12 A B C D E | 13 A B C D E | 14 A B C D E | 15 A B C D E | 16 A B C D E |
| 17 A B C D E | 18 A B C D E | 19 A B C D E | 20 A B C D E | 21 A B C D E | 22 A B C D E | 23 A B C D E | 24 A B C D E |
| 25 A B C D E | 26 A B C D E | 27 A B C D E | 28 A B C D E | 29 A B C D E | 30 A B C D E | | |

## TEST V. SENTENCE COMPLETIONS

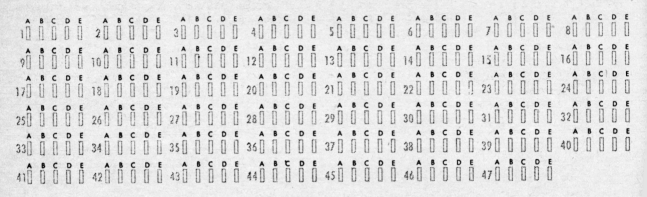

## TEST VI. QUANTITATIVE ABILITY

## TEST VII. PERCEPTUAL MOTOR ABILITY

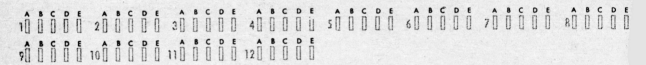

# TEST I. BIOMEDICAL SCIENCE

TIME: 65 Minutes*

DIRECTIONS: *For each of the following questions, select the choice which best answers the question or completes the statement.*

*Directions:* Choose the correct answer from the lettered choices.

1. Of the following, a disinfectant that liberates chlorine is
   (A) Dakin's solution
   (B) hydrogen peroxide
   (C) tricresol
   (D) Merthiolate.

2. Bacteria of decay may change dead leaves into which one of the following?
   (A) green manure      (B) humus
   (C) loam              (D) fungi.

3. True motility is present in bacteria that possess which one of the following?
   (A) cilia             (B) pseudopods
   (C) flagella          (D) cirri.

4. In the nitrogen cycle, the bacteria which changes proteins to ammonia are known as
   (A) bacteria of decay
   (B) denitrifying bacteria
   (C) nitrate bacteria
   (D) nitrogen-fixing bacteria.

5. Protista is a term that is used to include only
   (A) one-celled animals
   (B) unicellular plants
   (C) acellular organisms
   (D) multicellular organisms.

6. An eye is a light receptor in which the
   (A) rods distinguish color
   (B) visual purple is formed in the vitreous humor
   (C) blind spot contains only cones
   (D) fovea centralis has the most acute vision.

7. The transmission of impulses across synapses and myoneural junctions of the autonomic system depends on neurohumors such as
   (A) acetylcholine     (B) actomyosin
   (C) atropine          (D) avidin.

8. Organelles which serve as receptors in unicellular organisms are which one of the following?
   (A) myonemes          (B) chromatophores
   (C) flagella          (D) neurofibrils.

9. Muscular contractions known as tetany result from an undersecretion of the
   (A) thyroid           (B) parathyroid
   (C) adrenals          (D) thymus.

10. Of the following, the one which is an organ of equilibrium found in some invertebrates is the
    (A) labyrinth
    (B) cochlea
    (C) semicircular canal
    (D) statocyst.

11. Which of the following instruments can measure the activities of the cerebral cortex?
    (A) electroencephalograph
    (B) sphygmomanometer
    (C) pneumograph
    (D) electrocardiograph.

12. Of the following, the one which is a hormone produced in the pituitary gland that plays a role in growth is
    (A) luteotropin       (B) somatotropin
    (C) oxytocin          (D) vasopressin.

13. The parasympathetic system
    (A) speeds up the heart beat
    (B) is composed of chains of ganglia parallel to the spinal cord
    (C) produces cholinesterase to stimulate muscle contraction
    (D) opposes the action of the sympathetic system.

14. Which one of the following movements of plants illustrates the behavior of plant hormones?
    (A) rapid drooping of a mimosa plant

*The Science section of the DAT tests basic concepts and principles as well as the ability to show an understanding of chemical and biological methods and procedures.

(B) "sleep movements" of a clover
(C) leaf-closing movements of a Venus' flytrap
(D) turning of geranium leaves toward light.

15. Cyclosis may be demonstrated by using fresh slides of which one of the following?
(A) paramecium     (B) onion epidermis
(C) elodea leaf     (D) root tips.

16. The body of a complex fungus such a Rhizopus nigricans is called a
(A) rhizoid     (B) mycelium
(C) hypha     (D) stolon.

17. Which of the following statements does *not* apply to the tracheophytes?
(A) They possess vascular tissue
(B) The sporophyte generation is dominant over the gametophyte
(C) The embryo forms in an archegonium
(D) They are made up of mosses and ferns.

18. The process of building up complex carbohydrates from simple sugars is known as
(A) hydrolysis     (B) condensation
(C) peptide linkage     (D) induction.

19. Which one of the following organic compounds is *not* a polysaccharide?
(A) maltose     (B) starch
(C) cellulose     (D) glycogen.

20. Of the following, the most effective method of returning minerals to the soil is
(A) stripping
(B) terracing
(C) contour plowing
(D) crop rotation.

21. Which one of the following is the chief agent of erosion?
(A) running water     (B) air
(C) animals     (D) plants.

22. Human mutations caused by radiation from nuclear fall-out are expected to be produced mainly through the action of
(A) phosphorus $P^{32}$     (B) iodine $I^{131}$
(C) strontium $Sr^{90}$     (D) carbon $C^{14}$.

23. A common mold is used to show the effects of genes on enzyme production is the
(A) saprolegnia     (B) ergot
(C) aspergillus     (D) neurospora.

24. The 1961 Nobel Prize in Medicine for discoveries concerning the physical mechanism of stimulation within the cochlea was awarded to
(A) Lederberg     (B) Von Békésy
(C) Tatum     (D) Calvin.

25. Of the following, a plant which may play an important role in space travel is the
(A) spirogyra
(B) oedogonium
(C) chlamydomonas
(D) chlorella.

26. In which part of the cell is the middle lamella found?
(A) nucleoplasm     (B) cell wall
(C) cytoplasm     (D) cell membrane.

27. Which one of the following is used to identify the Feulgen reaction?
(A) xanthophylls     (B) DNA — proteins
(C) grana     (D) lipids.

28. From which one of the following embryonic tissues are the kidneys developed?
(A) blastopore     (B) ectoderm
(C) mesoderm     (D) endoderm.

29. The human fetus depends for most of its existence on a type of nutrition called
(A) trophoblastic     (B) hemotrophic
(C) embryotrophic     (D) blastocystic.

30. Of the following, the discovery which contributed most directly to the success of Salk's work was that involving
(A) successful tissue culture techniques
(B) crystallization of tobacco mosaic
(C) successful use of electrophoresis
(D) passing viruses through a porcelain filter.

31. A toxoid is used to produce immunity to which one of the following?
(A) smallpox     (B) poliomyelitis
(C) tuberculosis     (D) diphtheria.

32. Which one of the following diseases is water borne?
(A) undulant fever     (B) cholera
(C) malaria     (D) bubonic plague.

33. The vaccine known as BCG is used to produce immunity against
(A) tuberculosis     (B) typhoid
(C) malaria     (D) mumps.

34. Which one of the following is caused by the toxin found mainly in preserved foods, either home or commercially prepared?

(A) undulant fever
(B) botulism
(C) ptomaine poisoning
(D) bacillary dysentery.

35. Which one of the following first proposed the side chain theory of immunity?
(A) Koch      (B) Ehrlich
(C) Von Behring   (D) Park.

36. Oxygen may be prepared by pupils with greatest safety in the high school laboratory by employing which one of the following?
(A) $H_2O_2$ (3%) and $MnO_2$

(B) $KClO_3$ and $MNO_2$

(C) $KClO_3$

(D) $Na_2O_2$ and $H_2O$.

37. Of the following first aid measures, the most effective in case one inhales bromine vapor, is to
(A) swallow sodium thiosulfate solution
(B) breathe fresh air
(C) use glycerol
(D) breathe weak ammonia fumes.

38. Of the following hazardous mixtures, the one *not* used in high school classroom instruction is
(A) zinc dust and sulfur
(B) thermite
(C) potassium chlorate and charcoal
(D) hydrogen and air.

39. Of the following, the physical property *least* frequently used in chemistry instruction is
(A) taste      (B) odor
(C) solubility   (D) density.

40. Of the following, the reagent frequently used in gas analysis to absorb carbon monoxide is
(A) cuprous chloride
(B) calcium chloride
(C) pyrogallic acid
(D) sodium peroxide.

41. Of the following reagents, the one used to separate cupric ions from cadmium ions is
(A) ammonium hydroxide
(B) hydrogen sulfide
(C) sodium cyanide
(D) sodium thiocyanate.

42. The pH of a 0.3M solution of HCl is correctly expressed by

(A) log 3.3      (B) antilog 3.3
(C) 1/log 3.3    (D) log. 0.3.

43. A solution with pH = 2 is more acid than one with a pH = 6 by a factor of
(A) 4       (B) 12
(C) 400     (D) 10,000.

44. The addition of sodium acetate crystals to one liter of O.1 M acetic acid will produce a (n)
(A) increase in the value of $K_{eq}$
(B) decrease in the value of $K_{eq}$
(C) increase in the pH value
(D) decrease in sodium ion concentration.

45. The plastic "nylon" is best described as which one of the following?
(A) polymerized hydrocarbon
(B) polyamide
(C) polyester
(D) polyurethane.

46. The number of liters of air needed to burn completely 8 liters of acetylene is
(A) 40       (B) 60
(C) 80       (D) 100.

47. One would expect to find the term isotactic used in connection with which one of the following?
(A) plastics      (B) dyes
(C) textiles      (D) metals.

48. Of the following, a metallic compound which is increasing in importance as a lubricant is
(A) graphite
(B) iron oxide
(C) molybdenum disulfide
(D) tungsten oxide.

49. A monopropellant is a rocket fuel that combines within its molecule both fuel and oxidizing agent. Of the following, the substance that best fits this description is
(A) hydrogen peroxide
(B) fuming nitric acid
(C) nitromethane
(D) Decaborane.

50. Carbon dioxide is an illustration of a molecule which is
(A) polar with polar bonds
(B) non-polar with polar bonds
(C) non-polar with non-polar bonds
(D) polar with non-polar bonds.

# TEST II. INTERPRETATION OF SCIENCE READINGS

### TIME: 75 Minutes

*DIRECTIONS: Read each passage to get the general idea. Then reread the passage more carefully to answer the questions based on the passage. For each question read all choices carefully. Then select the answer you consider correct or most nearly correct. Blacken the answer space corresponding to your best choice, just as you would do on the actual examination.*

The isolation of crystalline leucine aminopeptidase from bovine lens is described. The yield of crystalline enzyme is 60—70% (with a more than 1000-fold purification.) At pH 8.0 (Tris buffer) and +4°, the enzyme is stable for months without loss of activity. Lyophilisation results in a loss of activity of about 40% after 3 months storage.

The crystalline enzyme is homogeneous in electrophoresis and ultracentrifugation. 100 $ul$ of a solution of recrystallized enzyme (2.7 mg protein per m$l$) were chromatographed on paper before and after 24 hr. incubation (37°); there was no additional ninhydrin positive material. In solution, the crystalline enzyme shows a pure protein spectrum, with a maximum of 281 m$u$ and a molar extinction of $2.8 \times 10^5$, assuming the molecular weight to be 326,000. Optimal conditions for enzyme determination were found with regard to pH, activators and pre-incubation. With L-leucinamide as substrate, the usual $C_1$-values were 150—180, corresponding to a specific gravity of 1395—1674 international enzyme units.

1.  The figures 60-70% in the second sentence of the first paragraph refer to the
    (A) purity of crystalline enzyme.
    (B) yield of crystalline enzyme.
    (C) loss of crystalline enzyme.
    (D) relative weight of crystalline enzyme.

2.  The purpose of the experiment was to
    (A) isolate crystalline leucine aminopeptidase from bovine lens.
    (B) test the stability of crystalline leucine aminopeptidase.
    (C) determine the effect of pH activators, and preincubation on the recrystallization of leucine aminopeptidase.
    (D) determine the $C_1$ values of leucine aminopeptidase.

3.  A solution of the recrystallized enzyme
    (A) contained 2.7 mg protein per ml.
    (B) did not react when chromatographed.
    (C) was incubated.
    (D) showed a substantial change in ninhydrin positive material.

4.  Lyophilisation
    (A) did not change the activity.
    (B) was 40% successful.
    (C) did not occur.
    (D) was allowed to occur over a period of 3 months.

The purity and molecular size of DNA isolated from microorganisms has been studied in relation to the method of extraction. In relation to this, a method was developed which permits the isolation of high-purity DNA, while largely avoiding sheering degradation. A comparison of this method was made on normal form, penicillin-induced spheroplasts, and on the stable L-form of *Proteus mirabilis* to determine the influence of cell wall polysaccharides and proteins on the isolated DNA purity; the best results were obtained with the L-form. The quality of the DNA samples was tested by extensive analysis (elementary analysis, chemical and physical-chemical methods). The polysaccharide and protein impurities were determined as monosaccharides, amino acids and hexosamines by a special hydrolysis technique, and the protein content determined according to Lowry. All samples showed a certain amount of residual protein, which had a characteristic amino acid composition. DNA, obtained by this method, had a mean molecular weight up to $50 \times 10^6$, ranging from $10—120 \times 10^6$. The base composition of the DNA samples was determined.

5. One advantage of the method developed for DNA isolation is that
   (A) large quantities of DNA could be isolated.
   (B) DNA purity could be regulated.
   (C) the molecular size of the DNA was desirable.
   (D) it avoided sheering degradation.

6. *Proteus mirabilis* was used in the experiment because it
   (A) is stable.
   (B) reacts with DNA.
   (C) was used to compare to the reaction of DNA on normal form, penicillin-induced spheroplasts.
   (D) is a polysaccharide.

7. A special hydrolysis technique was employed to
   (A) confirm results of chemical and physical-chemical techniques.
   (B) test for the presence of residual protein.
   (C) determine the polysaccharide and protein impurities.
   (D) determine the type of amino acid present.

8. The two most important factors studied in the experiment in relation to the isolation of DNA were
   (A) purity and feasibility of the method.
   (B) purity and molecular size.
   (C) purity and avoidance of sheering degradation.
   (D) amount of DNA yielded and molecular size.

---

The transition of a glow discharge from a stationary condition into other stationary or non-stationary conditions has been investigated in a number of experimental works.

As these experiments show, the glow discharge becomes unstable at certain values of the experimental parameters. The experimental results suggest a distinction of 2 types of instability.

Column instability has its origin in the mechanism of the column and can occur without a change in the cathodic discharge parts. This instability appears when a critical current value is exceeded, which is a function of the type of gas, pressure, and the radius of disharge.

Cathodic instability originates in the cathodic parts and induces, in general, an instability of the column.

The stability of the cathode parts of a glow discharge with respect to local current density disturbances is investigated. The cathodic region is described by the particle and momentum balances of the charge carriers and the boundary conditions at the cathode surface and the negative glow. The latter are formulated with the help of the coefficients $y$ and $\delta$. From a first order perturbation theory of the stationary mode we derive a dispersion relation. The evaluation of this equation using NYQUIST's theorem provides a criterion for the onset of the $y - \delta$ instability.

9. As stated in the first paragraph, a series of experimental studies has been devoted to investigations of
   (A) stationary glow-discharge.
   (B) stationary and instationary glow discharges.
   (C) the transition of a glow discharge from a stationary condition.
   (D) the breakdown of a stationary glow discharge.

10. According to the author, the relationhip of column instability to cathodic instability is that
    (A) they are not related.
    (B) the former does not influence the latter, but the latter influences the former.
    (C) they occur simultaneously.
    (D) they modify each other.

11. As stated in the last paragraph, the cathodic region is mainly described by
    (A) the coefficients $y$ and $\delta$.
    (B) the cathode surface and the negative glow.
    (C) impulses divided into small parts.
    (D) the particle and momentum balances of the charge carriers.

12. Nyquist's theorem is used
    (A) to yield a criterion for the onset of $y-\delta$ instability.
    (B) to yield a first-order perturbation theory.
    (C) for evaluating the first-order perturbation theory.
    (D) for evaluating the criterion for the instability.

---

Oxygen adsorption on W and Re was investigated employing the ionization of Cu and Ag. It was found that the adsorbed oxygen increased the work output of W by a maximum of 1.85 eV and that of Re a maximum of 1.75 eV, probably because of the formation of a monolayer. Using a statistical model, an adsorption equation for the chemisorption of oxygen was derived, which becomes the Langmuir equation when certain factors are neglected. The oxygen adsorption cannot, however, be adequately described by such an equation, because the energy of adsorption (Q) is not constant. Good agreement, on the oher hand, beween experiment and theory was achieved by an approximation equation in which several Langmuir adsorption equations are superimposed by varying energies of adsorption. According to this equation, oxygen is adsorbed on polycrystalline W with at least two discrete values of Q corresponding to two different levels of adsorption of about 3.3 eV and 4.8 eV. The energy of adsorption of Re assumes all values continuously until approximately 4 eV.

13. Oxygen adsorption on W and Re
    (A) is related to the ionization of Cu and Ag.
    (B) does not depend on the work output of W and Re.
    (C) increases the work output of W and Re.
    (D) forms a single layer on W.

14. The Langmuir adsorption equation
    (A) describes the experimental results.
    (B) does not adequately describe the adsorption on W and Re.
    (C) was used as a statistical model.
    (D) gives values for the adsorption of oxygen on Re.

15. The energy of adsorption
    (A) is derived from the Langmuir equation.
    (B) is a function of oxygen concentration.
    (C) is a varying quantity in these experiments.
    (D) decreases with increasing work output.

16. The values of 3.3 eV and 4.8 eV refer to
    (A) values of the energy of adsorption at which oxygen is adsorbed on W.
    (B) levels of energy of W work output.
    (C) upper and lower limits of energy adsorption.
    (D) mean values for the energy of adsorption of oxygen on W.

---

hold the hen's egg provided with a light conductor and keeping the required hatching temperature and humidity constant. This device is fitted into a tilting microscope. By a simple tilting movement the oblique position can be achieved in which the chorio-allantoid membrane with its capillary system touches the thin window (cover glass!) particularly closely without interference with the interior of the egg. Thus, the blood cells of the circulating blood stream are within reach even for powerful lenses with a short working distance.

Narrow passages in the capillary system and obstructions to the flow of blood all through the capillaries are especially frequent. These circulatory obstructions as well as the extremely narrow passages, together with the flow, impose a considerable mechanical strain on the blood cells.

17. According to the article, continuous microscopical observations of hatching hen's eggs
    (A) are not possible
    (B) are possible using fenestrated hen's eggs and a light conductor.
    (C) depend on the stage of development of the egg.
    (D) must destroy the egg.

18. The use of the tilting microscope
    (A) is not necessary.
    (B) is necessary to maintain constant temperature and humidity.
    (C) allows the chorio-allantoid membrane to be properly positioned.
    (D) might interfere with the interior of the egg.

19. Obstructions to the blood flow in the center of the capillaries
    (A) frequently occur.
    (B) are caused by the microscope used.
    (C) are not found.
    (D) are caused by narrow passages.

20. Narrow passages and circulatory obstructions
    (A) hinder the flow.
    (B) enhance the flow.
    (C) impose mechanical strain on the blood cells.
    (D) are not an important factor in determining the strain on blood cells.

---

Continuous microscopical observations over several days are made possible by means of fenestrated hen's eggs and a light conductor (of glass or plastic material) introduced into the fertilized hen's egg. A heatable work table is fitted with a container to

Eggs of *Culex pipiens* L. were irradiated by means of a micro-beam UV apparatus in various regions and at different stages in embryonic development. In this way definite areas of the embryo could either be destroyed or harmed by injury.

Irradiation of the polar plasm at the posterior end of the egg before blastele formation results in sterility of imagines. No sperm is formed in the testis, and in the ovaries neither egg nor nurse cells.

Irradiation immediately posterior to the cephalic fold, shortly after its formation, prevents the formation of maxillae. Dorsolateral irradiation anterior to the cephalic fold results in the lack of mandibles, eyes and antennae. Ventral irradiation in front of the cephalic fold results in no externally visible damage; however, the larvae are unable to hatch.

Irradiation of the posterior pole previous to elongation of the germ band causes defects of the hindmost abdominal segments; after elongation, mainly defects of the third abdominal segment. Irradiation experiments with individual clutches from 6½ to 8 hours after oviposition permitted to determine the onset and duration of germ band involution. Although variability is considerable involution never lasts longer than 1¼ hours (breeding temperature $25 \pm \frac{1}{2}°C$).

By irradiating a greater number of narrow stripes across the dorsal and ventral surface of the fully stretched-out embyo an approximate pattern of the position of primordia in the ninth hour of development was established.

Irradiation of the head region after embryonic evolution is completed causes a lack of the brain and corpus allatum complex. Since the abdomen develops normally, one may exclude hormonal influences of brain and (or) corpus allatum complex upon embryonic development. As a consequence of irradiation two different kinds of pigment formation were observed, i.e. pigment granules (dorsally beneath the integument) and lumps of pigment near the anus (between the anal papillae).

The eggs increase in length by 15 to 20% in the course of embryonic development.

Formation of the primitive groove can be observed in total preparations about 6 hours after oviposition. Previous to this, throughout the blastoderm stage, only a single layer of regular hexagonal cells is found. Shortly after the 6th hour there arise ventrally a number of secondary folds. Blastokinesis and dorsal involution of the embryo do not set in earlier than 6 hours and 20 min. after oviposition.

21. Eggs of *Culex pipiens L.* were irradiated
    (A) by various microbeam UV apparatus.
    (B) to destroy the eggs.
    (C) to localize and make visible definite areas of injury.
    (D) to stop growth at predetermined stages of embryo development.

22. Irradiation immediately posterior to the cephalic fold
    (A) prevents its formation.
    (B) prevents formation of maxillae.
    (C) results in the lack of mandibles, eyes and antennae.
    (D) has only a short-term effect.

23. Hormonal influence upon embryonic development
    (A) affects the brain and corpus allatum complex.
    (B) issues from the abdomen.
    (C) can be discounted.
    (D) issues from the brain and corpus allatum complex.

24. The last paragraph states that during the blastoderm stage
    (A) the primitive groove has formed.
    (B) six hours elapse.
    (C) a single layer of regular hexagonal cells is formed.
    (D) blastokinesis occurs.

---

During July, 1961, a continuous plankton catch from surface water was made between Durban and Cape Town; at the same time water temperature was registered.

The catch was subdivided into 12 plankton samples from contiguous areas of the ship's route.

The distance covered was divided into four areas with the aid of the thermograms.

The plankton volumes show a four- and sixfold increase in surface plankton during the night; the plankton density in the West was four times that in the East.

Phytoplankton blooms were found in two places near the point where there was a sharp drop in temperature. The species components of these blooms show that the cold water species are present as the main components in plankton blooms from the west coast of South Africa as far as east of the Agulhas Bank.

92 species of Copepods in plankton were identified; of these, 28 are recorded here for the first time for the South African seas. Their local occurrence and general distribution are compared with one other.

The abundance of Indopacific species, which characterize the fauna of the Agulhas Current, disappear from the coastal area as soon as the shelf starts broadening toward the Agulhas Bank.

Very few Indopacific species were found on the Agulhas Bank itself. Here, there seemed to be a strange plankton community; besides abundant cosmopolitan species, a surprising and apparently isolated colony of *Calanas finmarchicus* belongs to this community.

Over the western section of the Bank, and around the Cape of Good Hope, those species appear which form the huge zooplankton swarms that characterize the Benguela Current along the west coast of Sotuh Africa.

25. The plankton catch of July, 1961
    (A) was carried out on four different occasions.
    (B) captured 12 species of plankton.
    (C) took plankton from the surface water.
    (D) was not totally successful.

26. The plankton volume at night
    (A) was greater than that during the day.
    (B) was the same in the west and the east.
    (C) increased, because of the presence of phytoplankton blooms.
    (D) decreased, because of the lack of sunlight.

27. 92 species of Copepods identified
    (A) were of the cold water variety.
    (B) are found only in the west coast of South Africa.
    (C) contained some which had not been found before in this region.
    (D) are cosmopolitan.

28. The fauna of the Agulhas current
    (A) extends to the Agulhas Bank.
    (B) is characterized by abundant Indopacific species.
    (C) consists of several plankton communities.
    (D) consists of various zooplankton swarms.

---

1. The mechanism of the rowing apparatus of Gyrinidae is quantitatively analysed as a basis for the study of its strange movements on the water surface. Datas from high-frequency cinematographs (800 pictures/sec.) are combined for this purpose with dynamic data from flow experiments.

2. The functional-morphological, cinematic and hydromechanic features of the rowing apparatus are described and compared with those of Dytiseidae. The oars of *Gyrinus* and *Acilius* function in the same way but with different characteristics in anatomy and movements.

3. The dimensions of the legs and their single parts are measured. The morphological basics of increase of propulsion and decrease of counterdrive are determined. The changes in frontal area, surface and distance from the axis of rotation of the single rigid parts are most important.

4. Functional formation of rigid parts and muscles as well as attachment and spreading movements of swimming blades are discussed.

5. Cinematics of leg movement are described in detail and presented graphically quantitatively. They are divided into three phases of equal duration, but different function.

6. The hydromechanical role of single parts of the leg in generating thrust, especially with respect to the swimming blades is analysed. The swimming plades contribute 52% of the whole propulsion-force. The leg of *Gyrinus* is compared with the swimming hair carrying *Acilius*-leg.

7. Hydrodynamical specialties and efficiency factors of the rowing apparatus are investigated by graphical analysis. The counterthrust in drawing forward is only about $\frac{1}{40}$ of the thrust during the backward stroke. 96 % (!) of the swimming-power is changed into oar-stroking force; from this value again 87% is converted into thrust. So with a total efficiency factor of $n_R = 0,84$ the oar-leg of Gyrinus exceeds the comparable technical machines. *It is the best thrust apparatus in the animal kingdom making use of the resistance principle that is known.*

29. According to the first paragraph, the movements of *Gyrinus* on the water surface
    (A) has never been explained.
    (B) is quantitatively studied.
    (C) is shown on high-frequency cinematographs.
    (D) is investigated in terms of the mechanism of the rowing apparatus.

30. The functional-morphological features of the rowing apparatus of Dytiscidae
    (A) were investigated in detail.
    (B) are somewhat like those of *Gyrinus* and *Acilius*.
    (C) could not be investigated.
    (D) are unknown.

31 The figure 52% refers to
    (A) the role of the leg in generating thrust.
    (B) the effective propulsion force.
    (C) the contribution of the swimming blades to propulsion force.
    (D) the degree of superiority of the propulsion force generated by *Gyrinus* compared to that of *Acilius*.

32. In general, it can be said that
    (A) the efficiency of the oar-leg of *Gyrinus* is inexplicable.
    (B) 96% of the swimming power is dissipated.
    (C) the efficiency of the oar-leg of *Gyrinus* is better than most machines.
    (D) *Gyrinus* has an inefficient rowing apparatus.

# TEST III. VOCABULARY

TIME: 20 Minutes

*DIRECTIONS: In each of the following questions, one word
. . . a numbered word . . . is followed by four or five lettered
words or expressions. Choose the lettered word or expression
that has most nearly the opposite meaning of the numbered word.
Mark the letter preceding that word as the answer to the question.*

1. immutable
   (A) erudite        (B) abject
   (C) changeable     (D) fantastic
   (E) aural.

2. ductile
   (A) feted          (B) alluvial
   (C) stubborn       (D) abnormal
   (E) belabor.

3. fastidious
   (A) factitious     (B) absurd
   (C) indifferent    (D) sloppy
   (E) chary.

4. temerity
   (A) affinity       (B) cherubim
   (C) humility       (D) degenerate
   (E) celerity.

5. itinerant
   (A) animosity      (B) metaphor
   (C) perpetrator    (D) resident
   (E) cerebrum.

6. taciturn
   (A) malevolent     (B) loquacious
   (C) paltry         (D) opaque
   (E) morbid.

7. nefarious
   (A) grotesque      (B) virtuous
   (C) jovial         (D) pious
   (E) ceremonial.

8. obsequiousness
   (A) harbinger      (B) boldness
   (C) heredity       (D) quaff
   (E) honesty.

9. ostentation
   (A) emulsion       (B) languid
   (C) modesty        (D) kilogram
   (E) bey.

10. contention
    (A) equation      (B) oblivion
    (C) guild         (D) pacification
    (E) retrospect.

11. imputation
    (A) assiduity     (B) radiance
    (C) challis       (D) raiment
    (E) vindication.

12. benign
    (A) captious      (B) relevant
    (C) robot         (D) malevolent
    (E) precarious.

13. coherent
    (A) perspicacious (B) zephyr
    (C) wealthy       (D) chaotic
    (E) changeable

14. depredation
    (A) plethora      (B) gloss
    (C) restoration   (D) glamour
    (E) importation.

15. provocative
    (A) sedentary     (B) capricious
    (C) vindictive    (D) tawny
    (E) stimulating.

16. submission
    (A) authorization (B) defiiance
    (C) assignment    (D) defeat
    (E) labor.

17. affluent
    (A) immigrant     (B) conjunctive
    (C) insufficient  (D) filial
    (E) clandestine.

18. churlish
    (A) exiguous      (B) laudable
    (C) cheerful      (D) maternal
    (E) civilized.

S1219

19. symmetry
   - (A) invocation
   - (B) madrigal
   - (C) distortion
   - (D) satyr
   - (E) cilia.

20. dulcet
   - (A) extrinsic
   - (B) optimistic
   - (C) unanimous
   - (D) acerbate
   - (E) chiffonette.

21. irenic
   - (A) easily pleased
   - (B) sarcastic
   - (C) warlike
   - (D) non-ferrous
   - (E) lecherous.

22. mountebank
   - (A) one who lives in a valley
   - (B) an honest person
   - (C) sea gull
   - (D) beggar
   - (E) lectern.

23. acerbity
   - (A) cupidity
   - (B) amiability
   - (C) depredation
   - (D) insomnia
   - (E) facet.

24. expeditious
   - (A) lackadaisical
   - (B) unique
   - (C) ubiquitous
   - (D) epicurean
   - (E) portable.

25. perspicacity
   - (A) obtuseness
   - (B) argot
   - (C) dipsomania
   - (D) malediction
   - (E) kleptomania.

26. splenetic
   - (A) inane
   - (B) complaisant
   - (C) phlegmatic
   - (D) querulous
   - (E) sundered.

# TEST IV. VERBAL ANALOGIES

### TIME: 15 Minutes

*DIRECTIONS: In these test questions each of the two CAPI-TALIZED words have a certain relationship to each other. Following the capitalized words are other pairs of words, each designated by a letter. Select the lettered pair wherein the words are related in the same way as the two CAPITALIZED words are related to each other.*

## EXPLANATIONS OF KEY POINTS
## ARE GIVEN WITH THE ANSWERS

1. INFATUATION : LOVE ::
   - (A) youth : fancy
   - (B) obsession : interest
   - (C) June : wedding
   - (D) cupid : arrow
   - (E) romance : song

2. STOVE : KITCHEN ::
   - (A) window : bedroom
   - (B) sink : bathroom
   - (C) television : living room
   - (D) trunk : attic
   - (E) pot : pan

3. CELEBRATE : MARRIAGE ::
   - (A) announce : birthday
   - (B) report : injury
   - (C) lament : bereavement
   - (D) face : penalty
   - (E) kiss : groom

4. BUTTON : ZIPPER ::
   - (A) thread : needle
   - (B) cloth : material
   - (C) margarine : butter
   - (D) vitamin : health
   - (E) jacket : coat

5. NEGLIGENT : REQUIREMENT ::
   - (A) careful : position  (B) remiss : duty
   - (C) cautious : injury  (D) cogent : task
   - (E) easy : hard

6. GAZELLE : SWIFT ::
   - (A) horse : slow  (B) wolf : sly
   - (C) swan : graceful
   - (D) elephant : gray  (E) lion : tame

7. IGNOMINY : DISLOYALTY ::
   - (A) fame : heroism
   - (B) castigation : praise
   - (C) death : victory
   - (D) approbation : consecration
   - (E) derelict : martyr

8. SATURNINE : MERCURIAL ::
   - (A) Saturn : Venus
   - (B) Appenines : Alps
   - (C) redundant : wordy
   - (D) allegro : adagio
   - (E) heavenly : starry

9. ORANGE : MARMALADE ::
   - (A) potato : vegetable  (B) jelly : jam
   - (C) tomato : ketchup  (D) cake : picnic
   - (E) sandwich : ham

10. BANISH : APOSTATE ::
    - (A) punish : traitor
    - (B) request : assistance
    - (C) remove : result
    - (D) avoid : truce  (E) welcome : ally

11. CIRCLE : SPHERE ::
    - (A) square : triangle
    - (B) balloon : jet plane
    - (C) heaven : hell  (D) wheel : orange
    - (E) pill : drop

12. OPEN : SECRETIVE ::
    - (A) mystery : detective
    - (B) tunnel : toll
    - (C) forthright : snide
    - (D) better : best
    - (E) gun : mask

13. AFFIRM : HINT ::
    (A) say : deny  (B) assert : allege
    (C) confirm : reject
    (D) charge : insinuate
    (E) state : relate

14. THROW : BALL ::
    (A) kill : bullet  (B) shoot : gun
    (C) question : answer  (D) hit : run
    (E) stab : knife

15. SPEEDY : GREYHOUND ::
    (A) innocent : lamb
    (B) animate : animal
    (C) voracious : tiger  (D) clever : fox
    (E) sluggish : sloth

16. TRIANGLE : PYRAMID ::
    (A) cone : circle  (B) corner : angle
    (C) tube : cylinder
    (D) pentagon : quadrilateral
    (E) square : box

17. IMPEACH : DISMISS ::
    (A) arraign : convict
    (B) exonerate : charge
    (C) imprison : jail  (D) plant : reap
    (E) president : Johnson

18. EMULATE : MIMIC ::
    (A) slander : defame
    (B) praise : flatter
    (C) aggravate : promote
    (D) complain : condemn
    (E) express : imply.

19. PUPIL : CORNEA ::
    (A) teacher : pupil
    (B) page : print
    (C) peg : board
    (D) success : money
    (E) farm : kernel.

20. SQUARE : DIAMOND ::
    (A) cube : sugar
    (B) circle : ellipse
    (C) innocence : jewelry
    (D) rectangle : square
    (E) prizefight : baseball

21. WOODSMAN : AXE ::
    (A) mechanic : tool
    (B) soldier : sword.
    (C) draftsman : ruler
    (D) doctor : prescription
    (E) carpenter : saw

22. BIGOTRY : HATRED ::
    (A) sweetness : bitterness
    (B) segregation : integration
    (C) equality : government
    (D) sugar : grain
    (E) fanaticism : intolerance

23. ASSIST : SAVE ::
    (A) agree : oppose
    (B) rely : descry
    (C) help : aid.
    (D) declare : deny
    (E) request : command

24. 2 : 5 ::
    (A) 5 : 7        (B) 6 : 17
    (C) 6 : 15       (D) 5 : 14
    (E) 21 : 51.

25. DOUBLEHEADER : TRIDENT ::
    (A) twin : troika
    (B) ballgame : three bagger
    (C) chewing gum : toothpaste
    (D) freak : zoo
    (E) two : square.

26. BOUQUET : FLOWER ::
    (A) key : door       (B) air : balloon
    (C) skin : body      (D) chain : link
    (E) eye : pigment.

27. LETTER : WORD ::
    (A) club : people
    (B) homework : school
    (C) page : book
    (D) product : factory
    (E) picture : crayon.

28. 36 : 4 ::
    (A) 3 : 27  (B) 9 : 1  (C) 12 : 4
    (D) 12 : 4  (E) 5 : 2

29. GERM : DISEASE ::
    (A) trichinosis : pork
    (B) men : woman
    (C) doctor : medicine
    (D) war : destruction
    (E) biologist : cell

30. WAVE : CREST ::
    (A) pinnacle : nadir
    (B) mountain : peak
    (C) sea : ocean
    (D) breaker : swimming
    (E) island : archipelago

# TEST V. SENTENCE COMPLETIONS

### TIME: 15 Minutes

*DIRECTIONS: Each of the completion questions in this test consists of an incomplete sentence. Each sentence is followed by a series of lettered words, one of which best completes the sentence. Select the word that best completes the meaning of each sentence, and mark the letter of that word opposite that sentence.*

1. The _____ prowess of the pugilist _____ fear into his opponent.
   (A) redoubtable - instilled
   (B) supernatural - propelled
   (C) probing - prevented
   (D) pedagogic - conducted.

2. His _____ nature will aid him in attaining success in this difficult job.
   (A) imitative     (B) lackadaisical
   (C) persevering     (D) rotund.

3. Since he is a teacher of English, we would not expect him to be guilty of a _____.
   (A) solecism     (B) schism
   (C) stanchion     (D) freshet.

4. The servant's attitude was so _____ that it would have been _____ to anyone with an appreciation of sincerity.
   (A) natal - clear
   (B) hybrid - available
   (C) sycophantic - obnoxious
   (D) doleful - responsible.

5. One would expect a serf to _____ to a lord.
   (A) arrogate     (B) apprize
   (C) circumscribe     (D) truckle.

6. Any public officer who allows bribery to flourish should be subject to _____.
   (A) stringency     (B) vagary
   (C) stricture     (D) apologue.

7. The old man was so _____ that he refused to buy food.
   (A) parsimonious     (B) prescient
   (C) prolix     (D) affluent.

8. Our neighbor is so much disliked that we may well consider him a _____.
   (A) pariah     (B) latitudinarian
   (C) calumet     (D) cenotaph.

9. His _____ leads me to believe that he cannot be _____.
   (A) mendicity - injured
   (B) mendacity - trusted
   (C) catachresis - considered
   (D) baldric - trained.

10. In Hindu mythology, _____ referred to a _____ to earth.
    (A) autoclave - reference
    (B) dipsomania - prayer
    (C) divagation - bowing
    (D) avatar - descent.

11. In legislative investigations of _____ subjects, there will always be great risks that any standards set up will yield or be circumvented in one or another.
    (A) delicate     (B) innocuous
    (C) sublimal     (D) controversial
          (E) parsimonious.

12. One of the objects of statutes relating to judicial procedures is the separating of the _____ from the deciding function, and the provision of a measure of independence for the person who is called on to decide.
    (A) jurisprudence     (B) prosecuting
    (C) nonsensical     (D) superficial
          (E) mitigating.

13. In many cases injured persons find it impossible, through their personal initiative and ambition, to _____ themselves to the extent that they are enabled to pursue some work which will bring them a good living.
    (A) consecrate     (B) assimilate
    (C) rehabilitate     (D) coordinate
          (E) educate.

14. The principal object of the _____ law is to define crime and prescribe punishments.

(A) cure      (B) parole
(C) State      (D) Federal
          (E) penal.

15. It is the source of our constitutional rule that serious criminal charges must be made by _____ of a grand jury.
(A) indictment      (B) conviction
(C) consideration      (D) interrogation
          (E) amelioration.

16. In the long run, ideas are more powerful than more _____ weapons.
(A) lethal      (B) military
(C) atomic      (D) legal
          (E) tangible.

17. The Constitution provides that no person shall be twice put in _____ for the same offense.
(A) prison      (B) jeopardy
(C) the army      (D) coventry
          (E) court.

18. Compulsory education was instituted for the purpose of preventing _____ of young children, and guaranteeing them a minimum of education.
(A) malnutrition      (B) ignorance
(C) abuse      (D) exploitation
          (E) delinquency.

19. Any person who is in _____ while awaiting trial is considered innocent until he has been declared guilty.
(A) custody      (B) prison
(C) jeopardy      (D) suspicion
          (E) probation.

20. Certain employers, among them those employing fewer than four persons as well as non-profit making institutions, are _____ under the law, but may elect to become subject to the law.
(A) prohibited      (B) eliminated
(C) demoted      (D) exempted
          (E) mortified.

21. The day will come when _____ will look back upon us and our time with a sense of superiority.
(A) teachers      (B) posterity
(C) scientists      (D) ancestors
          (E) sophisticates.

22. Now, many years later, with the benefit of much _____, we see the activities in which these people engaged in a very unfavorable light.
(A) foresight      (B) education
(C) hindsight      (D) research
          (E) Federal aid.

23. A majority of the membership constitutes a _____ to do business in the Senate.
(A) forum      (B) quorum
(C) podium      (D) minority
          (E) malfeasance.

24. The fact that the locations were a mile and a half apart was welcomed by L'Enfant as conducing to ceremonial intercourse, and by the practical Washington as _____ the importunities of the legislature, a waste of time he suffered in New York and Philadelphia.
(A) creating      (B) mitigating
(C) multiplying      (D) relegating
          (E) implementing.

25. Practically anything can be done in either House by _____ consent except where the Constitution or the rules specifically prohibit the presiding officer from entertaining such a request.
(A) presidential      (B) parliamentary
(C) appropriate      (D) congressional
          (E) unanimous.

26. A "rider" is a (an) _____ provision incorporated in an appropriation bill, with the idea of "riding" through to enactment on the merits of the main measure.
(A) pusillanimous      (B) mandatory
(C) influential      (D) extraneous
          (E) macabre.

27. Monetary policy was _____ primarily through the flexible use of both open market operations and adjustments in the dicount rate.
(A) implemented      (B) controlled
(C) unified      (D) deliberated
          (E) associated.

28. While lenses and frames form the focus of operations, the company also makes a host of other _____ products such as artificial eyes and instruments used to correct ocular defects as well as eyeglass cases.
(A) panoramic      (B) corporate
(C) mutilated      (D) optimistic
          (E) ocular.

29. A minor legal _____ developed early when the legislature passed a new law.

    (A) impediment    (B) miscellany
    (C) diurnal        (D) morais
          (E) syncopation.

30. Short of a further major _____ of business conditions, it is difficult to see how inventory liquidation could continue at current rates much beyond mid-year.

    (A) infiltration    (B) delimitation
    (C) deterioration    (D) machination
          (E) obliteration.

# TEST VI. QUANTITATIVE ABILITY

### TIME: 60 Minutes

*DIRECTIONS: For each of the following questions, select the choice which best answers the question or completes the statement.*

## EXPLANATIONS ARE GIVEN WITH THE ANSWERS
## WHICH FOLLOW THE QUESTIONS

1. Of the following, the one that is *not* a meaning of ⅔ is

   (A) 1 of the 3 equal parts of 2
   (B) 2 of the 3 equal parts of 1
   (C) 2 divided by 3
   (D) a ratio of 2 to 3
   (E) 4 of the 6 equal parts of 2

2. If the average weight of boys of John's age and height is 105 lbs. and if John weighs 110% of average, then John weighs

   (A) 110 lbs.          (B) 110.5 lbs.
   (C) 106.05 lbs.       (D) 126 lbs.
            (E) 115½ lbs.

3. On a house plan on which 2 inches represents 5 feet, the length of a room measures 7½ inches. The actual length of the room is

   (A) 12½ feet          (B) 15¾ feet
   (C) 17½ feet          (D) 18¾ feet
            (E) 13¾ feet

*Questions 4-7 are to be answered with reference to the following diagram.*

The figure shown in the diagram is made of pieces of plastic, each piece half a centimeter thick and one centimeter wide.

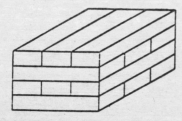

4. What is the volume of the figure?

   (A) 12 cu cm
   (B) 18 cu cm
   (C) 27 cu cm
   (D) 36 cu cm
   (E) Cannot be determined from the given information

5. How many pieces are touched by at least 8 other pieces?

   (A) 1              (B) 2
   (C) 3              (D) 4
            (E) 5

6. If all the pieces had been cut from one strip of plastic, how long a piece of ½ cm × 1 cm material would have been required?

   (A) 15 cm
   (B) 18 cm
   (C) 27 cm
   (D) 12 cm
   (E) 36 cm

7. What is the total surface in square centimeters of all the pieces?

   (A) 10
   (B) 18
   (C) 72
   (D) 120
   (E) 42

S1346

*Questions 8-12 are to be answered with reference to the graph-chart below.*

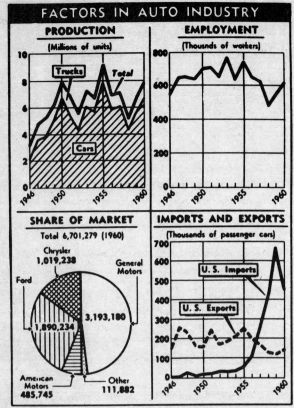

FACTORS IN AUTO INDUSTRY

PRODUCTION (Millions of units) — Trucks, Total, Cars — 1946 1950 1955 1960

EMPLOYMENT (Thousnds of workers) — 1946 1950 1955 1960

SHARE OF MARKET
Total 6,701,279 (1960)
Chrysler 1,019,238
General Motors 3,193,180
Ford 1,890,234
American Motors 485,745
Other 111,882

IMPORTS AND EXPORTS (Thousands of passenger cars) — U.S. Imports, U.S. Exports — 1946 1950 1955 1960

8. The number of auto workers in 1960 was about what per cent of the peak year of employment?

   (A) 55%
   (B) 70%
   (C) 80%
   (D) 88%
   (E) 95%

9. These auto industry graphs and charts will not be able to tell you the following for the 1946-1960 period:

   (A) how employment in one year compared with employment in another year
   (B) the percent of production that trucks have constituted
   (C) the breakdown of the Chrysler Company types of cars which have been sold
   (D) the number of U.S.-made passenger cars marketed abroad
   (E) how many passenger cars were produced

10. In 1960, the exports of cars made up approximately what part of the import-export total?

    (A) one-eighth
    (B) one-seventh
    (C) one-fourth
    (D) one-third
    (E) one-half

11. General Motors and Ford combined have about what per cent of the entire market?

    (A) 50%
    (B) 60%
    (C) 75%
    (D) 85%
    (E) 90%

12. The years in which the number of passenger car imports and exports were a) about the same and b) farthest apart were

    (A) 1955 and 1950
    (B) 1957 and 1959
    (C) 1946 and 1957
    (D) 1960 and 1959
    (E) 1960 and 1957

13. ABCD is a parallelogram, and DE = EC

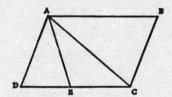

What is the ratio of triangle ADE to the area of the parallelogram?

    (A) 1:2
    (B) 1:3
    (C) 2:5
    (D) 1:4
    (E) cannot be determined from the given information

14. If pencils are bought at 35 cents per dozen and sold at 3 for 10 cents the total profit on 5½ dozen is

    (A) 25 cents
    (B) 27½ cents
    (C) 28½ cents
    (D) 31½ cents
    (E) 35 cents

15. Of the following, the one which may be used correctly to compute $26 \times 3\frac{1}{2}$ is

   (A) $(26 \times 30) + (26 \times \frac{1}{2})$
   (B) $(20 \times 3) + (6 \times 3\frac{1}{2})$
   (C) $(20 \times 3\frac{1}{2}) + (6 \times 3)$
   (D) $(20 \times 3) + (26 \times \frac{1}{2}) + (6 \times 3\frac{1}{2})$
   (E) $(26 \times \frac{1}{2}) + (20 \times 3) + (6 \times 3)$

16. It costs 31 cents a square foot to lay linoleum. To lay 20 square yards of linoleum it will cost

   (A) $16.20
   (B) $18.60
   (C) $62.80
   (D) $62.00
   (E) $55.80

*Questions 17-21 are to be answered with reference to the following explanation and table.*

Ten judges were asked to judge the relative sweetness of five compounds (A, B, C, D, and E) by the method of paired comparisons. In judging each of the possible pairs they were required to state unequivocally which of the two compounds was the sweeter—a judgment of equality or no difference was not permitted.

The results of their judgments are summarized in the table below. In studying the table, note that each cell entry shows the number of comparisons in which the "row" compound was judged to be sweeter than the "column" compound.

|   | A | B | C | D | E |
|---|---|---|---|---|---|
| A |   | 5 | 8 | 10 | 2 |
| B | 5 |   | 3 | 9 | 6 |
| C | 2 | 7 |   | 7 | 8 |
| D | 0 | 1 | 3 |   | 4 |
| E | 8 | 4 | 2 | 6 |   |

17. How many comparisons did each judge make?

   (A) 5
   (B) 10
   (C) 15
   (D) 20
   (E) 25

18. Which compound was judged to be sweetest?

   (A) A
   (B) B

(C) C
(D) D
(E) E

19. Which compound was judged to be least sweet?

   (A) A
   (B) B
   (C) C
   (D) D
   (E) E

20. Which of the following statements is most nearly correct?

   (A) There was almost perfect agreement among the ten judges.
   (B) The clearest discrimination was between B and C.
   (C) The judges were not expert in discriminating sweetnesses.
   (D) Compound D was most clearly discriminated from the other four compounds.
   (E) Compounds C and E were judged to have the same sweetness.

21. Between which two compounds was the discrimination least consistent?

   (A) A and D
   (B) B and E
   (C) C and E
   (D) C and D
   (E) A and B

22. A piece of wood 35 feet, 6 inches long was used to make 4 shelves of equal length. The length of each shelf was

   (A) 9 feet, 1½ inches
   (B) 8 feet, 10½ inches
   (C) 7 feet, 10½ inches
   (D) 7 feet, 1½ inches
   (E) 6 feet, 8½ inches

23. A class punch ball team won 2 games and lost 10. The fraction of its games won is correctly expressed as

   (A) 1/6
   (B) 1/5
   (C) 4/5
   (D) 5/6
   (E) 1/10

24. 10 to the fifth power may correctly be expressed as

    (A) $10 \times 5$
    (B) $5^{10}$
    (C) $5\sqrt{10}$
    (D) $10 \times 10 \times 10 \times 10 \times 10$
    (E) $10^{10} \div 10^2$

25. The total cost of 3½ pounds of meat at $1.10 a pound and 20 oranges at $.60 a dozen will be

    (A) $4.65
    (B) $4.85
    (C) $5.05
    (D) $4.45
    (E) none of these

*Questions 26-28 are to be answered with reference to the following number system:*

The following symbols are used in the same fashion as Roman numerals are used.

$$I = |$$
$$V = \cap$$
$$X = ?$$
$$L = \Gamma$$
$$C = \emptyset$$
$$D = \bigcirc$$
$$M = \&$$

For example, $?|\cap = 14$.

Thousands are indicated by drawing a line over the symbol. For example, $\overline{\cap} = 5000$.

26. $\overline{?\,\emptyset\,\Gamma}$ equals ?

    (A) 1915
    (B) 10,315
    (C) 10,915
    (D) 10,150
    (E) 11,050

27. $4(10^4) + 5(10^3) + 4(100)$ is represented by

    (A) [symbols]
    (B) [symbols]
    (C) [symbols]
    (D) [symbols]
    (E) [symbols]

28. Select the correct expression for [symbols]

    (A) $1,000,000 + 100 + 2,000 + 100,000 + 2$
    (B) $2(10^6) + 2(10^4) + 10 + 1,000 + 2$
    (C) $2(100) + 2(10^3) + 5(10) + 10(1000,000) + 2$
    (D) $10^6 + 50(10,000) + 2,000 + 2$
    (E) $100 \times 10^5 + 5 \times 10^5 + 20 \times 10^2 + 2 \times 10^1$

29. The total number of eighths in two wholes and three fourths is

    (A) 11
    (B) 14
    (C) 19
    (D) 22
    (E) 24

30. The difference between one hundred five thousand eighty-four and ninety-three thousand seven hundred nine is

    (A) 37,215
    (B) 12,131
    (C) 56,294
    (D) 56,375
    (E) 11,375

31. A recipe for a cake calls for 2½ cups of milk and 3 cups of flour. With this recipe, a cake was baked using 14 cups of flour. How many cups of milk were required?

    (A) 10⅓
    (B) 10¾
    (C) 11
    (D) 11⅗
    (E) 11⅔

*Questions 32-34 are to be answered with reference to the following explanation and diagram.*

A cube may be rotated about any one of its three axes, a, b, or c. The rotation of the cube 90° about "a" in the direction of the arrow may be denoted by $a$; the rotation of the cube 90° about "b" in the direction of the arrow by $b$; and rotation of the cube 90° about "c" in the direction of the arrow by $c$.

If operation $a$ is performed twice, the whole operation may be indicated as $a^2$; if three times, as $a^3$; etc. Similarly, the same holds for $b$ and $c$. If operation $b$ is performed, and then $c$, the result is $bc$.

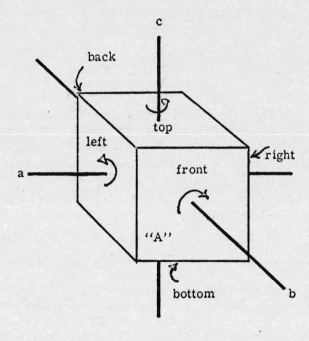

32. After the operation $a^3b$, where is face "A"?

(A) back
(B) bottom
(C) left
(D) top
(E) right

33. Where was the face which is on the bottom after the operation bc before the operation?

(A) back
(B) left
(C) right
(D) top
(E) bottom

34. Which operation leaves the cube in the same position as it is after $a^2b^2c^2$?

(A) $(bc)^2$
(B) $b^3c^3$
(C) $c^4$
(D) $c^3ba^3$
(E) $(ab)^3$

35. What would be the marked price of an article if the cost was $12.60 and the gain was 10% of the selling price?

(A) $13.66
(B) $13.86
(C) $11.34
(D) $12.48
(E) $14.00

36. A certain type of board is sold only in lengths of multiples of 2 feet from 6 ft. to 24 ft. A builder needs a large quantity of this type of board in 5½ foot lengths. For minimum waste, the lengths to be ordered should be

(A) 6 ft.
(B) 12 ft.
(C) 24 ft.
(D) 22 ft.
(E) 18 ft.

37. The tiles in the floor of a bathroom are 15/16 inch squares. The cement between the tiles is 1/16 inch. There are 3240 individual tiles in this floor. The area of the floor is

(A) 225 sq. yds.
(B) 2.5 sq. yds.
(C) 250 sq. ft.
(D) 22.5 sq. yds.
(E) 225 sq. ft.

38. A group of 15 children received the following scores in a reading test: 36 36 30 30 30 29 27 27 27 26 26 26 26 18 13. What was the median score?

(A) 25.4
(B) 26
(C) 27
(D) 30
(E) 24.5

*Questions 39-43 are to be answered with reference to the following diagram and explanation.*

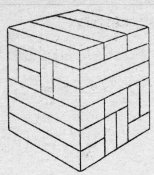

The 6-inch cube shown in the diagram is made up of pieces each 1 inch thick, 2 inches wide, and 6 inches long. Each block is painted in three colors, red, blue, and yellow according to its position as shown in the diagram. The top side of each block is red. The bottom side of each piece is blue, and the vertical sides are yellow.

39. How many 1 × 2 × 6 blocks are there in the 6-inch cube?
    (A) 15
    (B) 18
    (C) 27
    (D) 36
    (E) 24

40. How many square inches of block are painted blue?
    (A) 150
    (B) 316
    (C) 210
    (D) 256
    (E) 180

41. What is the largest number of plane surfaces of other blocks touched by the plane surfaces of any one block?
    (A) 8
    (B) 11
    (C) 13
    (D) 15
    (E) 16

42. How many square inches of blue surface are touching red surfaces?
    (A) 94
    (B) 108
    (C) 144
    (D) 196
    (E) 216

43. Which arrangement of the blocks, forming a 6-inch cube, painted in the fashion described in the paragraph, would require the smallest possible area of yellow paint?
    (A) all blocks laid with a 2 × 6 side horizontal
    (B) all blocks laid with a 1 × 6 side horizontal
    (C) all blocks laid with a 1 × 2 end horizontal
    (D) all blocks laid with a 1 × 2 side vertical
    (E) the arrangement makes no difference

44. Of the following the one that is *not* equivalent to 376 is
    (A) (3 × 100) + (6 × 10) + 16
    (B) (2 × 100) + (17 × 10) + 6
    (C) (3 × 100) + (7 × 10) + 6
    (D) (2 × 100) + (16 × 10) + 6
    (E) (2 × 100) + (7 × 10) + 106

45. A man bought a TV set that was listed at $160. He was given successive discounts of 20% and 10%. The price he paid was
    (A) $112.00
    (B) $115.20
    (C) $119.60
    (D) $129.60
    (E) $118.20

46. The total length of fencing needed to enclose a rectangular area 46 feet by 34 feet is
    (A) 26 yards 1 foot
    (B) 26⅔ yards
    (C) 52 yards 2 feet
    (D) 53⅓ yards
    (E) 37⅔ yards

47. Mr. Jones' income for a year is $15,000. He pays 15% of this in federal taxes and 10% of the remainder for state taxes. How much is left?
    (A) $12,750
    (B) $ 9,750
    (C) $14,125
    (D) $13,500
    (E) $11,475

# TEST VII. PERCEPTUAL MOTOR ABILITY

### TIME: 20 Minutes

*DIRECTIONS: Each question in this test consists of a numbered picture showing a piece of cardboard that is to be folded. The dotted lines show where folds are to be made. The problem is to choose the lettered picture, A, B, C, or D which would be made by folding the cardboard in the numbered picture. For each question blacken the space on your answer sheet corresponding to the letter of the best answer.*

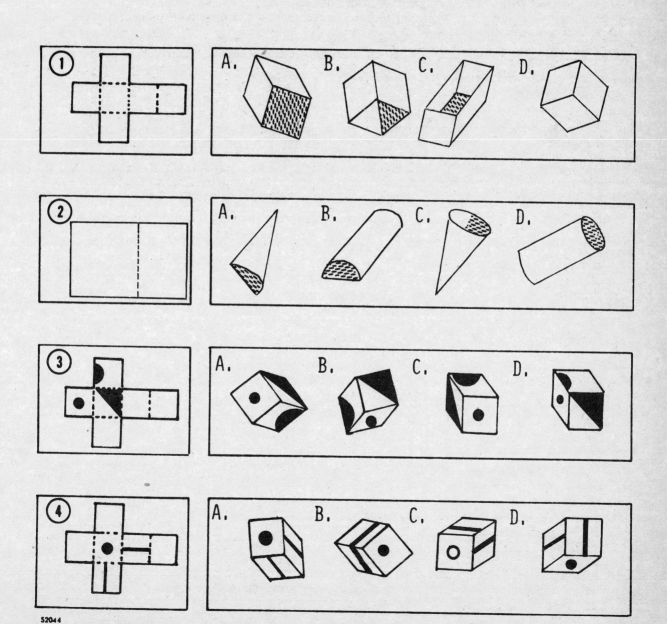

S2044

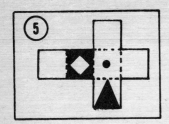
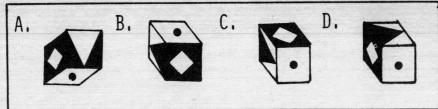

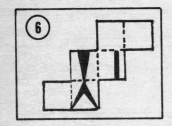
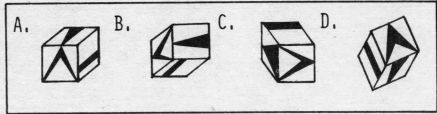

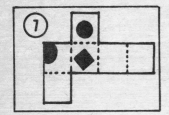
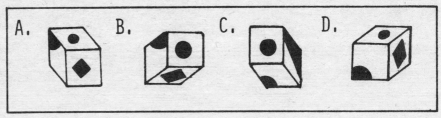

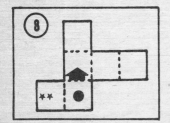
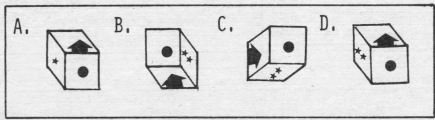

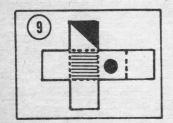
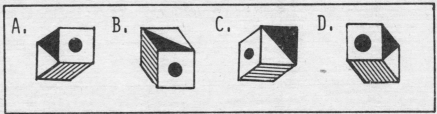

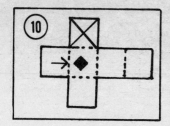

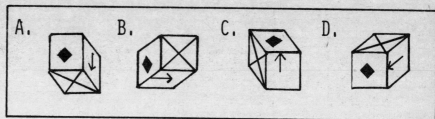

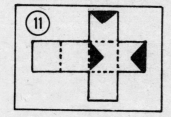

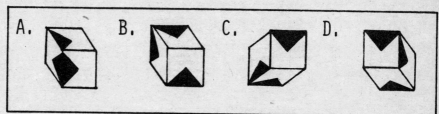

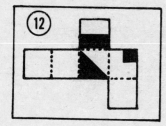

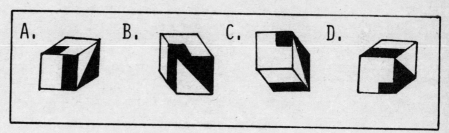

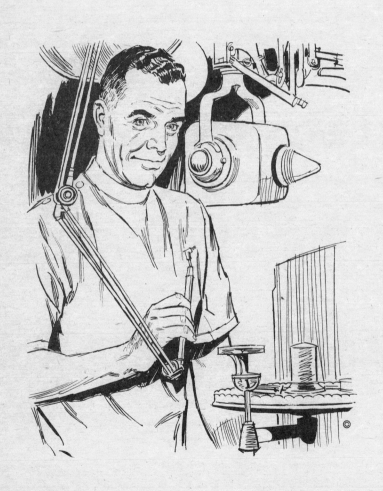

# AFTER TAKING EXAMINATION I.

*STEP ONE — Check all your answers with the Correct Answers that follow. Then compare your total score with the Unofficial Percentile Ranking Table below. This Table will give you a reasonably good idea of how you stand with others taking the Exam. For example, if your percentile ranking is 61, according to your score, you are superior to 60% and inferior to 39% of those who have taken the Exam. Your percentile ranking on the Examination is a major factor in determining your eligibility.*

## PERCENTILE RANKING TABLE
### (unofficial)

| Approximate Percentile Ranking | Score On Test | Approximate Percentile Ranking | Score On Test |
|---|---|---|---|
| 99 | 225–227 | 69 | 161–162 |
| 98 | 222–224 | 68 | 159–160 |
| 97 | 219–221 | 67 | 157–158 |
| 96 | 216–218 | 66 | 155–156 |
| 95 | 213–215 | 65 | 153–154 |
| 94 | 211–212 | 64 | 151–152 |
| 93 | 209–210 | 63 | 149–150 |
| 92 | 207–208 | 62 | 147–148 |
| 91 | 205–206 | 61 | 145–146 |
| 90 | 203–204 | 60 | 143–144 |
| 89 | 201–202 | 59 | 140–142 |
| 88 | 199–200 | 58 | 137–139 |
| 87 | 197–198 | 57 | 134–136 |
| 86 | 195–196 | 56 | 131–133 |
| 85 | 193–194 | 55 | 128–130 |
| 84 | 191–192 | 54 | 125–127 |
| 83 | 189–190 | 53 | 122–124 |
| 82 | 187–188 | 52 | 119–121 |
| 81 | 185–186 | 51 | 116–118 |
| 80 | 183–184 | 50 | 113–115 |
| 79 | 181–182 | 49 | 110–112 |
| 78 | 179–180 | 48 | 107–109 |
| 77 | 177–178 | 47 | 104–106 |
| 76 | 175–176 | 46 | 101–103 |
| 75 | 173–174 | 45 | 98–100 |
| 74 | 171–172 | 44 | 95–97 |
| 73 | 169–170 | 43 | 92–94 |
| 72 | 167–168 | 42 | 89–91 |
| 71 | 165–166 | 41 | 86–88 |
| 70 | 163–164 | 0–40 | 0–85 |

*STEP TWO — Use the results of the Examination you have just taken to diagnose yourself. Pinpoint the areas in which you show the greatest weakness. Fill in the Diagnostic Table to spotlight the subjects in which you need the most practice.*

| DIAGNOSTIC TABLE FOR EXAMINATION I. | | | |
|---|---|---|---|
| SUBJECT TESTED | QUESTIONS ANSWERED CORRECTLY ON EXAM | | |
| | Strong | Average | Weak |
| TEST I. BIOMEDICAL SCIENCE | 41–50 | 26–40 | 20–25 |
| TEST II. INTERPRETATION OF SCIENCE READINGS | 23–32 | 17–22 | 10–16 |
| TEST III. VOCABULARY | 17–26 | 13–16 | 7–12 |
| TEST IV. VERBAL ANALOGIES | 21–30 | 16–20 | 10–15 |
| TEST V. SENTENCE COMPLETIONS | 21–30 | 16–20 | 10–15 |
| TEST VI. QUANTITATIVE ABILITY | 39–47 | 24–38 | 19–23 |
| TEST VII. PERCEPTUAL MOTOR ABILITY | 10–12 | 8–9 | 6–7 |

*STEP THREE*—Use the following Check List to establish areas that require the greatest application on your part. One check (√) after the item means moderately weak; *two checks (√ √) means* seriously weak.

| Area of Weakness | Check Below | Area of Weakness | Check Below |
|---|---|---|---|
| BIOLOGY | | VERBAL ANALOGIES | |
| CHEMISTRY | | SENTENCE COMPLETIONS | |
| SCIENCE READINGS | | MATHEMATICS | |
| SYNONYMS | | SPATIAL PROBLEM SOLVING | |
| OPPOSITES | | | |

*STEP FOUR* — The Pinpoint Practice chapters which follow provide all the drill material you need for every phase of the Examination. Plan your attack systematically. Concentrate on your weaknesses. Answer the practice questions in these areas. As you will discover, the material is presented so that the areas tested in the actual exam are individually treated in this book.

*STEP FIVE* — When you have strengthened yourself sufficiently where strengthening is necessary, take the other Examinations in the book. Again place yourself under strict testing conditions. We have every confidence that you will do better on the following Exams than you did on this one, if you've followed our suggestions for eliminating "soft spots." Now, please get to work.

# CORRECT ANSWERS FOR PREDICTIVE EXAMINATION I.

*(Please try to answer the questions on your own before looking at our answers. You'll do much better on your test if you follow this rule.)*

## TEST I. BIOMEDICAL SCIENCE

| | | | | | | | |
|---|---|---|---|---|---|---|---|
| 1. A | 8. A | 15. C | 21. A | 27. B | 33. A | 39. A | 45. B |
| 2. B | 9. B | 16. B | 22. C | 28. C | 34. B | 40. A | 46. D |
| 3. C | 10. D | 17. D | 23. D | 29. B | 35. C | 41. C | 47. A |
| 4. A | 11. A | 18. B | 24. B | 30. A | 36. A | 42. C | 48. C |
| 5. A | 12. B | 19. A | 25. D | 31. D | 37. B | 43. D | 49. C |
| 6. D | 13. D | 20. D | 26. B | 32. B | 38. C | 44. C | 50. C |
| 7. A | 14. D | | | | | | |

## TEST II. INTERPRETATION OF SCIENCE READINGS

| | | | | | | | |
|---|---|---|---|---|---|---|---|
| 1. B | 5. D | 9. C | 13. C | 17. B | 21. C | 25. C | 29. D |
| 2. A | 6. C | 10. B | 14. B | 18. C | 22. B | 26. A | 30. B |
| 3. A | 7. C | 11. D | 15. C | 19. A | 23. C | 27. C | 31. C |
| 4. D | 8. B | 12. C | 16. A | 20. C | 24. C | 28. B | 32. C |

## TEST III. VOCABULARY

| | | | | | | | |
|---|---|---|---|---|---|---|---|
| 1. C | 5. D | 9. C | 12. D | 15. A | 18. C | 21. C | 24. A |
| 2. C | 6. B | 10. D | 13. D | 16. B | 19. C | 22. B | 25. A |
| 3. D | 7. B | 11. E | 14. C | 17. C | 20. D | 23. B | 26. B |
| 4. C | 8. B | | | | | | |

## TEST IV. VERBAL ANALOGIES

| | | | | | | | |
|---|---|---|---|---|---|---|---|
| 1. B | 5. B | 9. C | 13. D | 17. A | 21. E | 25. A | 28. B |
| 2. B | 6. C | 10. E | 14. B | 18. B | 22. E | 26. D | 29. D |
| 3. C | 7. A | 11. D | 15. E | 19. A | 23. E | 27. C | 30. B |
| 4. C | 8. D | 12. C | 16. E | 20. B | 24. C | | |

# TEST IV. EXPLANATORY ANSWERS

*Elucidation, clarification, explication and a little help with the fundamental facts covered in the Previous Test. These are the points and principles likely to crop up in the form of questions on future tests.*

1. **(B)** An infatuation is an extreme form of love; an obsession is an extreme form of interest.

2. **(B)** A stove is an essential part of a kitchen; a sink is an essential part of a bathroom.

3. **(C)** You happily celebrate a marriage; you sorrowfully lament a bereavement.

4. **(C)** A button may be used instead of a zipper; margarine may be used instead of butter. Note that a jacket is a *type* of coat.

5. **(B)** A person may be negligent in meeting a requirement; he may similarly be remiss in performing his duty.

6. **(C)** A gazelle is known to be swift; a swan is known to be graceful.

7. **(A)** One falls into ignominy if he shows disloyalty; one gains fame if he shows heroism.

8. **(D)** Saturnine and mercurial are antonyms; so are allegro and adagio.

9. **(C)** Marmalade is made from oranges; ketchup is made from tomatoes.

10. **(E)** An apostate is banished (sent away); an ally is welcomed (brought in).

11. **(D)** All four are round: circle, sphere, wheel, and orange.

12. **(C)** Open is the opposite of secretive; forthright is the opposite of snide.

13. **(D)** When you affirm, you are direct—when you hint, you are indirect; when you charge, you are direct—when you insinuate, you are indirect.

14. **(B)** One throws a ball and one shoots a gun.

15. **(E)** A greyhound is proverbially speedy; on the other hand, a sloth is proverbially sluggish.

16. **(E)** A triangle is a three-sided plane figure—a pyramid is a three-sided solid figure; a square is a four-sided plane figure—a box is a four-sided solid figure.

17. **(A)** To impeach is to charge or challenge—if the impeachment proceedings are successful, the charged person is dismissed; to arraign is to call into court as a result of accusation—if the accusation is proved correct, the arraigned person is convicted.

18. **(B)** To emulate is to do things similar to what another person does—to mimic is to do exactly what another person does; to praise is to speak well of another person—to flatter is to praise excessively. Moreover, all four words indicate a favorable attitude toward some person.

19. **(A)** The pupil and the cornea are essential parts of the eye; the teacher and the pupil are essential parts of the class.

20. **(B)** A diamond is a partially "compressed" square; an ellipse is a partially "compressed" circle.

21. **(E)** A woodsman cuts with an axe; a carpenter cuts with a saw.

22. **(E)** Bigotry breeds hatred; fanaticism breeds intolerance.

23. **(E)** When you assist, you help—when you save, you help a great deal; when you request, you ask—when you command, you are very strong in what you ask for.

24. **(C)** 2½ times 2 = 5; 2½ times 6 = 15.

25. **(A)** A doubleheader has two parts—a trident has three teeth; a twin is two of a kind—a troika is a vehicle drawn by three horses.

26. **(D)** A flower is part of a bouquet; a link is part of a chain.

27. **(C)** Letters make up a word; pages make up a book.

28. **(B)** 36 = 9 times 4; 9 = <u>9</u> times 1.

29. **(D)** A germ often causes disease; a war often causes destruction.

30. **(B)** The top of the wave is the crest; the top of the mountain is the peak.

## TEST V. SENTENCE COMPLETIONS

| | | | | | | | |
|---|---|---|---|---|---|---|---|
| 1. A | 5. D | 9. B | 13. C | 17. B | 21. B | 25. E | 28. E |
| 2. C | 6. C | 10. D | 14. E | 18. D | 22. C | 26. D | 29. A |
| 3. A | 7. A | 11. D | 15. A | 19. A | 23. B | 27. A | 30. C |
| 4. C | 8. A | 12. B | 16. E | 20. D | 24. B | | |

## TEST VI. QUANTITATIVE ABILITY

| | | | | | | | |
|---|---|---|---|---|---|---|---|
| 1. E | 7. D | 13. D | 19. D | 25. B | 31. E | 37. B | 43. A |
| 2. E | 8. C | 14. B | 20. D | 26. D | 32. C | 38. C | 44. D |
| 3. D | 9. C | 15. E | 21. E | 27. C | 33. C | 39. B | 45. B |
| 4. B | 10. C | 16. E | 22. B | 28. D | 34. C | 40. E | 46. D |
| 5. B | 11. C | 17. B | 23. A | 29. D | 35. E | 41. B | 47. E. |
| 6. E | 12. B | 18. A | 24. D | 30. E | 36. D | 42. C | |

## TEST VI. EXPLANATORY ANSWERS

*Elucidation, clarification, explication and a little help with the fundamental facts covered in the Previous Test. These are the points and principles likely to crop up in the form of questions on future tests.*

1. **(E)** 4 of the 6 equal parts of 2 means
$$\frac{4}{6} \times 2, \text{ or } \frac{4}{3}.$$

2. **(E)** 110% of 105 is 1.1 × 105, or 115.5

3. **(D)** This is a proportion: 2 inches: 7½ inches = 5 feet: x, so x = 18¾ feet.

4. **(B)** The horizontal edges are each 3 cm. long, and the vertical edges are 2 cm. long. Therefore, the volume is 3 × 3 × 2, or 18 cc.

5. **(B)** The only pieces that touch eight other pieces are the shaded ones in this diagram:

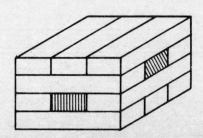

6. **(E)** In order to have a volume of 18 cc., the piece of material must be ½ cm. × 1 cm. × 36 cm.

7. **(D)** Each piece has two faces which are 1 cm. × ½ cm., or ½ sq. cm., two faces which are 1 cm. × 3 cm., or 3 sq. cm., and two faces which are ½ cm. × 3 cm., or 1½ sq. cm. The surface area of each piece is therefore 10 sq. cm. Since there are 12 such pieces, the total area is 120 sq. cm.

8. **(C)** The employment in the peak year was about 750,000, while the employment in 1960 was about 600,000. 600,000 is about 80% of 750,000.

9. **(C)** The only mention of Chrysler cars is their total production, not a breakdown of their types of cars.

10. **(C)** In 1960, the U.S. exported about 150,000 cars, and imported 450,000. 150,000 is about ¼ of the total, 600,000.

11. **(C)** General Motors had a little under 50%, and Ford had a little over 25%, so their sum was about 75%.

12. **(B)** In 1957, both were about 200,000 while in 1959, imports were close to 700,000, while exports fell nearly to 100,000.

13. **(D)** The area of triangle ADE equals the area of triangle AEC, since they have the same base and altitude. The area of triangle ABC equals that of triangle ADC, since the diagonal of a parallelogram divides it equally.

14. **(B)** At 3 for 10¢, one dozen pencils cost 40¢, so the profit on each dozen is 5¢. With 5½ dozen, the profit is 27½¢.

15. **(E)** $26 \times 3\frac{1}{2} = (26 \times 3) + (26 \times \frac{1}{2})$ by the distributive law. $26 \times 3 = (20 \times 3) + (6 \times 3)$ by the distributive law. Therefore, $26 \times 3\frac{1}{2} = (26 \times \frac{1}{2}) + (20 \times 3) + (6 \times 3)$.

16. **(E)** 20 square yards equals 180 square feet. At 31¢ per square foot, it will cost $55.80.

17. **(B)** Each compound is compared with all the others, giving 20, but since each comparison has been counted twice, we divide by 2 to give 10.

18. **(A)** A was judged sweeter 25 times.

19. **(D)** D was judged sweeter only 8 times.

20. **(D)** The other compounds were judged sweeter 25, 23, 24, and 20 times, while D was judged sweeter only 8 times.

21. **(E)** 5 judges called A sweeter, and 5 called B sweeter.

22. **(B)** 35 feet, 6 inches equals 426 inches. One-fourth of this is 106½ inches, or 8 feet, 10½ inches.

23. **(A)** Out of 12 total games, two were won. Thus, the fraction is 2/12, or 1/6.

24. **(D)** $10^5$ is defined as $10 \times 10 \times 10 \times 10 \times 10$, or 100,000. $10 \times 5 = 50$; $5^{10} = 25^5$; $5\sqrt{10}$ is between 1 and 2; and $10^{10} \div 10^2 = 10^8$.

25. **(B)** $3\frac{1}{2} \times \$1.10 = \$3.85$. At 60¢ a dozen, one orange costs 5¢, and 20 cost $1.00. The total is $4.85.

26. **(D)** ⳋⳋⳋ° = XCL = 10,150.

27. **(C)** $4(10^4) + 5(10^3) + 4(100) = 45,400 =$

𝓃ⵏ𝓒𝓒𝓒𝓒

28. **(D)** ⳤⳡ‖ ‖ = 1,502,002 = $10^6$ + 50(10,-000) + 2,000 +2.

29. **(D)** $2\frac{3}{4} \div \frac{1}{8} = \frac{11}{4} \div \frac{1}{8} = \frac{11}{4} \times 8 = 22$

30. **(E)** 105,084 − 93,709 = 11,375.

31. **(E)** This is a proportion → $2\frac{1}{2} : 3 = x : 14$; $x = {}^{35}\!/_3$, or 11⅔.

32. **(C)** After a³, "A" is on the bottom. After this, then b; "A" moves to the left.

33. **(C)** Starting on the right, b brings the face in question to the bottom, and c then leaves it in the same position.

34. **(C)** $a^2b^2c^2$ returns the cube to its original position, and so does $c^4$.

35. **(E)** If the gain was 10% of the selling price, then $12.60 was 90% so 100% was equal to $14.00.

36. **(D)** There will be no waste if the lengths are multiples of 5½ feet. This occurs between 6 and 24 only for 22 feet.

37. **(B)** Each tile, including half of the cement around it, has an area of 1 square inch. 3240 square inches equals 22.5 square feet, or 2.5 square yards.

38. **(C)** A median score is the middle score when all scores are arranged in ascending or descending order. This is 27 here.

39. **(B)** The volume of the large cube is $6^3$, or 216 cubic inches. Each $1'' \times 2'' \times 6''$ block has a volume of 12 cubic inches. Dividing, there are 18 cubes.

40. **(E)** 12 blocks have their $2'' \times 6''$ faces painted blue. 6 more have their $1'' \times 6''$ faces painted blue. The total area of blue is 180 sq. in.

41. **(B)** The shaded block touches 11 other blocks.

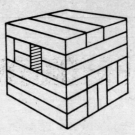

42. **(C)** All the blue surface touches red surface, except for the 36 square inches on the bottom of the cube. Since 180 square inches are blue (see #40), 144 of these touch red surfaces.

43. **(A)** It is required to have the least possible vertical area. This is obtained when the $2'' \times 6''$ side is horizontal, leaving only $1'' \times 2''$ and $1'' \times 6''$ sides to be vertical.

44. **(D)** $(2 \times 100) + (16 \times 10) + 6 = 200 + 160 + 6 = 366$.

45. **(B)** After the 20% discount, the price was $128. After the 10% discount, the price was $115.20.

46. **(D)** The perimeter of a $46' \times 34'$ rectangle is 160 feet, which equals 53⅓ yards.

47. **(E)** After the 15% deduction, $12,750 is left. After the 10% is deducted from $12,750, $11,475 is left. Note that you cannot simply deduct 25% from the $15,000.

# TEST VII. PERCEPTUAL MOTOR ABILITY

| | | | | | | | |
|---|---|---|---|---|---|---|---|
| 1. D | 3. D | 5. C | 7. B | 9. A | 10. C | 11. B | 12. A |
| 2. B | 4. A | 6. A | 8. D | | | | |

# II. PREDICTIVE PRACTICE EXAMINATION

*This Examination is very much like the one you'll take. It was constructed by professionals who utilized all the latest information available. They derived a series of Tests which neatly cover all the subjects you are likely to encounter on the actual examination. Stick to business; follow all instructions closely; and score yourself objectively. If you do poorly . . . review. If necessary, take this Examination again for comparison.*

**TOTAL TIME: 4 hours 30 minutes. In order to create the climate of the test to come, that's precisely what you should allow yourself . . . no more, no less. Use a watch and keep a record of your time, especially since you may find it convenient to take the test in several sittings.**

In making up the Tests we predict for your exam, great care was exercised to prepare questions having just the difficulty level you'll encounter on your exam. Not easier; not harder, but just what you may expect.

The various subjects expected on your exam are represented by separate Tests. Each Test has just about the number of questions you may find on the actual exam. And each Test is timed accordingly.

The questions on each Test are represented exactly on the special Answer Sheet provided. Mark your answers on this sheet. It's just about the way you'll have to do it on the real exam.

As a result you have an Examination which simulates the real one closely enough to provide you with important training.

Proceed through the entire exam without pausing after each Test. Remember that you are taking this Exam under actual battle conditions, and therefore you do not stop until told to do so by the proctor.

Correct answers for all the questions in all the Tests of the Exam appear at the end of the Exam, after the suggestions for self diagnosis and further study.

# II. PREDICTIVE PRACTICE EXAMINATION

| ANALYSIS AND TIMETABLE: PREDICTIVE PRACTICE EXAMINATION | |
| --- | --- |
| *Since the number of questions for each test may vary on different forms of the actual examination, the time allotments below are flexible.* | |
| *SUBJECT TESTED* | *Time Allowed* |
| TEST I. BIOMEDICAL SCIENCE | 65 Minutes |
| TEST II. INTERPRETATION OF SCIENCE READINGS | 75 Minutes |
| TEST III. VOCABULARY | 20 Minutes |
| TEST IV. VERBAL ANALOGIES | 15 Minutes |
| TEST V. SENTENCE COMPLETIONS | 15 Minutes |
| TEST VI. QUANTITATIVE ABILITY | 60 Minutes |
| TEST VII. PERCEPTUAL MOTOR ABILITY | 20 Minutes |

# ANSWER SHEET FOR PREDICTIVE EXAMINATION II.

*(Please make every effort to answer the questions on your own before looking at these answers. You'll make faster progress by following this rule.)*

## TEST I. BIOMEDICAL SCIENCE

| | | | | | | | |
|---|---|---|---|---|---|---|---|
| 1 A B C D E | 2 A B C D E | 3 A B C D E | 4 A B C D E | 5 A B C D E | 6 A B C D E | 7 A B C D E | 8 A B C D E |
| 9 A B C D E | 10 A B C D E | 11 A B C D E | 12 A B C D E | 13 A B C D E | 14 A B C D E | 15 A B C D E | 16 A B C D E |
| 17 A B C D E | 18 A B C D E | 19 A B C D E | 20 A B C D E | 21 A B C D E | 22 A B C D E | 23 A B C D E | 24 A B C D E |
| 25 A B C D E | 26 A B C D E | 27 A B C D E | 28 A B C D E | 29 A B C D E | 30 A B C D E | 31 A B C D E | 32 A B C D E |
| 33 A B C D E | 34 A B C D E | 35 A B C D E | 36 A B C D E | 37 A B C D E | 38 A B C D E | 39 A B C D E | 40 A B C D E |
| 41 A B C D E | 42 A B C D E | 43 A B C D E | 44 A B C D E | 45 A B C D E | | | |

## TEST II. INTERPRETATION OF SCIENCE READINGS

| | | | | | | | |
|---|---|---|---|---|---|---|---|
| 1 A B C D E | 2 A B C D E | 3 A B C D E | 4 A B C D E | 5 A B C D E | 6 A B C D E | 7 A B C D E | 8 A B C D E |
| 9 A B C D E | 10 A B C D E | 11 A B C D E | 12 A B C D E | 13 A B C D E | 14 A B C D E | 15 A B C D E | 16 A B C D E |
| 17 A B C D E | 18 A B C D E | 19 A B C D E | 20 A B C D E | 21 A B C D E | 22 A B C D E | 23 A B C D E | 24 A B C D E |
| 25 A B C D E | 26 A B C D E | 27 A B C D E | 28 A B C D E | 29 A B C D E | 30 A B C D E | 31 A B C D E | 32 A B C D E |
| 33 A B C D E | 34 A B C D E | 35 A B C D E | 36 A B C D E | 37 A B C D E | 38 A B C D E | 39 A B C D E | 40 A B C D E |

## TEST III. VOCABULARY

| | | | | | | | |
|---|---|---|---|---|---|---|---|
| 1 A B C D E | 2 A B C D E | 3 A B C D E | 4 A B C D E | 5 A B C D E | 6 A B C D E | 7 A B C D E | 8 A B C D E |
| 9 A B C D E | 10 A B C D E | 11 A B C D E | 12 A B C D E | 13 A B C D E | 14 A B C D E | 15 A B C D E | 16 A B C D E |
| 17 A B C D E | 18 A B C D E | 19 A B C D E | 20 A B C D E | 21 A B C D E | 22 A B C D E | 23 A B C D E | 24 A B C D E |
| 25 A B C D E | 26 A B C D E | 27 A B C D E | 28 A B C D E | 29 A B C D E | 30 A B C D E | | |

## TEST IV. VERBAL ANALOGIES

| | | | | | | | |
|---|---|---|---|---|---|---|---|
| 1 A B C D E | 2 A B C D E | 3 A B C D E | 4 A B C D E | 5 A B C D E | 6 A B C D E | 7 A B C D E | 8 A B C D E |
| 9 A B C D E | 10 A B C D E | 11 A B C D E | 12 A B C D E | 13 A B C D E | 14 A B C D E | 15 A B C D E | 16 A B C D E |
| 17 A B C D E | 18 A B C D E | 19 A B C D E | 20 A B C D E | 21 A B C D E | 22 A B C D E | 23 A B C D E | 24 A B C D E |
| 25 A B C D E | 26 A B C D E | 27 A B C D E | 28 A B C D E | 29 A B C D E | 30 A B C D E | | |

## TEST V. SENTENCE COMPLETIONS

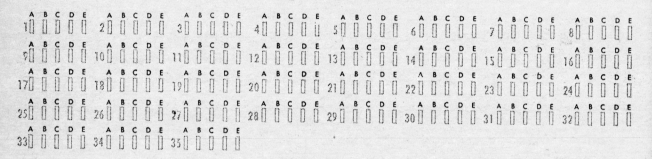

## TEST VI. QUANTITATIVE ABILITY

## TEST VII. PERCEPTUAL MOTOR ABILITY

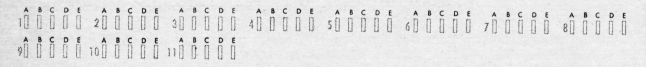

# TEST I. BIOMEDICAL SCIENCE

TIME: 65 Minutes*

*DIRECTIONS: For each of the following questions, select the choice which best answers the question or completes the statement.*

1. The development of unfertilized daphnia eggs is an example of
   (A) maturation
   (B) metamorphosis
   (C) parthenogenesis
   (D) ontogeny.

2. Meiosis occurs during the
   (A) abnormal division of cancer cells
   (B) animals cell division
   (C) plant cell division
   (D) formation of haploid cells.

3. Alternation of generation in plants refers to the
   (A) alternation of diploid and haploid generations
   (B) alternation of mature and immature forms
   (C) alternation of apospory and apogamy
   (D) seasonal growth cycle.

4. Abiogenesis can best be described as
   (A) gamete formation
   (B) asexual reproduction
   (C) evolution
   (D) spontaneous generation.

5. During its development, the cat embryo obtains its food through the
   (A) yolk sac          (B) placenta
   (C) ova               (D) albumen.

6. The suction-tension theory seems to explain
   (A) transpiration in plants
   (B) movement of nutrients in phloem
   (C) cohesion of water molecules in xylem
   (D) transport of water by plants.

7. In vertebrates, blood cells which carry oxygen are known as
   (A) leucocytes        (B) erythrocytes
   (C) thrombocytes      (D) monocytes

8. Which one of the following does *not* describe a phase of blood clotting?
   (A) Vitamin K is involved in prothrombin formation by the liver
   (B) Thrombokinase is released by blood platelets after an injury
   (C) Prothrombin combines with thrombokinase and sodium ions to form thrombin
   (D) Thrombin unites with fibrinogen to form fibrin.

9. A systolic blood pressure normal for a high school boy would be closest to which one of the following?
   (A) 100               (B) 125
   (C) 150               (D) 175.

10. The digestive hormone that stimulates the emptying of the gall bladder is
    (A) cholecystokinin  (B) pancreatin
    (C) enterogastrone   (D) gastrin.

11. Which one of the following statements does *not* apply to enzymes?
    (A) They are all made of an apoenzyme and a coenzyme.
    (B) They are usually not specific in their effect.
    (C) They lose their stability at high temperatures.
    (D) They can function outside of living cells.

12. The liver is an organ which
    (A) receives blood from the hepatic vein
    (B) produces the enzyme erepsin
    (C) contains Kupffer cells that absorb fat globules
    (D) carries on diapedesis.

13. The air we inhale when we take a deep breath is called
    (A) tidal air
    (B) supplemental air
    (C) complemental air
    (D) residual air.

*The Science section of the DAT tests basic concepts and principles as well as the ability to show an understanding of chemical and biological methods and procedures.

14. Of the following, the blood cells which are *not* manufactured in the red bone marrow are the
    (A) lymphocytes    (B) granulocytes
    (C) red blood cells    (D) blood platelets.

15. The following vitamins are members of the B complex, with the exception of
    (A) riboflavin    (B) pantothenic acid
    (C) inositol    (D) tocopherol.

16. It has been discovered in working with blood groups that
    (A) type O people can serve as universal recipients
    (B) cross matching is unnecessary if people have the same blood type
    (C) the agglutinogens are found in the red blood corpuscles
    (D) type A is the rarest group.

17. The energy for muscular contraction and flagella movement seems to come from
    (A) oxygen in the environment
    (B) ATP breakdown
    (C) DNA control
    (D) glycogen synthesis.

18. Bleeding gums is generally associated with a deficiency of
    (A) thiamin    (B) folic acid
    (C) ascorbic acid    (D) niacin.

19. Recent research with radioactive oxygen indicates that during photosynthesis
    (A) all oxygen released comes from the water molecule
    (B) whole water molecules are used in making carbohydrates
    (C) all oxygen released comes from the carbon dioxide molecule
    (D) oxygen released from a cell comes from both the $CO_2$ and $H_2O$.

20. Which one of the following statements does *not* apply to aerobic metabolism?
    (A) Pyruvic acid combines with two hydrogens to form lactic acid.
    (B) Carbon compounds are decarboxylated.
    (C) Acetic acid combines with oxaloacetic acid to form citric acid.
    (D) Carbon compounds are dehydrogenated.

21. The movement of materials through a cell membrane against a concentration gradient is called

    (A) diffusion
    (B) osmosis
    (C) active transport
    (D) Brownian movement.

22. Photosynthetic phosphorylation means that
    (A) photolysis has occurred in the light reaction
    (B) $CO_2$ incorporation has taken place in the dark reaction
    (C) ADP has been changed to ATP
    (D) $H_2O$ is split in the grana of the chloroplasts.

23. Which one of the following terms includes all the others?
    (A) alga    (B) fungus
    (C) thallophyte    (D) slime mold.

24. Which of the following developed the system of binomial nomenclature?
    (A) Linnaeus    (B) John Ray
    (C) Spemann    (D) Driesch.

25. Which one of the following statements does *not* apply to the euglenophytes?
    (A) They are partly plant-like and partly animal-like.
    (B) They have active locomotion.
    (C) Many carry on mixotrophic nutrition.
    (D) True cell walls are usually present.

26. Which one of the following pairs of animal groups consists of two groups belonging to the same phylum?
    (A) myriapods and leeches
    (B) slugs and earthworms
    (C) sand dollars and clams
    (D) tarantulas and barnacles.

27. Which one of the following represents a monocotyledonous family of plants?
    (A) legumes    (B) water lilies
    (C) grasses    (D) roses.

28. Which one of the following is arranged in a correct sequence?
    (A) family, genus, phylum, order
    (B) order, family, species, variety
    (C) phylum, order, genus, family
    (D) kingdom, order, species, genus.

29. Which one of the following is used as a mold inhibitor in the preparation of a Drosophila culture medium?

(A) ninhydrin    (B) nipagen
(C) pyridoxin    (D) glycine.

30. The osmotic effect of water in the paramecium is controlled by the
    (A) cell membrane
    (B) pellicle
    (C) macronucleus
    (D) contractile vacuoles.

31. Intracellular digestion occurs exclusively in which one of the following?
    (A) molds    (C) carnivorous plants
    (B) sponges    (D) echinoderms.

32. The excretory organs of insects are called
    (A) green glands
    (B) nephridia
    (C) Malpighian tubules
    (D) glomeruli.

33. An open type blood circulation is found in all of the following *except* the
    (A) earthworms    (B) insects
    (C) crustacea    (D) mollusks.

34. In which one of the following groups of animals is there found a gastrovascular cavity used for both ingestion and egestion?
    (A) protozoa and sponges
    (B) sponges and hydroids
    (C) coelenterates and flatworms
    (D) flatworms and annelids.

35. The smallest mammal known is a species of
    (A) mole    (B) shrew
    (C) vole    (D) lemming.

36. The radioactive disintegration of $_{14}Si^{27}$ yields $_{13}Al^{27}$ and a(n)
    (A) proton    (B) neutron
    (C) positron    (D) electron.

37. Which one of the following elements is proproduced by irradiating a bismuth target with high energy helium ions?
    (A) californium    (B) astatine
    (C) americium    (D) niobium.

38. The barium ion may be separated from strontium ions by employing
    (A) $Na_2CO_3$ and $HCl$
    (B) $K_4Fe(CN)_6$ and $NH_4NO_3$
    (C) $(NH_4)_2CO_3$ and $NH_4OH$
    (D) $K_2CrO_4$ and $HC_2H_3O_2$.

39. The reagent dimethylglyoxime is used in a confirmatory test for the element
    (A) iron    (B) calcium
    (C) nickel    (D) cobalt.

40. The group reagent for the silver group in qualitative analysis is
    (A) $H_2S$    (B) $H_2S + NH_3$
    (C) $(NH_4)_2CO_3$    (D) $HCl$.

41. If a halide soluble in water gave a white precipitate when dilute nitric acid and a solution of sodium chloride were added, the original salt was silver
    (A) chloride    (B) bromide
    (C) fluoride    (D) iodide.

42. Since lead has an atomic weight of 207.2 and a density of 11.4 g/c.c, its atomic volume is
    (A) 1.13 c.c.    (B) 9.1 c.c.
    (C) 18.2 c.c.    (D) 36.4 c.c.

43. A Tyndall effect would most likely be observed in which one of the following?
    (A) solution    (B) precipitate
    (C) sol    (D) solvent.

44. Of the following, the metal that does *not* give a red flame test is
    (A) lithium    (B) barium
    (C) strontium    (D) rubidium.

45. Assuming that n = energy level, quantum mechanics postulates that the electron population of any energy level in an atom is limited to
    (A) $2n$    (B) $2n^2$
    (C) $2n^2 + 2$    (D) $2n^2 - 2$.

# TEST II. INTERPRETATION OF SCIENCE READINGS

## TIME: 75 Minutes

*DIRECTIONS: Read each passage to get the general idea. Then reread the passage more carefully to answer the questions based on the passage. For each question read all choices carefully. Then select the answer you consider correct or most nearly correct. Blacken the answer space corresponding to your best choice, just as you would do on the actual examination.*

Where a metal is bombarded by gas ions, it is known that such treatment causes the ejection of metal atoms from the surface. This effect is described as cathode-sputtering, a name given a hundred years ago to a phenomenon first observed in a gas discharge between two (cold) electrodes. Our experiments have been carried out using monoenergetic rare-gas ions striking the surface perpendicularly. The ion energy varied between 50 and 1500 eV. Chapter I contains a general review of the most important literature treating this problem. The apparatus used, as well as a few measurements directed towards determining the average energy and energy spread of the bombarding ions, is described in chapter II. The detection of atoms freed by ion bombardment is indicated in chapter III. Conjointly with a review of the methods of detection used by other researchers, we include a more extensive description of our own method wherein the quantity of sputtered metal, collected on a glass plate, is determined from the optical transmission of glass plate and metal layer. This chapter also contains a comparison between the structures of silver (and copper) layers formed by evaporation and by sputtering respectively. The results of the sputtering experiments are set out in chapter IV. For polycrystalline silver, the relationship between the sputtering yield (atoms/ion) and the energy of the colliding rare-gas ions (40-250 eV) has been determined. For bombardment of monocrystalline copper by the above ions, (now however at energies up to 1500 eV), the angular distribution of the sputtered material has been measured. There appears to be a preferential ejection of atoms in the $<110>$ and $<100>$ lattice directions. The distribution of sputtering intensity among different preferential ejection directions depends upon ion species and energy. On the basis of our results and data from recent literature, some qualitative observations are made in chapter V regarding the phenomena occurring in an ion-bombarded metal lattice. The appearance of preferential ejection directions and of a relationship between angular distribution and the energy of the colloding ions can, from a consideration of the above-mentioned theoretical aspects, be understood.

1. "Cathode-sputtering"

   (A) is minimized in the present work
   (B) was a rare phenomenon
   (C) was described a hundred years ago
   (D) is still theoretical

2. This problem

   (A) has never been treated by anyone else
   (B) involves middle dispersion
   (C) required hitherto totally unknown apparatus
   (D) has its own bibliography

3. The silver layers are formed by

   (A) sputtering only
   (B) evaporation only
   (C) an initial introduction of copper only
   (D) all of the above

4. The distribution of sputtering intensity
   (A) depends on many variables
   (B) enters diverse directions
   (C) is irrelevant to the conclusions
   (D) is related to the ion and its energy

In the second part of this work, the accent is on the importance of the contribution to the emission of particles of certain solar centers (repetitive centers) which give rise to several type IV bursts and to several SSC's: the variations of the efficiency of these centers during the present solar cycle as well as their distribution on the sun and their importance for the appearance of "privileged regions" are underlined.

Subsequently the study of the radio sources associated with solar centers of activity makes it possible to distinguish between two groups of centers: those which give rise to the type IV bursts and which are at the origin of the geophysical corpuscular emission, and those which do not lead to any special activity. Among the active centers, those called "repetitive centers" are associated with a strong characteristic radio-emission on centimeter wave-lengths: certain hypothesis aimed at interpreting this effect are envisaged.

Finally in a last chapter, an examination of the morphology of the optical centers reveals certain properties, related to the structure of the local magnetic field. A geometric parameter is defined which is characteristic of the solar sun spot groups in which occur the flares which are associated with meter wavelength radio-emissions, and with the ejection of high energy particles.

5. The "repetitive centers"

   (A) give rise to various bursts
   (B) furnish a handy definition
   (C) are relegated to a second place
   (D) resemble corpuscles

6. Repetitive centers

   (A) do not interpenetrate
   (B) are not associated with radio emissions
   (C) are one kind of active center
   (D) prevent further analysis

7. There are two groups of centers:

   (A) those associated and those not associated with radio centers
   (B) those which are and those which are not present in the current solar cycle
   (C) the active centers and the repetitive centers
   (D) those which do and those which do not lead to a certain activity

8. In the last chapter, certain properties are

   (A) ejected in high energy particles
   (B) formed
   (C) revealed
   (D) discussed again

Having recalled the different observations of the red shifts observed in the solar spectrum, in different points of the disk, the author reviews the different phenomena of which any interpretation must take account, namely: The Einstein effect (effect to a gravitational field, called often the "slowing down of clocks"), the Lindholm effect (effect of collisions on the atomic energy levels, the Van der Waals interaction law being assumed valid), the Spitzer effect (effect of collisions, when the distances between the atoms are too small for the Van der Waals law to be valid), the Findlay-Freundlich effect (photon-photon interactions), and finally all sorts of Doppler effects, due to radial or non-radial motions, compensating themselves in an incomplete way, either because of the thermodynamical heterogeneities of the photosphere or because of the effects of optical or geometrical "roughness."

A special study is made of the Lindholm effect. The effective depth of formation of this effect is calculated, after the numerical resolution of the problem of transfer in an atmosphere where successive layers provoke differing spectral line shifts. This notion of depth of formation may very much simplify the calculations, even if one must introduce the near-collisions which Spitzer thinks to be essential.

The effects of geometrical and of optical roughness are calculated in the case of radical motions. The center-to-limb variation of shifts which is deduced cannot, by itself, explain the observed facts; but its order of magnitude is such that it is impossible not to take it into account.

The summing-up of this study concludes the paper in orienting future research in clearly defined directions: physical study of the collision effects; study of non-radial motions, and of the influence of roughness phenomena on their observed effects.

9. Any interpretation of the phenomena observed must

   (A) take into account previous observations
   (B) be tentative
   (C) depend on the sun
   (D) depend on redness

10. Van der Walls' law is valid

   (A) according to Spitzer
   (B) following Doppler
   (C) only when certain distances exist between atoms
   (D) only after a gravitational field exists

11. The notion of depth of formation

    (A) fatally weakens the calculation
    (B) does not complicate the calculations
    (C) hastens near-collisions
    (D) is irrelevant to Spitzer

12. In the conclusion of this study, the author

    (A) reveals Chinese research
    (B) balances the five effects
    (C) studies non-radial motions
    (D) outlines future research

---

This work is mainly concerned with the emission of particles from the Sun, which is directly related to important geophysical phenomena such as sudden commencement of geomagnetic storms (SSC) and exceptional variation of the intensity of cosmic rays.

This work is divided into two parts:

The first is devoted, partly to the solar events which give rise to the sudden commencement, geomagnetic storms, and partly to the study of the transit time, from the SUN to the earth of the corresponding disturbances.

The second part concerns the study of the centers on the SUN responsible for such events.

Certain new results are presented. In particular it is established that there is a statistical relationship between the Sun-earth transit-time for the disturbances responsible for sudden commencement storms and the radio energy emitted by the associated type IV bursts.

This relation in turn makes it possible to study the role of certain secondary factors. Thus two important effects, relative to the influence of conditions in interplanetary space on the time of transit have been brought to light. A disturbance which follows, within a few days on a first disturbance crosses interplanetary space under conditions such that it propagates faster than the initial disturbance. Also the conditions encountered by the second disturbances are much more regular than those encountered by the first.

This relation between transit time and energy of the burst also makes it possible to suggest a model for the disturbance. This model is characterized by weak directivity.

13. The study of the emission of particles from the sun is

    (A) carried beyond earlier beginnings

(B) limited
(C) the topic principally dealt with
(D) exceptional

14. Geomagnetic storms are

    (A) responsible for telling events
    (B) caused by solar events
    (C) provocative
    (D) transitory

15. There is a statistical relationship between

    (A) transit time and radio energy
    (B) the Sun and the Earth
    (C) sudden beginnings and weak conclusions
    (D) responsibility and association

16. A second disturbance propagates faster than an initial disturbance when it

    (A) is more regular than the first
    (B) takes place shortly after the first
    (C) is a bigger disturbance
    (D) meets two important conditions

---

Three groups of Wistar CF rats are put on three types of diets immediately after weaning: *diet LP* containing only threshold amounts of linoleic acid, as far as lipids are concerned, *diet S* containing 20 p. 100 lard and *diet T* 20 p. 100 sunflower oil. The whole experiment lasts 6 months in the course of which animals are killed at regular intervals. The fatty acid composition of reserve tryglycerides (perirenal and epididymal tissues) is studied on the one hand, and on the other hand the structure of these triglycerides, making use of the specificity of position of pancreatic lipase which hydrolyzes first the primary ester bonds of glycerol.

There are differences in composition between the triglycerides of perirenal fat and those of perigenital tissue. Nevertheless the influence of diet has the same effect, in both cases. We have studied more especially the *perigenital triglycerides*.

In rats on the lard diet these triglycerides show only very slight modifications; those of rats fed with sunflower oil increase progressively their linoleic acid content (more than 50 moles p. 100 after 5 months), at the expense of oleic and palmitic acids mainly. In animals on the lipid-deprived diet, receiving only the minimum of essential fatty acids, the oleic acid content of reserve triglycerides increases in the course of time; palmitic acid content is constant but higher than in the other groups.

The structure of the glycerides conforms to the general scheme admitted for most natural fats: the saturated fatty acids are attached preferentially at the external positions, the unsaturated acids at the inernal position. However, when an unsaturated acid is present to the extent of more than one third of the molecules, it is also located partially at the external positions. After prolonged ingestion of sunflower oil there seems to be competition between oleic and linoleic chains (80 p. 100 of total fatty acids) for the central position, although this position seems to be occupied preferentially by linoleic acid.

17. The experiments were carried out on

 (A) adult rats
 (B) young rats
 (C) six month old rats only
 (D) both (a) and (b)

18. The rats on diet T

 (A) lost oleic and palmitic acids
 (B) did not change much
 (C) lost sunflower oil
 (D) received lard

19. Among rats on the lipid-deprived diet

 (A) more died
 (B) the minimum of essential fatty acid was reduced
 (C) no particular changes were noted
 (D) a constant palmitoleic acid constant existed

20. After a prolonged T diet

 (A) rats prefer an LP diet
 (B) position competition exists
 (C) the oleic chains dominate the central position
 (D) 80% of the total fatty acids is contained in $\frac{1}{3}$ of the molecules

---

We have shown the interest of the spectrophotometric method for the determination of calcium in biological media. After recalling the existence of a few interfering ions, we have determined more precisely the role of pH, sulfates and above all phosphates, in order to examine the different procedures liable to obviate the influence of these factors.

In serum and cerebrospinal fluid the spectro-

photometric method gives directly the calcium content from a sample of 1,5 or 3 ml. The results are comparable with those given by chemical methods, but the rapidity is considerably greater.

The peculiar inorganic composition of urine and feces constitutes a major obstacle to the direct measurement of the element, for the spectrophotometric determinations show an important depression, the decrease in transmission being about 20 to 25 p. 100.

A direct determination, after suitable dilution and acidification aiming at the dissolution of all forms of calcium, makes possible rough estimate of calcium present. A second determination, after addition of a known amount of this ion, enables one to know exactly the interference of the medium with the determination. A simple calculation then makes possible the determination of the real quantity of calcium.

These two successive determinations restore its reliability and precision to the spectrophotometric determination of calcium in urine and feces without losing much of its rapidity.

21. The understanding of the role of pH., sulfates and phosphates is necessary

 (A) for the modern student in biology
 (B) to discuss all ions
 (C) to regulate their influence
 (D) to reduce overdoses of calcium

22. In paragraph two, the author states that the great utility of the spectrophotometric method resides in

 (A) its newness
 (B) its chemical accuracy
 (C) the limitless possibilities of its use
 (D) the speed of its results

23. The direct measurement of calcium is difficult because of the
 (A) inorganic composition of the matter under study
 (B) modifications necessary to the method of study
 (C) chemical reactions
 (D) direct interference by certain ions

24. Paragraph five states that the steps in paragraph four

 (A) reduce the fidelity of the determination

(B) greatly reduce the rapidity of the spectrophotometric determination
(C) does not greatly reduce the rapidity of the determination
(D) are bothersome but necessary

---

It has been shown previously that crude extracts of Teleostean pituitaries capable of stimulating intensely the thyroid of Teleosteans, has no action on the thyroid of Mammalians; this zoological specificity suggested the existence of physico-chemical differences between TSHs of various origins, and we have therefore undertaken the purification and physico-chemical study of TSH from a Teleostean.

We have been able to purify partially the factor possessing thyrotropic activity towards Teleosteans from eel pituitaries by filtration on Sephadex gels and chromatographies on CMC and DEAEC. In the course of the different steps of purification, this factor behaves like a protein with physico-chemical properties analogous to those of Mammalian TSH. It has been possible to achieve a degree of purification similar to that obtained in the case of Mammalians.

The final product, like crude pituitary extracts, is inactive on Mammalians at doses which stimulate intensely the thyroid of Teleosteans. Several of its physico-chemical properties have been determined and compared with those of Mammalian TSHs; molecular size is of the same order, probably a little larger for eel TSH.

Analysis of amino-acids present shows up some important differences, particularly a low relative cystine and amino-sugar content of eel TSH.

The hypothesis of a relation between these facts and the zoological specificity of the Teleostean hormone is proposed.

25. Throughout the purification, the factor purified

    (A) was not understood by the author
    (B) resisted partial filtration
    (C) behaved in a way similar to that of a certain protein
    (D) resisted all purification

26. The action of the crude extracts chosen indicates a relationship between

    (A) the origin of the extract and what it will act upon
    (B) all thyroid reactions
    (C) intensity and purity
    (D) all of the above

27. The author was able to determine

    (A) the molecular size of various mammalian TSHs.
    (B) the dosage which stimulated mammalian thyroids
    (C) various properties of eel TSH
    (D) the importance of a larger molecular size for eel TSH

28. The cystine and amino-sugar content of eel TSH is

    (A) related to that of mammalians
    (B) lower than that of mammalians
    (C) not important
    (D) supposed hypothetically

---

It was therefore by indirect methods that De Nobele succeeded in showing that the germ he had isolated—and under such difficult conditions—was the cause of the serious gastro-intestinal poisonings of July 1898 at Aertrijcke and that this germ differs from all those previously isolated during similar epidemics. His works proves that he was a remarkably able technician, a tenacious and thorough investigator and a precursor several years ahead of his fellow bacteriologists. He grasped the practical importance of his findings and brought it out several times. On the other hand, he abstained from theoretic matters, for he had most probably too precise a mind to get lost in speculations which were liable to make even less clear those things which were already so unclear at that time. That wise man was content to communicate his findings and to draw formal conclusions from them without superfluous remarks. But the facts which he recorded in the two memoirs we discussed have never been weakened nor contradicted.

In conclusion, we must point out that De Nobele, who was very modest, never boasted of his discovery. It is only fitting that the homage he deserves be accorded him.

29. The germ isolated by De Nobele

    (A) had been present in earlier epidemics
    (B) was isolated only indirectly
    (C) was isolated only under trying conditions
    (D) produced few illnesses

30. De Nobele's work shows him to be

    (A) thorough
    (B) concerned with mentally sick people
    (C) wonderfully human
    (D) concerned with death

31. If De Nobele avoided theory it was because he felt that

    (A) theoreticians were held in disrepute
    (B) theory lacked the possibility of ever being demonstrated
    (C) nothing could be gained by it
    (D) theory might only confuse an unclear field

32. The author thinks it fitting that

    (A) one overlook the errors of De Nobele
    (B) one praise De Nobele's work
    (C) one point out the vanity of pioneering
    (D) De Nobele's facts were ironically weak but the conclusions solid

---

As the world's population grows, the part played by man in influencing plant life becomes more and more important. In old and densely populated countries, as in central Europe, man determines almost wholly what shall grow and what shall not grow. In such regions, the influence of man on plant life is in large measure a beneficial one. Laws, often centuries old, protect plants of economic value and preserve soil fertility. In newly settled countries the situation is unfortunately quite the reverse. The pioneer's life is too strenuous a one for him to think of posterity.

Some years ago Mt. Mitchell, the highest summit east of the Mississippi, was covered with a magnificent forest. A lumber company was given full rights to fell the trees. Those not cut down were crushed. The mountain was left a wasted area where fire would rage and erosion would complete the destruction. There was no stopping the devastating foresting of the company, for the contract had been given. Under a more enlightened civilization this could not have happened. The denuding of Mt. Mitchell is a minor chapter in the destruction of lands in the United States; and this country is by no means the only or chief sufferer. China, India, Egypt, and East Africa all have their thousands of square miles of waste land, the result of man's indifference to the future.

Deforestation, grazing, and poor farming are the chief causes of the destruction of land fertility. Wasteful cutting of timber is the first step. Grazing then follows lumbering in bringing about ruin. The Caribbean slopes of northern Venezuela are barren wastes owing first to ruthless cutting of forests and then to destructive grazing. Hordes of goats have roamed these slopes until only a few thorny acacias and cacti remain. Erosion completed the desvastation. What is there illustrated on a small scale is the story of vast areas in China and India, countries where famines are of regular occurrence.

Man is not wholly to blame, for Nature is often merciless. In parts of India and China, plant life, when left undisturbed by man, cannot cope with either the disastrous floods of wet seasons or the destructive winds of the dry season. Man has learned much; prudent land management has been the policy of the Chinese people since 2700 B. C., but even they have not learned enough.

When the American forestry service was in its infancy, it met with much opposition from legislators who loudly claimed that the protected land would in one season yield a crop of cabbages of more value than all the timber on it. Herein lay the fallacy, that one season's crop is all that need be thought of. Nature, through the years, adjusts crops to the soil and to the climate. Forests usually occur where precipitation exceeds evaporation. If the reverse is true, grasslands are found; and where evaporation is still greater, desert or scrub vegetation alone survives. The phytogeographic map of a country is very similar to the climatic map based on rainfall, evaporation, and temperature. Man ignores this natural adjustment of crops and strives for one "bumper" crop in a single season; he may produce it, but "year in and year out the yield of the grassland is certain, that of the planted fields, never."

Man is learning; he sprays his trees with insecticides and fungicides; he imports ladybugs to destroy aphids; he irrigates, fertilizes, and rotates his crops; but he is still indifferent to many of the consequences of his short-sighted policies. The great dust storms of the western United States are proof of this indifference.

In spite of the evidence to be had from this country, the people of other countries, still in the pioneer stage, farm as wastefully as did our own pioneers. In the interiors of Central and South

American Republics, natives fell superb forest trees and leave them to rot in order to obtain virgin soil for cultivation. Where the land is hillside, it readily washes and after one or two seasons is unfit for crops. So the frontier farmer pushes back into the primeval forest, moving his hut as he goes, and fells more monarchs to lay bare another patch of ground for his plantings to support his family. Valuable timber which will require a century to replace is destroyed and the land laid waste to produce what could be supplied for a pittance.

How badly man can err in his handling of land is shown by the draining of extensive swamp areas, which to the uninformed would seem to be a very good thing to do. One of the first effects of the drainage is the lowering of the water-table, which may bring about the death of the dominant species and leave to another species the possession of the soil, even when the difference in water level is little more than an inch. Frequently, bog country will yield marketable crops of cranberries and blueberries but, if drained, neither these nor any other economic plant will grow on the fallow soil. Swamps and marshes have their drawbacks but also their virtues. When drained they may leave waste land, the surface of which rapidly erodes to be then blown away in dust blizzards disastrous to both man and wild beasts.

33. The best title for this passage is
    (A) How to Increase Soil Productivity
    (B) Conservation of Natural Resources
    (C) Man's Effect on Soil
    (D) Soil Conditions and Plant Growth.

34. A policy of good management is sometimes upset by
    (A) the indifference of man
    (B) centuries-old laws
    (C) floods and winds
    (D) grazing animals.

35. Areas in which the total amounts of rain and snow falling on the ground are greater than that which is evaporated will support
    (A) forests          (C) scrub vegetation
    (B) grasslands       (D) no plants.

36. Pioneers do not have a long range view on soil problems since they
    (A) are not protected by laws
    (B) live under adverse conditions
    (C) use poor methods of farming
    (D) must protect themselves from famine.

37. Phytogeographic maps are those that show
    (A) areas of grassland
    (B) areas of bumper crops
    (C) areas of similar climate
    (D) areas of similar plants.

38. The basic cause of frequent famines in China and India is probably due to
    (A) allowing animals to roam wild
    (B) drainage of swamps
    (C) over-grazing of the land
    (D) destruction of forests.

39. With a growing world population, the increased need for soil for food production may be met by
    (A) draining unproductive swamp areas
    (B) legislating against excess lumbering
    (C) trying to raise bumper crops each year
    (D) irrigating desert areas.

40. What is meant by "the yield of the grassland is certain; that of the planted field, never" is that
    (A) it is impossible to get more than one bumper crop from any one cultivated area
    (B) crops, planted in former grassland, will not give good yields
    (C) through the indifference of man, dust blizzards have occurred in former grasslands
    (D) if man does not interfere, plants will grow in the most suitable environment.

# TEST III. VOCABULARY

## TIME: 20 Minutes

*DIRECTIONS: For each question in this test, select the appropriate letter preceding the word which is most nearly the same in meaning as the italicized word in each sentence.*

1. abnegation
   - (A) renunciation
   - (B) failure to conform to rule
   - (C) utter humiliation
   - (D) sudden departure.

2. abortive
   - (A) decadent
   - (B) failing to succeed
   - (C) carrying off surreptitiously
   - (D) degrading.

3. amorphous
   - (A) sleep-inducing
   - (B) powdered
   - (C) shapeless
   - (D) crystalline.

4. argot
   - (A) medicinal root
   - (B) wooden shoe
   - (C) jargon
   - (D) semi-precious stone.

5. artificer
   - (A) mimic
   - (B) artistic worker
   - (C) copyist of works of art
   - (D) curator.

6. Barmecide feast
   - (A) Lucullan repast
   - (B) murder at the dinner table
   - (C) false appearance of plenty
   - (D) hearty meal eaten by a condemned man.

7. barouche
   - (A) conveyance
   - (B) vestment
   - (C) headgear
   - (D) thicket.

8. billingsgate
   - (A) speech at the medieval English court
   - (B) coarse language
   - (C) insecure enclosure
   - (D) stevedore's hook.

9. blench
   - (A) dredge
   - (B) clean
   - (C) shrink
   - (D) blow (as glass).

10. caisson
    - (A) capital letter
    - (B) structure in which men can work on river bottoms
    - (C) ideograph
    - (D) type of cheese.

11. lees
    - (A) scuppers awash
    - (B) dregs
    - (C) onions
    - (D) meadows.

12. livid
    - (A) gray-blue
    - (B) tense
    - (C) wrathful
    - (D) flushed.

13. lumbar pertains to
    - (A) weight
    - (B) a crosspiece
    - (C) a joint
    - (D) the loins.

14. maculate
    - (A) produce conformity by violent means
    - (B) scheme
    - (C) stain
    - (D) reduce to a pulp by crushing or kneading.

15. mare's-nest
    - (A) imaginary discovery that brings ridicule on the claimant
    - (B) eyrie
    - (C) well-padded stall
    - (D) horse van.

16. maverick
    - (A) heavy cudgel
    - (B) orator
    - (C) opponent
    - (D) unbranded animal.

17. mawkish
    - (A) fumbling
    - (B) sickening
    - (C) awkward
    - (D) surly.

18. **mayhem**
    (A) maiming     (B) murder
    (C) fate     (D) irresolution.

19. **mendicity**
    (A) deceit     (B) hypocrisy
    (B) haggling     (D) begging.

20. **mephitic**
    (A) intoxicating     (B) noxious
    (C) soporific     (D) tubercular.

21. **eclectic**
    (A) selecting     (B) secular
    (C) clerical     (D) provincial.

22. **egregious**
    (A) friendly     (B) eminent
    (C) niggardly     (D) infamous.

23. **ephemeral**
    (A) frightening     (B) weak
    (C) transient     (D) ethereal.

24. **equivocal**
    (A) corresponding     (B) hidden
    (C) uncertain     (D) average.

25. **eschew**
    (A) copy     (B) digest
    (C) avoid     (D) despise.

26. **esurient**
    (A) certain     (B) hungry
    (C) luxurious     (D) foolish.

27. **exorcise**
    (A) bring back to life
    (B) make a pact with the devil
    (C) wring the hands
    (D) drive off an evil spirit.

28. **factitious**
    (A) accurate     (B) treacherous
    (C) sham     (D) argumentative.

29. **flagellate**
    (A) scold     (B) whip
    (C) decorate     (D) scorn.

30. **halcyon**
    (A) peaceful     (B) healthy
    (C) pastoral     (D) musical.

# TEST IV. VERBAL ANALOGIES

## TIME: 15 Minutes

*DIRECTIONS: In these test questions each of the two CAPITALIZED words have a certain relationship to each other. Following the capitalized words are other pairs of words, each designated by a letter. Select the lettered pair wherein the words are related in the same way as the two CAPITALIZED words are related to each other.*

## EXPLANATIONS OF KEY POINTS BEHIND THESE QUESTIONS ARE GIVEN WITH THE ANSWERS

1. CONTROL : ORDER ::
   (A) discipline : school
   (B) teacher : pupil
   (C) disorder : climax
   (D) anarchy : chaos
   (E) government : legislator.

2. WOOD : CARVE ::
   (A) trees : sway
   (B) paper : burn
   (C) clay : mold
   (D) pipe : blow
   (E) statue : model.

3. STATE : BORDER ::
   (A) nation : state
   (B) flag : loyalty
   (C) Idaho : Montana
   (D) planet : satellite
   (E) property : fence.

4. SOLDIER : REGIMENT ::
   (A) navy : army
   (B) lake : river
   (C) star : constellation
   (D) amphibian : frog
   (E) flock : geese.

5. APOGEE : PERIGEE
   (A) dog : pedigree.
   (B) opposite : composite
   (C) paradoxical : incredible
   (D) effigy : statue
   (E) inappropriate : apposite

6. ASYLUM : REFUGEE ::
   (A) flight : escape.
   (B) peace : war

   (C) lunatic : insanity
   (D) accident : injury
   (E) destination : traveler

7. WORRIED : HYSTERICAL ::
   (A) hot : cold
   (B) happy : ecstatic
   (C) peeved : bitter
   (D) frozen : cold
   (E) ice : frost.

8. WORD : CHARADE ::
   (A) phrase : act
   (B) idea : philosophy
   (C) fun : party
   (D) message : code
   (E) graph : chart.

9. PLAYER : TEAM ::
   (A) fawn : doe
   (B) book : story
   (C) ball : bat
   (D) fish : school
   (E) tennis : racket.

10. BANANA : BUNCH ::
    (A) city : state
    (B) world : earth
    (C) president : nation
    (D) people : continent
    (E) universe : planet.

11. MOTH : CLOTHING ::
    (A) egg : larva
    (B) suit : dress
    (C) hole : repair
    (D) stigma : reputation
    (E) mouse : closet.

12. LINCOLN : NEBRASKA ::
    (A) Washington : D. C.
    (B) Trenton : New Jersey
    (C) New York : U. S.
    (D) Chicago : New York
    (E) city : state.

13. BUZZ : HUM ::
    (A) noise : explosion
    (B) reverberation : peal
    (C) tinkle : clang
    (D) echo : sound
    (E) crack : whip.

14. BOXER : GLOVES ::
    (A) swimmer : water
    (B) librarian : glasses
    (C) businessman : bills
    (D) fruit : pedlar.
    (E) bacteriologist : microscope

15. DECISION : CONSIDERATION ::
    (A) gift : party
    (B) plea : request
    (C) greed : charity
    (D) conference : constitution.
    (E) fulfillment : wish

16. DELUSION : MIRAGE ::
    (A) haunter : specter
    (B) imagination : concentration
    (C) dream : reality
    (D) mirror : glass
    (E) desert : oasis.

17. FRANCE : EUROPE ::
    (A) Australia : New Zealand
    (B) Paris : France
    (C) Israel : Egypt
    (D) Algeria : Africa
    (E) India : Pakistan

18. INSULT : INVULNERABLE ::
    (A) success : capable
    (B) poverty : miserable
    (C) purchase : refundable
    (D) assault : impregnable
    (E) research : difficult.

19. POISON : DEATH ::
    (A) book : pages
    (B) music : violin
    (C) kindness : cooperation
    (D) life : famine
    (E) nothing : something.

20. ROCK : SLATE ::
    (A) wave : sea
    (B) mineral : ore
    (C) swimmer : male
    (D) lifeguard : beach
    (E) boat : kayak.

21. LAW : CITIZEN ::
    (A) democracy : communism
    (B) weapon : peace
    (C) reins : horse
    (D) gangster : policeman
    (E) tyranny : despot.

22. JOY : ECSTASY ::
    (A) admiration : love
    (B) weather : humidity
    (C) happiness : sorrow
    (D) life : hope
    (E) youth : frolic.

23. LARCENY : GRAND ::
    (A) theft : daring
    (B) apple : red
    (C) pepper : bitter
    (D) silence : peaceful
    (E) school : elementary.

24. ANTISEPTIC : GERMS ::
    (A) bullet : death
    (B) mosquitos : disease
    (C) lion : prey
    (D) doctor : medicine
    (E) streptococcus : throat.

25. HORSE : RIDE ::
    (A) sharpener : sharpen
    (B) purchase : make
    (C) use : reuse
    (D) break : crack
    (E) sing : song.

26. MYSTERY : CLUE ::
    (A) key : door
    (B) fruit : bowl
    (C) test : study
    (D) detective : crime
    (E) fry : pan.

27. PENCIL : SHARPEN ::
    (A) knife : cut
    (B) carpenter : build
    (C) blow : puff.
    (D) well : fill
    (E) wood : saw

28. GARBAGE : SQUALOR ::
    (A) filth : cleanliness
    (B) fame : knowledge
    (C) diamonds : magnificence
    (D) color : brush
    (E) mayor : governor.

29. MYTH : STORY ::
    (A) fiction : reality
    (B) bonnet : hat

    (C) literature : poetry
    (D) flower : redness
    (E) stencil : paper.

30. DUNCE : CLEVER ::
    (A) idiot : stupid
    (B) courage : fearful
    (C) help : weak
    (D) worry : poor
    (E) cucumber : soft.

# TEST V. SENTENCE COMPLETIONS

### TIME: 15 Minutes

*DIRECTIONS: Each of the completion questions in this test consists of an incomplete sentence. Each sentence is followed by a series of lettered words, one of which best completes the sentence. Select the word that best completes the meaning of each sentence, and mark the letter of that word opposite that sentence.*

1. An _____ study should reveal the influence of environment on man.
   (A) ecumenical      (B) endemic
   (C) ecological      (D) epigraphic.

2. The researcher in the field of _____ was interested in race improvement.
   (A) euthenics       (B) euthanasia
   (C) euphuism        (D) euphonics.

3. _____ concerns itself with _____ of plants.
   (A) etiology . . . eating
   (B) ethnology . . . drying
   (C) etiolation . . . blanching
   (D) epistemology . . . collecting.

4. Through a _____ circumstance, we unexpectedly found ourselves on the same steamer with Uncle Harry.
   (A) fortuitous      (B) fetid
   (C) friable         (D) lambent.

5. I had a terrible night caused by an _____ during my sleep.
   (A) epilogue        (B) insipidity
   (C) insouciance     (D) incubus.

6. The Romans depended on the _____ for the _____ of their homes.
   (A) lares . . . protection
   (B) caries . . . painting
   (C) aborigines . . . blessing
   (D) mores . . . erection.

7. In the study of grammatical forms, the _____ is very helpful.
   (A) syllogism
   (B) mattock
   (C) paradigm
   (D) pimpernel.

8. The _____ method is used to _____ admission.
   (A) plutonic . . . offer
   (B) Socratic . . . elicit
   (C) sardonic . . . bar
   (D) Hippocratic . . . prepare.

9. They had a wonderful view of the bay through the _____.
   (A) nadir           (B) behemoth
   (C) oriel           (D) fiat.

10. There is no reason to insult and _____ the man simply because you do not agree with him.
    (A) depict          (B) enervate
    (C) defame          (D) distort.

11. Dealers complying with our prices in fair trade states have been placed in a (an) _____ competitive position when located next to non-fair trade areas or in states where it has become increasingly difficult to secure injunctions promptly or adequate penalties to enforce them.
    (A) sensational
    (B) multilateral
    (C) unicameral
    (D) untenable
    (E) categorical.

12. Although there is reason to expect an improvement in business conditions, at least a seasonal rise would be necessary to show that the _____ of the slump has been passed.
    (A) nadir           (B) minority
    (C) majority        (D) economics
              (E) cycle.

13. The appearance of corruption in Washington clearly shows the need for closer scrutiny and stricter _____ for men chosen to direct our government.
    (A) discipline    (B) grading
    (C) coercion    (D) criteria
        (E) decisions.

14. It took great political courage for the President to face down the _____ farm lobby clamoring aggressively for greater handouts and to veto a bill to freeze farm price supports.
    (A) nefarious    (B) militant
    (C) democratic    (D) unconstitutional
        (E) communistic.

15. The strenuousness of the 102-hour week is further _____ when it is compared to the police forces in our American cities.
    (A) accentuated    (B) demoralized
    (C) inculcated    (D) cauterized
        (E) anaesthetized.

16. The meeting between this man of means and vision and the needy young architect came at an _____ moment when the needs of the country were greatest.
    (A) enlightened    (B) usurious
    (C) ominous    (D) auspicious
        (E) inspiring.

17. The gifted young man was soon _____ with local architects, helping with various minor civil commissions.
    (A) commiserating    (B) scintillating
    (C) luxuriating    (D) undulating
        (E) collaborating.

18. Objectives may be _____, the mistake may be nothing worse than excessive zeal, yet if all similar plans were adopted, the employees' predicament would be a sorry one.
    (A) subversive    (B) laudable
    (C) nugatory    (D) compensatory
        (E) precarious.

19. Specifically our proposal would be to establish sufficient journeyman level positions so that when capability and performance is achieved by individuals they would _____ achieve journeyman level positions.
    (A) derisively
    (B) never
    (C) automatically
    (D) consequently
    (E) eventually.

20. _____ of qualitative research on readers is costing newspapers considerable linage.
    (A) Accuracy    (B) Delicacy
    (C) Monotony    (D) Paucity
        (E) Simplicity.

21. As often with those who spend themselves in the agony of revolutionizing set patterns, many of the _____ for which he broke ground were left to be fully realized by others.
    (A) foundations    (B) initiations
    (C) collaborations    (D) provocations
        (E) innovations.

22. Attendance of museums and galleries increases by leaps and bounds, new exhibition facilities _____ and possession of works of art is becoming a badge of cultural honor.
    (A) proliferate    (B) coagulate
    (C) asphyxiate    (D) conglomerate
        (E) simulate.

23. A _____ statement shows the Toronto Star Ltd.'s net operating revenue for the year ending Sept. 30, 1957, as $1,596,403, as compared with $2,016,024 the previous year.

    (A) mercenary    (B) notarized
    (C) economic    (D) financial
        (E) judicial.

24. One of the clearest affirmations of the confidence which fifteenth-century intellectuals felt in the _____ of their art, their sense of belonging to a momentous epoch, their joy in conquest and spiritual discovery, is a letter written in May 1473.
    (A) consanguinity    (B) rejuvenation
    (C) juxtaposition    (D) rectitude
        (E) multiplicity.

25. While the government asks its employees to back a (an) _____ budget on the ground that the City must conserve every possible penny to make both ends meet, it does not say what the employees must do to make both ends meet.
    (A) meticulous    (B) inconspicuous
    (C) austerity    (D) sententious
        (E) meritorious.

26. It has come to the attention of the court that a newspaper recently published a series of photographs _____ taken during a session.
    (A) judiciously    (B) notoriously
    (C) economically    (D) patiently
        (E) surreptitiously.

27. Even as many of them _____ their pledges of support, their actions belie their words.
    (A) conform    (B) renege
    (C) reiterate    (D) decline
            (E) remand.

28. Jones has continued his _____ with athletics in pictures of football, lacrosse and boxing.
    (A) sensation    (B) tension
    (C) schizophrenia    (D) metamorphosis
            (E) preoccupation.

29. There has been an almost _____ fear of inflation which has been especially terrifying to people who live on unearned income exclusively.
    (A) neurotic    (B) salubrious
    (C) sadistic    (D) concomitant
            (E) puerile.

30. We would certainly be _____ if we did not report the error.
    (A) malaise    (B) derelict
    (C) consonant    (D) nominative
            (E) eleemosynary.

# TEST VI. QUANTITATIVE ABILITY

## TIME: 60 Minutes

*DIRECTIONS: For each of the following questions, select the choice which best answers the question or completes the statement.*

### EXPLANATIONS ARE GIVEN WITH THE ANSWERS
### WHICH FOLLOW THE QUESTIONS

1. Which one of these quantities is the smallest?

    (A) $\frac{1}{5}$      (B) $\frac{7}{9}$

    (C) .76      (D) $\frac{5}{7}$

    (E) $\frac{9}{11}$

**DO YOUR FIGURING HERE**

2. A girl earns twice as much in December as in each of the other months. What part of her entire year's earnings does she earn in December?

    (A) $\frac{2}{11}$

    (B) $\frac{2}{13}$

    (C) $\frac{3}{14}$

    (D) $\frac{1}{6}$

    (E) $\frac{1}{7}$

3. If $x = -1$, then $3x^3 + 2x^2 + x + 1 =$

    (A) $-1$

    (B) $1$

    (C) $-5$

    (D) $5$

    (E) $2$

4. How many twelfths of a pound are equal to $83\frac{1}{3}\%$ of a pound?

    (A) 5

    (B) 10

    (C) 12

    (D) 14

    (E) 16

5. An equilateral triangle 3 inches on a side is cut up into smaller equilateral triangles one inch on a side. What is the greatest number of such triangles that can be formed?

    (A) 3

    (B) 6

    (C) 9

    (D) 12

    (E) 15

S1346

6.  If $\dfrac{a}{b} = \dfrac{3}{5}$, then $15a =$

   (A)  3b
   (B)  5b
   (C)  6b
   (D)  9b
   (E)  15b

7.  A square 5 units on a side has one vertex at the point (1, 1). Which one of the following points *cannot* be diagonally opposite vertex?

   (A)  (6, 6)
   (B)  (− 4, 6)
   (C)  (− 4, − 4)
   (D)  (6, − 4)
   (E)  (4, − 6)

8.  Five equal squares are placed side by side to make a single rectangle whose perimeter is 372 inches. Find the number of square inches in the area of one of these squares.

   (A)  72
   (B)  324
   (C)  900
   (D)  961
   (E)  984

9.  Which is the smallest of the following numbers?

   (A)  $\sqrt{3}$

   (B)  $\dfrac{1}{\sqrt{3}}$

   (C)  $\dfrac{\sqrt{3}}{3}$

   (D)  ⅓

   (E)  $\dfrac{1}{3\sqrt{3}}$

10.  In the figure, what percent of the area of rectangle PQRS is shaded?

   (A)  20

   (B)  25

   (C)  30

   (D)  33⅓

   (E)  40

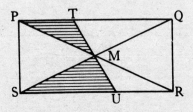

11. $\frac{1}{6}$ of an audience consisted of boys and $\frac{1}{3}$ of it consisted of girls. What percent of the audience consisted of children?

   (A) 66⅔
   (B) 50
   (C) 37½
   (D) 40
   (E) 33⅓

**DO YOUR FIGURING HERE**

12. One wheel has a diameter of 30 inches and a second wheel has a diameter of 20 inches. The first wheel traveled a certain distance in 240 revolutions. In how many revolutions did the second wheel travel the same distance?

   (A) 120
   (B) 160
   (C) 360
   (D) 420
   (E) 480

13. If x and y are two different real numbers and $rx = ry$, then r =

   (A) 0
   (B) 1
   (C) $\frac{x}{y}$
   (D) $\frac{y}{x}$
   (E) $x - y$

14. If $\frac{m}{n} = \frac{5}{6}$, then what is $3m + 2n$?

   (A) 0
   (B) 2
   (C) 7
   (D) 10
   (E) cannot be determined from the information given.

15. If $x > 1$, which of the following increase(s) as x increase(s)?

   I. $x - \frac{1}{x}$

   II. $\frac{1}{x^2 - x}$

   III. $4x^3 - 2x^2$

   (A) only I
   (B) only II
   (C) only III
   (D) only I and III
   (E) I, II, and III

16. In the figure, PQRS is a parallelogram, and ST = TV = VR. What is the ratio of the area of triangle SPT to the area of the parallelogram?

(A) ⅙

(B) ⅕

(C) ⅓

(D) ²⁄₇

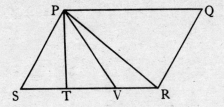

(E) cannot be determined from the information given

17. One angle of a triangle is 82°. The other two angles are in the ratio 2:5. Find the number of degrees in the smallest angle of the triangle.

(A) 14
(B) 25
(C) 28
(D) 38
(E) 82

18. If a boy can mow a lawn in t minutes, what part can he do in 15 minutes?

(A) t — 15

(B) $\dfrac{t}{15}$

(C) 15t

(D) 15 — t

(E) $\dfrac{15}{t}$

19. A typist uses lengthwise a sheet of paper 9 inches by 12 inches. She leaves a 1-inch margin on each side and a 1½ inch margin on top and bottom. What fractional part of the page is used for typing?

(A) ²¹⁄₂₂
(B) ⁷⁄₁₂
(C) ⁵⁄₉
(D) ¾
(E) ⁵⁄₁₂

20. It takes a boy 9 seconds to run a distance of 132 feet. What is his speed in miles per hour?

(A) 8
(B) 9
(C) 10
(D) 11
(E) 12

21. A rectangular sign is cut down by 10% of its height and 30% of its width. What percent of the original area remains?

    (A) 30
    (B) 37
    (C) 57
    (D) 70
    (E) 63

DO YOUR FIGURING HERE

22. How many of the numbers between 100 and 300 begin or end with 2?

    (A) 20
    (B) 40
    (C) 180
    (D) 100
    (E) 110

23. If Mary knows that y is an integer greater than 2 and less than 7 and John knows that y is an integer greater than 5 and less than 10, then Mary and John may correctly conclude that

    (A) y can be exactly determined
    (B) y may be either of 2 values
    (C) y may be any of 3 values
    (D) y may be any of 4 values
    (E) there is no value of y satisfying these conditions

24. The area of a square is $49 x^2$. What is the length of a diagonal of the square?

    (A) 7x
    (B) $7x \sqrt{2}$
    (C) 14x
    (D) $7x^2$
    (E) $\dfrac{7x}{\sqrt{2}}$

25. In the figure, MNOP is a square of area 1, Q is the mid-point of MN, and R is the mid-point of NO. What is the ratio of the area of triangle PQR to the area of the square?

    (A) ¼

    (B) ⅓

    (C) ¹⁄₁₆

    (D) ⅜

    (E) ½

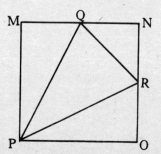

26. If a rectangle is 4 feet by 12 feet, how many two-inch tiles would have to be put around the outside edge to completely frame the rectangle?

(A) 32
(B) 36
(C) 192
(D) 196
(E) 200

**DO YOUR FIGURING HERE**

27. One-tenth is what part of three-fourths?

(A) $^{40}\!/_3$
(B) $^3\!/_{40}$
(C) $^{15}\!/_2$
(D) $\frac{1}{8}$
(E) $^2\!/_{15}$

28. The area of square PQRS is 49. What are the coordinates of Q?

(A) $\dfrac{(7\sqrt{2},\ 0)}{2}$

(B) $\dfrac{(0,\ 7\ \sqrt{2})}{2}$

(C) $(0,\ 7)$

(D) $(7,\ 0)$

(E) $(0,\ 7\ \sqrt{2})$

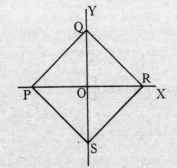

29. Village A has a population of 6800, which is decreasing at a rate of 120 per year. Village B has a population of 4200, which is increasing at a rate of 80 per year. In how many years will the population of the two villages be equal?

(A) 9
(B) 11
(C) 13
(D) 14
(E) 16

30. The average of 8 numbers is 6; the average of 6 other numbers is 8. What is the average of all 14 numbers?

(A) 6
(B) $6^6\!/_7$
(C) 7
(D) $7^2\!/_7$
(E) $8^1\!/_7$

31. If x is between 0 and 1, which of the following increases as x increases?

    I. $1 - x^2$
    II. $x - 1$
    III. $\dfrac{1}{x^2}$

    (A) I and II
    (B) II and III
    (C) I and III
    (D) II only
    (E) I only

32. In the formula $T = 2\sqrt{\dfrac{L}{g}}$, g is a constant.

    By what number must L be multiplied so that T will be multiplied by 3?

    (A) 3
    (B) 6
    (C) 9
    (D) 12
    (E) $\sqrt{3}$

33. Three circles are tangent externally to each other and have radii of 2 inches, 3 inches, and 4 inches respectively. How many inches are in the perimeter of the triangle formed by joining the centers of the three circles?

    (A) 9
    (B) 12
    (C) 15
    (D) 18
    (E) 21

34. If a circle of radius 10 inches has its radius decreased 3 inches, what percent is its area decreased?

    (A) 9
    (B) 49
    (C) 51
    (D) 70
    (E) 91

35. If a hat cost $4.20 after a 40% discount, what was its original price?

    (A) $2.52
    (B) $4.60
    (C) $5.33
    (D) $7.00
    (E) $10.50

# TEST VII. PERCEPTUAL MOTOR ABILITY

### TIME: 20 Minutes

*DIRECTIONS: Each question in this test consists of a numbered picture showing a piece of cardboard that is to be folded. The dotted lines show where folds are to be made. The problem is to choose the lettered picture, A, B, C, or D which would be made by folding the cardboard in the numbered picture. For each question blacken the space on your answer sheet corresponding to the letter of the best answer.*

*Correct key answers to all these test questions will be found at the end of the test.*

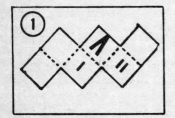
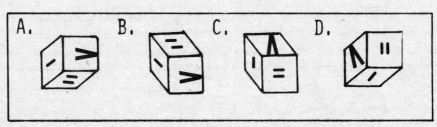

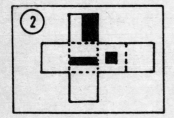
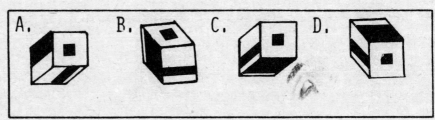

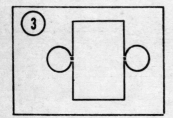
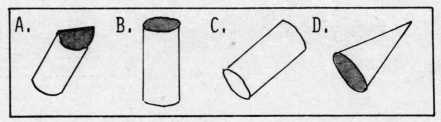

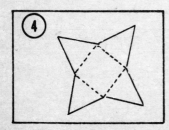
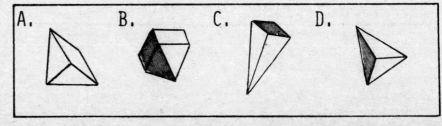

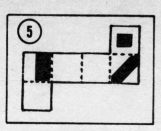    

**5.** A. B. C. D.

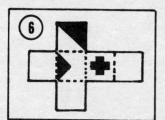 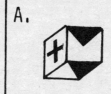 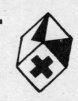  

**6.** A. B. C. D.

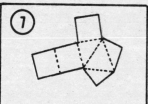  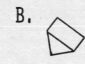  

**7.** A. B. C. D.

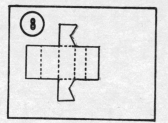   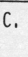  

**8.** A. B. C. D.

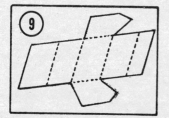 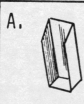 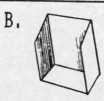 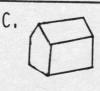 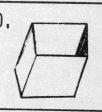

**9.** A. B. C. D.

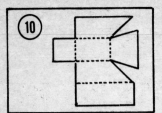

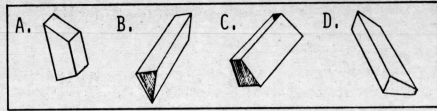

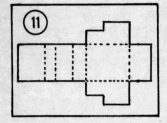

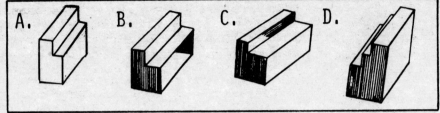

# AFTER TAKING EXAMINATION II.

*STEP ONE — Check all your answers with the Correct Answers that follow. Then compare your total score with the Unofficial Percentile Ranking Table below. This Table will give you a reasonably good idea of how you stand with others taking the Exam. For example, if your percentile ranking is 61, according to your score, you are superior to 60% and inferior to 39% of those who have taken the Exam. Your percentile ranking on the Examination is a major factor in determining your eligibility.*

## PERCENTILE RANKING TABLE
### (unofficial)

| Approximate Percentile Ranking | Score On Test | Approximate Percentile Ranking | Score On Test |
|---|---|---|---|
| 99 | 219–221 | 69 | 153–154 |
| 98 | 216–218 | 68 | 151–152 |
| 97 | 213–215 | 67 | 149–150 |
| 96 | 210–212 | 66 | 147–148 |
| 95 | 207–209 | 65 | 145–146 |
| 94 | 204–206 | 64 | 143–144 |
| 93 | 201–203 | 63 | 141–142 |
| 92 | 199–200 | 62 | 139–140 |
| 91 | 197–198 | 61 | 137–138 |
| 90 | 195–196 | 60 | 135–136 |
| 89 | 193–194 | 59 | 133–134 |
| 88 | 191–192 | 58 | 130–132 |
| 87 | 189–190 | 57 | 127–129 |
| 86 | 187–188 | 56 | 124–126 |
| 85 | 185–186 | 55 | 121–123 |
| 84 | 183–184 | 54 | 118–120 |
| 83 | 181–182 | 53 | 115–117 |
| 82 | 179–180 | 52 | 112–114 |
| 81 | 177–178 | 51 | 109–111 |
| 80 | 175–176 | 50 | 106–108 |
| 79 | 173–174 | 49 | 103–105 |
| 78 | 171–172 | 48 | 100–102 |
| 77 | 169–170 | 47 | 97–99 |
| 76 | 167–168 | 46 | 94–96 |
| 75 | 165–166 | 45 | 91–93 |
| 74 | 163–164 | 44 | 88–90 |
| 73 | 161–162 | 43 | 85–87 |
| 72 | 159–160 | 42 | 82–84 |
| 71 | 157–158 | 41 | 79–81 |
| 70 | 155–156 | 0–40 | 0–78 |

*STEP TWO — Use the results of the Examination you have just taken to diagnose yourself. Pinpoint the areas in which you show the greatest weakness. Fill in the Diagnostic Table to spotlight the subjects in which you need the most practice.*

## DIAGNOSTIC TABLE FOR EXAMINATION II.

| SUBJECT TESTED | QUESTIONS ANSWERED CORRECTLY ON EXAM | | |
|---|---|---|---|
| | Strong | Average | Weak |
| TEST I. BIOMEDICAL SCIENCE | 37–45 | 24–36 | 19–23 |
| TEST II. INTERPRETATION OF SCIENCE READINGS | 34–40 | 22–33 | 10–21 |
| TEST III. VOCABULARY | 21–30 | 16–20 | 10–15 |
| TEST IV. VERBAL ANALOGIES | 21–30 | 16–20 | 10–15 |
| TEST V. SENTENCE COMPLETIONS | 21–30 | 16–20 | 10–15 |
| TEST VI. QUANTITATIVE ABILITY | 24–35 | 18–23 | 11–17 |
| TEST VII. PERCEPTUAL MOTOR ABILITY | 9–11 | 7–8 | 5–6 |

*STEP THREE—Use the following Check List to establish areas that require the greatest application on your part. One check ( √ ) after the item means* moderately *weak; two checks ( √ √ ) means* seriously weak.

| Area of Weakness | Check Below | Area of Weakness | Check Below |
|---|---|---|---|
| BIOLOGY | | VERBAL ANALOGIES | |
| CHEMISTRY | | SENTENCE COMPLETIONS | |
| SCIENCE READINGS | | MATHEMATICS | |
| SYNONYMS | | SPATIAL PROBLEM SOLVING | |
| OPPOSITES | | | |

*STEP FOUR — The Pinpoint Practice chapters which follow provide all the drill material you need for every phase of the Examination. Plan your attack systematically. Concentrate on your weaknesses. Answer the practice questions in these areas. As you will discover, the material is presented so that the areas tested in the actual exam are individually treated in this book.*

*STEP FIVE — When you have strengthened yourself sufficiently where strengthening is necessary, take the other Examinations in the book. Again place yourself under strict testing conditions. We have every confidence that you will do better on the following Exams than you did on this one, if you've followed our suggestions for eliminating "soft spots." Now, please get to work.*

# CORRECT ANSWERS FOR PREDICTIVE EXAMINATION II.

*(Please make every effort to answer the questions on your own before looking at these answers. You'll make faster progress by following this rule.)*

## TEST I. BIOMEDICAL SCIENCE

| | | | | | | | |
|---|---|---|---|---|---|---|---|
| 1. C | 7. B | 13. C | 19. A | 25. D | 31. D | 36. C | 41. C |
| 2. D | 8. D | 14. A | 20. A | 26. D | 32. C | 37. B | 42. C |
| 3. A | 9. B | 15. D | 21. C | 27. C | 33. A | 38. D | 43. C |
| 4. D | 10. A | 16. C | 22. C | 28. B | 34. C | 39. C | 44. B |
| 5. B | 11. B | 17. B | 23. C | 29. B | 35. B | 40. D | 45. B |
| 6. D | 12. C | 18. C | 24. A | 30. D | | | |

## TEST II. INTERPRETATION OF SCIENCE READINGS

| | | | | | | | |
|---|---|---|---|---|---|---|---|
| 1. C | 6. D | 11. B | 16. B | 21. C | 26. C | 31. D | 36. B |
| 2. D | 7. C | 12. D | 17. B | 22. D | 27. C | 32. B | 37. D |
| 3. B | 8. C | 13. C | 18. A | 23. A | 28. B | 33. C | 38. D |
| 4. D | 9. A | 14. B | 19. D | 24. C | 29. C | 34. C | 39. B |
| 5. A | 10. C | 15. A | 20. B | 25. A | 30. A | 35. A | 40. D |

## TEST III. VOCABULARY

| | | | | | | |
|---|---|---|---|---|---|---|
| 1. A | 5. B | 9. C | 13. D | 17. B | 21. A | 25. C | 28. C |
| 2. B | 6. C | 10. B | 14. C | 18. A | 22. D | 26. B | 29. B |
| 3. C | 7. A | 11. B | 15. A | 19. D | 23. C | 27. D | 30. A |
| 4. C | 8. B | 12. A | 16. D | 20. B | 24. C | | |

## TEST IV. VERBAL ANALOGIES

| | | | | | | |
|---|---|---|---|---|---|---|
| 1. D | 5. E | 9. D | 13. C | 17. D | 21. C | 25. B | 28. C |
| 2. C | 6. E | 10. A | 14. E | 18. D | 22. A | 26. C | 29. B |
| 3. E | 7. B | 11. D | 15. E | 19. C | 23. E | 27. E | 30. B |
| 4. C | 8. D | 12. B | 16. A | 20. E | 24. C | | |

# TEST IV. EXPLANATORY ANSWERS

*Elucidation, clarification, explication and a little help with the fundamental facts covered in the Previous Test.*

1. **(D)** Control results in order; anarchy results in chaos.

2. **(C)** One creates something by carving wood; one creates something by molding clay.

3. **(E)** A border separates one state from another; a fence separates one property from another.

4. **(C)** A soldier is part of a regiment; a star is part of a constellation.

5. **(E)** Apogee and perigee are opposites; so are inappropriate and apposite.

6. **(E)** A refugee seeks asylum; a traveler seeks a destination.

7. **(B)** One who is greatly worried may become hysterical; one who is very happy may well be ecstatic.

8. **(D)** A word may be disguised by a charade; a message may be disguised by a code.

9. **(D)** A player is part of a team; a fish is part of a school.

10. **(A)** A banana is one of several bananas in a bunch; a city is one of several cities in a state.

11. **(D)** A moth will injure clothing; a stigma will injure a reputation.

12. **(B)** Lincoln is the capital of Nebraska; Trenton is the capital of New Jersey.

13. **(C)** The words buzz and hum are onomatopoetic; so are the words tinkle and clang.

14. **(E)** A boxer uses gloves in his profession; a bacteriologist uses a microscope in his profession.

15. **(E)** Consideration is a likely preliminary before making a decision; a wish is preliminary to the fulfillment of that wish.

16. **(A)** A delusion is a mirage; a haunter is a specter.

17. **(D)** France is a country in Europe; Algeria is a country in Africa.

18. **(D)** A person who is invulnerable cannot be hurt by an insult; a city which is impregnable cannot be hurt by an assault.

19. **(C)** Poison often results in death; kindness often results in cooperation.

20. **(E)** Slate is a type of rock; a kayak is a type of boat.

21. **(C)** Law controls the citizen; reins control the horse.

22. **(A)** Joy is a milder form of ecstasy; admiration is a milder form of love.

23. **(E)** A level of larceny is grand larceny; a level of school is elementary school.

24. **(C)** An antiseptic kills germs; a lion kills his prey.

25. **(B)** You ride a horse and you make a purchase.

26. **(C)** One employs a clue to solve a mystery; one employs study to succeed on a test.

27. **(E)** One sharpens a pencil and one saws wood.

28. **(C)** Garbage leads to a condition of squalor; diamonds lead to a condition of magnificence.

29. **(B)** A myth is a type of story; a bonnet is a type of hat.

30. **(B)** One who is a dunce is certainly not clever; one who has courage is certainly not fearful.

## TEST V. SENTENCE COMPLETIONS

| | | | | | | | |
|---|---|---|---|---|---|---|---|
| 1. C | 5. D | 9. C | 13. D | 17. E | 21. E | 25. C | 28. E |
| 2. A | 6. A | 10. C | 14. B | 18. B | 22. A | 26. E | 29. A |
| 3. C | 7. C | 11. D | 15. A | 19. C | 23. D | 27. C | 30. B |
| 4. A | 8. B | 12. A | 16. D | 20. D | 24. D | | |

## TEST VI. QUANTITATIVE ABILITY

| | | | | | | | |
|---|---|---|---|---|---|---|---|
| 1. D | 6. D | 11. B | 16. A | 20. C | 24. B | 28. B | 32. C |
| 2. B | 7. E | 12. C | 17. C | 21. E | 25. D | 29. C | 33. D |
| 3. A | 8. D | 13. A | 18. E | 22. E | 26. D | 30. B | 34. C |
| 4. B | 9. E | 14. E | 19. B | 23. A | 27. E | 31. D | 35. D |
| 5. C | 10. B | 15. D | | | | | |

## TEST VII. PERCEPTUAL MOTOR ABILITY

| | | | | | | | |
|---|---|---|---|---|---|---|---|
| 1. A | 3. C | 5. B | 7. A | 8. B | 9. C | 10. A | 11. A |
| 2. D | 4. A | 6. D | | | | | |

# III. PREDICTIVE PRACTICE EXAMINATION

*This professionally-written Examination enables you to display and exercise the important test-taking abilities leading to high scores . . . judgment, coolness, and flexibility. The various Tests fairly represent the actual exam. They should help in jogging your memory for all kinds of useful and relevant information which might otherwise be lost to you in achieving the highest exam rating possible.*

TOTAL TIME: 4 hours 30 minutes . In order to create the climate of the test to come, that's precisely what you should allow yourself . . . no more, no less. Use a watch and keep a record of your time, especially since you may find it convenient to take the test in several sittings.

Although copies of past exams are not released, we were able to piece together a fairly complete picture of the forthcoming exam.

A principal source of information was our analysis of official announcements going back several years.

Critical comparison of these announcements, particularly the sample questions, revealed the testing trend; foretold the important subjects, and those that are likely to recur.

The various subjects expected on your exam are represented by separate Tests.

The questions on each Test are represented exactly on the special Answer Sheet provided. Mark your answers on this sheet. It's just about the way you'll have to do it on the real exam.

As a result you have an Examination which simulates the real one closely enough to provide you with important training.

Correct answers for all the questions in all the Tests of the Exam appear at the end of the Exam, after the suggestions for self diagnosis and further study.

Don't cheat yourself by looking at these answers while taking the Exam. They are to be compared with your own answers *after* the time limit is up.

Then you may convert your answers to a percentage score for each Test, using the score boxes we provide. You'll also be able to compare your performance with that of others who have taken the Exam. In addition, you'll get a few ideas for further study which can save you a lot of valuable time.

# III. PREDICTIVE PRACTICE EXAMINATION

| ANALYSIS AND TIMETABLE: PREDICTIVE PRACTICE EXAMINATION | |
| --- | --- |
| *Since the number of questions for each test may vary on different forms of the actual examination, the time allotments below are flexible.* | |
| *SUBJECT TESTED* | *Time Allowed* |
| TEST I. BIOMEDICAL SCIENCE | 65 Minutes |
| TEST II. INTERPRETATION OF SCIENCE READINGS | 75 Minutes |
| TEST III. VOCABULARY | 20 Minutes |
| TEST IV. VERBAL ANALOGIES | 20 Minutes |
| TEST V. SENTENCE COMPLETIONS | 15 Minutes |
| TEST VI. QUANTITATIVE ABILITY | 60 Minutes |
| TEST VII. PERCEPTUAL MOTOR ABILITY | 20 Minutes |

# ANSWER SHEET FOR PREDICTIVE EXAMINATION III.

## TEST I. BIOMEDICAL SCIENCE

## TEST II. INTERPRETATION OF SCIENCE READINGS

## TEST III. VOCABULARY

## TEST IV. VERBAL ANALOGIES

# TEST V. SENTENCE COMPLETIONS

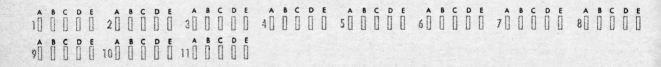

| | A B C D E | | A B C D E | | A B C D E | | A B C D E | | A B C D E | | A B C D E | | A B C D E | | A B C D E |
|---|---|---|---|---|---|---|---|---|---|---|---|---|---|---|---|
| 1 | | 2 | | 3 | | 4 | | 5 | | 6 | | 7 | | 8 | |
| 9 | | 10 | | 11 | | 12 | | 13 | | 14 | | 15 | | 16 | |
| 17 | | 18 | | 19 | | 20 | | | | | | | | | |

# TEST VI. QUANTITATIVE ABILITY

| | A B C D E | | A B C D E | | A B C D E | | A B C D E | | A B C D E | | A B C D E | | A B C D E | | A B C D E |
|---|---|---|---|---|---|---|---|---|---|---|---|---|---|---|---|
| 1 | | 2 | | 3 | | 4 | | 5 | | 6 | | 7 | | 8 | |
| 9 | | 10 | | 11 | | 12 | | 13 | | 14 | | 15 | | 16 | |
| 17 | | 18 | | 19 | | 20 | | 21 | | 22 | | 23 | | 24 | |
| 25 | | 26 | | 27 | | 28 | | 29 | | 30 | | 31 | | 32 | |
| 33 | | 34 | | 35 | | | | | | | | | | | |

# TEST VII. PERCEPTUAL MOTOR ABILITY

| | A B C D E | | A B C D E | | A B C D E | | A B C D E | | A B C D E | | A B C D E | | A B C D E | | A B C D E |
|---|---|---|---|---|---|---|---|---|---|---|---|---|---|---|---|
| 1 | | 2 | | 3 | | 4 | | 5 | | 6 | | 7 | | 8 | |
| 9 | | 10 | | 11 | | | | | | | | | | | | | |

# TEST I. BIOMEDICAL SCIENCE

## TIME: 65 Minutes

*DIRECTIONS: For each of the following questions, select the choice which best answers the question or completes the statement.*

1. The best fuel for use in present fuel cells is
   1. carbon
   2. hydrogen
   3. kerosene
   4. sodium

2. The term "systolic" would probably be found in an article on
   1. abstract mathematics
   2. heart research
   3. plastics
   4. soil conservation

3. A klystron is most closely related to a
   1. bevatron
   2. mho
   3. mitochondria
   4. vacuum tube

4. The newly accepted standard for the weight of the chemical elements is
   1. carbon-12
   2. hydrogen
   3. oxygen
   4. sodium

5. A thanatocoenose is
   1. an assemblage of dead plants and animals
   2. an extinct reptile
   3. a preserving fluid
   4. used in the study of protozoans

6. The light sensitive pigment found in all plants is
   1. indigo
   2. melanin
   3. phytochrome
   4. rhodopsin

7. Canal rays are
   1. directed beams of light
   2. positive particles issuing from a perforated cathode
   3. topographical features of Mars
   4. related to sharks

8. Which of the following was the nation's number one cause of death in 1960?
   1. accidents
   2. cancer
   3. heart disease
   4. pneumonia

9. An amphiprotic substance would be
   1. $HSO_4$
   2. $NH_3$
   3. NaCl
   4. NaOH

10. Which of the following causes hyperopia?
    1. increased fluid pressure on the eye
    2. lengthened focal length of eye lens
    3. shortened focal length of eye lens
    4. uneven curvature of the cornea

11. An anthropologist believes that the first man from outer space to be seen by earth men will be bimanous, quadrupedal hexapods. Such outer space men will
    1. have four limbs
    2. have six feet
    3. have two hands
    4. not be bilaterally symmetrical

12. Pyroclastic cones are
    1. for measuring subterranean pressure
    2. for measuring temperature
    3. rocket nose cones
    4. cones of volcanic ejecta

13. The Milky Way Galaxy, to which the earth and sun belong is a huge
    1. concave disc
    2. diffuse globule
    3. doughnut-shaped pattern
    4. spiral with three arms

14. A springtail is classified as
    1. a coelenterate
    2. a mollusk
    3. an annelid
    4. an arthropod

15. The liquid hydrogen bubble chamber was developed by
    1. Donald Glaser
    2. Edward Purcell
    3. William Shockley
    4. C. C. Wilson

16. Maser principles would most likely be discussed in an article on
    1. genetics
    2. long distance communications
    3. psychology
    4. zoology

17. *Zinjanthropus boisei* has been estimated to have lived 1,750,-000 years ago. By what dating method was this estimate made?
    1. carbon-14
    2. neon-sodium
    3. nitrogen-krypton
    4. potassium-argon

18. High purity beryllium relative to ordinary beryllium is more
    1. brittle
    2. chemically active
    3. dense
    4. ductile

19. The key to heredity appears to be in
    1. amino acids
    2. cell nuclei
    3. molecules of deoxyribonucleic acid
    4. protein content of cells

20. The physical membrane of erythrocytes possesses a highly selective permeability, being freely permeable to
    1. all anions
    2. calcium or barium ions
    3. fats
    4. sugar

21. Chelation compounds are used for
    1. anesthetics
    2. experiments with nucleic acids
    3. investigating sensory thresholds of insects
    4. sequestering metallic ions

22. Electron spin resonance is used to
    1. investigate atomic structure
    2. measure radiation in the Van Allen belts
    3. measure the charge of an electron
    4. study free radicals

23. Which of the following is a means of fitting a line to a particular set of points?
    1. Cartesian method
    2. integration
    3. method of least squares
    4. Poisson distribution

24. Neoplastic refers to
    1. cancer
    2. facial surgery
    3. glass
    4. polystyrene

25. The Rousseau diagram is used to find
    1. average candle power
    2. dielectric constant
    3. moment of inertia
    4. Norton equivalent

## SECTION A

The theory of spontaneous generation is an old one, having its origins with Aristotle and Lucretius. It remained in fashion until the 17th century, supported by the work of one Van Helmont, who reported, after an actual, if not carefully controlled experiment, the spontaneous generation of mice from dirty undergarments and wheat. The theory was dealt its death blow, however, two hundred years later, by Pasteur.

Since the days of Pasteur we have come far towards the secret of life, and are perhaps on the verge of a final answer. Viruses are believed by some to be the simplest elements of life, and amino acids, basic constituents of the virus' protein jacket, have been synthesized under conditions approximating those in the earth's atmosphere two billion years ago. It may be soon possible to synthesize nucleic acids, the other major components of viruses, which possess on their own properties of infection, reproduction, and mutation.

## QUESTIONS ON SECTION A

26. In this section, the theory of spontaneous generation is
    1. given wholehearted support
    2. placed in proper historical context
    3. shown to be impossible
    4. shown to be possible for viruses

27. According to the section,
    1. because of their simplicity, viruses will be the first living material to be synthesized
    2. enzymes contain both viruses and some proteins
    3. nucleic acids could have been formed in the primeval atmosphere
    4. viruses' second component, nucleic acids, have not been successfully synthesized

28. Which of the following is the best expression of the meaning of the phrase "secret of life?"
    1. proof that spontaneous generation does take place
    2. synthesis of material having all the characteristics of a living organism
    3. fertilization of mammalian ova outside the animal body
    4. development of mutations

## SECTION B

The diagram shows a cube. Each corner has been identified by a letter. Corner E is not shown, but its location is the one corner not shown in the diagram. The cube has a 1″ side.

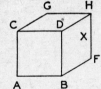

## QUESTIONS ON SECTION B

29. The distance from A to D is
    1. $\sqrt{1}$ inches
    2. $\sqrt{2}$ inches
    3. $\sqrt{3}$ inches
    4. $\sqrt{4}$ inches

30. There is a dot X on the BDHF face of the cube. Let the cube rotate 180° in a clockwise direction on an axis running through A and H, the
    1. cube will be standing on corner C
    2. dot X will appear in the plane where face ABCD is now shown
    3. dot X will be in the plane where face CDGH is now shown
    4. cube will return to its position as shown in the diagram

31. If the cube be rotated 270° counter clockwise on an axis going through the centers of faces ABCD and EFGH, and then is rotated 90° on an axis going through the centers of faces CDGH and ABEF, the face which contains point X will be
    1. at the top or bottom of the cube
    2. at the right side of the cube
    3. at the back or front of the cube
    4. at the left side of the cube

32. If the cube is successively rotated 180° on axes going through the center of faces ABCD and EFGH, faces AECG and BFDH, and faces CDGH and ABEF, where will the face containing point X be?
    1. It will return to the position from which it started.
    2. Where face AECG was at the start of the operation.
    3. Where face EFGH was at the start of the operation.
    4. Where face ABEF was at the start of the operation.

## SECTION C

The behavior of a nonuniform field can best be understood by considering first the simpler case of a uniform field, such as the one between a pair of flat parallel metal plates that are oppositely charged. A charged body freely suspended between the plates — for example, in a nonconducting liquid — will move parallel to the field, toward the plate bearing the opposite charge. A neutral body, on the other hand, is not impelled in either direction; it stays put.

Even though it appears to ignore the field, the neutral body is not completely unaffected. It acquires, in effect, a negative charge on the side facing the positive electrode and a positive charge on the side facing the negative electrode. The reason for this polarization, as it is called, is that the atoms composing the neutral body are made up of separate electric charges — positive nuclei and negative electrons. Under the influence of the outside field the electrons and nuclei are pulled in opposite directions, so that the center of negative charge no longer coincides with the center of positive charge. . . .

The net effect is an excess of positive charge on one part of the body and an equal excess of negative charge on the other. Therefore, the two sides of the gross body are pulled in opposite directions by the field. Since the charges are equal and the field is the same on both sides, the opposing forces exactly cancel.

If, however, the field is made stronger on one side than the other, the forces are no longer in balance, and the body is pulled in the direction of the stronger field. The effect can be demonstrated with electrodes in the form of a pair of concentric cylinders.

## QUESTIONS ON SECTION C

33. A neutral particle is placed in a nonuniform field. The particle moves toward
    1. one of the electrodes, but insufficient information is given to determine toward which one it moves
    2. the larger electrode (outer)
    3. the smaller electrode (inner)
    4. whichever electrode is closer

34. An alpha particle is placed in a nonuniform field. The particle moves toward
    1. one of the electrodes, but insufficient information is given to determine toward which one it moves
    2. the larger electrode
    3. the smaller electrode
    4. whichever electrode is closer

35. A neutral particle is placed in a nonuniform field. The polarity of the electrodes is then suddenly reversed. The particle
    1. becomes ionized
    2. continues moving in the same direction as before the polarity was changed
    3. is unaffected by the change in polarity
    4. reverses its direction

36. Since the extent of polarization caused by an electric field varies for different substances, some substances move more rapidly in a nonuniform field than do others. On the basis of this principle, devices have been constructed which separate different components of a mixture by creating a nonuniform electric field.
    1. These devices can operate on alternating current only.
    2. These devices can operate on both direct and alternating current.
    3. These devices can operate on direct current only.
    4. Insufficient information has been given to determine the type of current necessary.

37. In a given field
    1. all materials are polarized to the same degree
    2. no polarization takes place
    3. all neutral bodies are polarized
    4. some materials are polarized, and some are not

## SECTION D

The differential chain block, shown in the diagram, consists of two sheaves, A and B, A being a double sheave having diameters R and r. The multiplying power of this mechanism depends upon the ratio of these diameters. If they are equal, the pull P will not move the weight, and the efficiency of the mechanism will be zero percent, but the theoretical mechanical advantage is infinity. A slight difference in radii will produce a very large lifting effort, although the efficiency may still be very low. The sheaves are made with link pockets so that the chain fits nicely into the circumference, and is restrained from slipping. Furthermore, the chain is endless, and the mechanism is self-locking by virtue of the friction intentionally allowed on the journals.

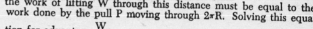

In explanation of the chain block, if the pull P revolves sheave A one revolution, the vertical chain at a is lowered through a distance to $2\pi r$, while the side b is raised the distance $2\pi R$. The net vertical displacement of the sheave B is $\pi(R-r)$ upward. With no friction considered, the the work of lifting W through this distance must be equal to the work done by the pull P moving through $2\pi R$. Solving this equation for advantage $\frac{W}{P}$,

$$\frac{W}{P} = \frac{2R}{R-r}.$$

Applying the mechanical efficiency e to this equation, the actual mechanical advantage is

$$\frac{W}{P} = \frac{2\,Re}{R-r}$$

These chain blocks are built in different sizes for hoisting loads from one-quarter ton to three or four tons, by hand. On account of the self-locking feature depending on friction, the average mechanical efficiency of this device is only about 30%.

## QUESTIONS ON SECTION D

38. Which of the following statements is true? When the pull P revolves sheave A two revolutions, and sheaves A and B have the same diameter, then
    1. if R = r, sheave B can only rotate in place
    2. if R > r, sheave B will be lowered
    3. if R < r, sheave B will be raised
    4. for any values of R and r, sheave B will be neither lowered nor raised

39. The multiplying power of the mechanism is
    1. a function of the ratio of R and r
    2. limited by the amount of pull a man can exert
    3. lowered by the amount of friction present
    4. the same as the mechanical advantage

40. As sheave B is raised through the use of the mechanism
    1. the chain loop of P will become larger
    2. the chain loop of P will become smaller
    3. the chain loop of P will remain the same size
    4. no information is available to show relationship of length of the chain loop of P and travel of sheave B

41. If R = 10 inches and r = 8 inches, how much will sheave B be raised by 10 complete revolutions of sheave A?
    1. $8\pi$ inches
    2. $18\pi$ inches
    3. $20\pi$ inches
    4. $25\pi$ inches

42. Using the equation for mechanical advantage given, and assuming that mechanical efficiency is 40%, what is the advantage of a differential chain block in which the diameters of the double sheave are 20 and 15, and the diameter of sheave B is 10?
    1. 2.4
    2. 2.8
    3. 3.2
    4. 3.6

## SECTION E

The table shows some radioactive isotopes, the kind of radiation emitted and their half-life. (Half-life is the time required for the disintegration of half of the atoms in a sample of some specific radioactive substance.)

| ISOTOPE | RADIATION EMITTED | HALF-LIFE |
|---|---|---|
| Nitrogen-16 | beta and gamma | 7.4 seconds |
| Sulfur-37 | beta and gamma | 5 minutes |
| Sodium-24 | beta and gamma | 15 hours |
| Gold-108 | beta and gamma | 2.7 days |
| Iodine-131 | beta and gamma | 8 days |
| Iron-59 | beta and gamma | 45 days |
| Cobalt-60 | beta and gamma | 5.2 years |
| Strontium-90 | beta | 28 years |
| Radium-226 | alpha and gamma | 1,620 years |
| Carbon-14 | beta | 5,600 years |
| Chlorine-36 | beta | 310,005 years |
| Uranium-235 | alpha, beta, gamma and neutrons | 710 million years |

## QUESTIONS ON SECTION E

43. Which of the following statements is most nearly correct?
    1. The greater the number of kinds of radiation emitted, the longer the half-life of the isotope.
    2. Filtering out the beta radiation and leaving the gamma rays will decrease the half-life of sulfur-37.
    3. Carbon-14 cannot be used for dating archeological artifacts more than 5,600 years old.
    4. There appears to be some relationship between kind of radiation emitted and length of half-life.

44. Which of the isotopes listed below has a half-life nearest the time required for iodine-131 to have expended 63/64 of its radiation?
    1. sodium-24
    2. gold-108
    3. iron-59
    4. cobalt-60

45. How long does it take a radioactive isotope to lose at least 99% of its radioactivity?
    1. two half-lives
    2. four half-lives
    3. seven half-lives
    4. fifteen half-lives

## TEST II. INTERPRETATION OF SCIENCE READINGS

### TIME: 75 Minutes

*DIRECTIONS: Read each passage to get the general idea. Then reread the passage more carefully to answer the questions based on the passage. For each question read all choices carefully. Then select the answer you consider correct or most nearly correct. Blacken the answer space corresponding to your best choice, just as you would do on the actual examination.*

*Reading Passage 1*

As the world's population grows, the part played by man in influencing plant life becomes increasingly greater. In old and densely populated countries, as in central Europe, man determines almost wholly what shall grow and what shall not grow. In such regions, the influence of man on plant life is in large measure a beneficial one. Laws, often centuries old, protect plants of economic value and preserve soil fertility. In newly settled countries the situation is unfortunately quite the reverse. The pioneer's life is too strenuous for him to think of posterity.

Some years ago Mt. Mitchell, the highest summit east of the Mississippi, was covered with a magnificent forest. A lumber company was given full rights to fell the trees. Those not cut down were crushed. The mountain was left a wasted area where fire would rage and erosion complete the destruction. There was no stopping the devastating foresting of the company, for the contract had been given. Under a more enlightened civilization this could not have happened. The denuding of Mt. Mitchell is a minor chapter in the destruction of lands in the United States; and this country is by no means the only sufferer. China, India, Egypt, and East Africa all have their thousands of square miles of wasteland, the result of man's indifference to the future.

Deforestation, grazing, and poor farming are the chief causes of the destruction of land fertility. Wasteful cutting of timber is the first step. Grazing then follows lumbering in bringing about ruin. The Caribbean slopes of northern Venezuela are barren wastes owing first to ruthless cutting of forests and then to destructive grazing. Hordes of goats have roamed these slopes until only a few thorny acacias and cacti remain. Erosion completed the devastation. What is there illustrated on a small scale is the story of vast areas in China and India, countries where famines are of regular occurrence.

Man is not wholly to blame, for Nature is often merciless. In parts of India and China, plant life, when left undisturbed by man, cannot cope with either the disastrous floods of wet seasons or the destructive winds of the dry season. Man has learned much; prudent land management has been the policy of the Chinese people since 2700 B. C., but even they have not learned enough.

When the American forestry service was in its infancy, it met with much opposition from legislators who loudly claimed that the protected land would in one season yield a crop of cabbages of more value than all the timber on it.

Herein lay the fallacy, that one season's crop is all that need be thought of. Nature, through the years, adjusts crops to the soil and to the climate. Forests usually occur where precipitation exceeds evaporation. If the reverse is true, grasslands are found; and where evaporation is still greater, desert or scrub vegetation alone survives. The phytogeographic map of a country is very similar to the climatic map based on rainfall, evaporation, and temperature. Man ignores this natural adjustment of crops and strives for one "bumper" crop in a single season; he may produce it, but "year in and year out the yield of the grassland is certain, that of the planted fields, never."

Man is learning; he sprays his trees with insecticides and fungicides; he imports ladybugs to destroy aphids; he irrigates, fertilizes, and rotates his crops; but he is still indifferent to many of the consequences of his short-sighted policies. The great dust storms of the western United States are proof of this indifference.

In spite of the evidence to be had from this country, the people of other countries, still in the pioneer stage, farm as wastefully as did our own pioneers. In the interiors of Central and South American Republics natives fell superb forest trees and leave them to rot in order to obtain virgin soil for cultivation. Where the land is hillside, it readily washes and after one or two seasons is unfit for crops. So the frontier farmer pushes back into the primeval forest, moving his hut as he goes, and fells more monarchs to lay bare another patch of ground for his plantings to support his family. Valuable timber which will require a century to replace is destroyed and the land laid waste to produce what could be supplied for a pittance.

How badly man can err in his handling of land is shown by the draining of extensive swamp areas, which to the uninformed would seem to be a very good thing to do. One of the first effects of the drainage is the lowering of the water-table, which may bring about the death of the dominant species and leave to another species the possession of the soil, even when the difference in water level is little more than an inch. Frequently, bog country will yield marketable crops of cranberries and blueberries but, if drained, neither these nor any other economic plant will grow on the fallow soil. Swamps and marshes have their drawbacks but also their virtues. When drained they may leave waste land the surface of which rapidly erodes to be then blown away in dust blizzards disastrous to both man and wild beasts.

1. The best title for this passage might be

    (A) How to Increase Soil Productivity
    (B) Conservation of Natural Resources
    (C) Man's Effect on Soil
    (D) Soil Conditions and Plant Growth.

2. A policy of good management is sometimes upset by

    (A) the indifference of man
    (B) centuries-old laws
    (C) floods and winds
    (D) grazing animals.

3. Areas in which the total amounts of rain and snow falling on the ground are greater than that which is evaporated will support

    (A) forests
    (B) grasslands
    (C) scrub vegetation
    (D) no plants

4. Pioneers do not have a long range view on soil problems since they

    (A) are not protected by laws
    (B) live under averse conditions
    (C) use poor methods of farming
    (D) must protect themselves from famine.

5. Phytogeographic maps are those that show

    (A) areas of grassland
    (B) areas of bumper crops
    (C) areas of similar climate
    (D) areas of similar plants.

6. The basic cause of frequent famines in China and India is probably due to

    (A) allowing animals to roam wild
    (B) drainage of swamps
    (C) over-grazing of the land
    (D) destruction of forests.

7. With a growing world population the increased need for soil for food production might be met by

    (A) draining unproductive swamp areas
    (B) legislating against excess lumbering
    (C) trying to raise bumper crops each year
    (D) irrigating desert areas.

8. What is meant by "the yield of the grasslands is certain; that of the planted field, never" is that

    (A) it is impossible to get more than one bumper crop from any one cultivated area
    (B) crops, planted in former grasslands will not give good yields
    (C) through the indifference of man, dust blizzards have occurred in former grasslands
    (D) if man does not interfere, plants will grow in the most suitable environment.

9. The first act of prudent land management might be to

    (A) prohibit drainage of swamps
    (B) use irrigation and crop rotation in planted areas
    (C) increase use of fertilizers
    (D) prohibit excessive forest lumbering.

10. The results of good land management may usually be found in

    (A) heavily populated areas
    (B) areas not given over to grazing
    (C) underdeveloped areas
    (D) ancient civilizations.

11. Long-range programs of soil management are possible only in

    (A) young nations
    (B) ancient civilizations
    (C) those nations with an agricultural economy
    (D) those nations which want it.

*Reading Passage II*

Of all the physical changes that have been and are now taking place on the surface of the earth, the sea and its shores have been the scene of the greatest stability. The dry land has seen the rise, the decline, and even the disappearance of vast hordes of various types and forms within times comparatively recent, geologically speaking; but life in the sea is today virtually what it was when many of the forms now extinct on land had not yet been evolved. Also, it may be parenthetically stated here, the marine habitat has been biologically the most important in the evolution and development of life on this planet. Its rhythmic influence can still be traced in those animals whose ancestors have long since left that realm to abide far from their primary haunts. For it is now generally held as an accepted fact that the shore area of an ancient sea was the birthplace of life.

Still, despite the primitive conditions still maintained in the sea, its shore inhabitants show an amazing diversity; while their adaptive characters are perhaps not exceeded in refinement by those that distinguish the dwellers of dry land. Why is this diversity manifest? We must look for an answer into the physical factors obtaining in that extremely slender zone surrounding the continents, marked by the rise and fall of the tides.

It will be noticed by the most casual observer that on any given seashore the area exposed between the tide marks may be roughly divided into a number of levels each characterized by a certain assemblage of animals. Thus in proceeding from high—to low-water mark, new forms constantly become predominant while other forms gradually drop out. Now, provided that the character of the substratum does not change, these differences in the types of animals are determined almost exlusively by the duration of time that the individual forms may remain exposed to the air without harm. Indeed, so regularly does the tidal rhythm act on certain animals (the barnacles, for instance), that certain species have come to require a definite period of exposure in order to maintain themselves, and will die out if kept continuously submerged. Although there are some forms that actually require periodic exposure, the number of species inhabiting the shore that are able to endure exposure every twelve hours, when the tide falls, is comparatively few.

With the alternate rise and fall of the tides, the successive areas of the tidal zone are subjected to force of wave-impact. In certain regions the waves often break with considerable force. Consequently, wave-shock has had a profound influence on the structure and habits of shore animals. It is characteristic of most shore animals that they shun definitely exposed places, and seek shelter in nooks and crannies and such refuges as are offered under stones and seaweed; particularly is this true of those forms living on rock and other firm foundations. Many of these have a marked capacity to cling closely to the

*Reading Passage II (cont'd)*

substratum; some, such as anemones and certain snails, although without the grasping organs of higher animals, have special powers of adhesion; others, such as sponges and sea squirts, remain permanently fixed, and if torn loose from their base are incapable of forming a new attachment. But perhaps the most significant method of solving the problem presented by the surf has been in the adaptation of body-form to minimize friction. This is strikingly displayed in the fact that seashore animals are essentially flattened forms. Thus, in the typically shore forms the sponges are of the encrusting type, the non-burrowing worms are leaflike, the snails and other mollusks are squat forms and are without the spines and other ornate extensions such as are often produced on the shells of many mollusks in deeper and quieter waters. The same influence is no less marked in the case of the crustaceans; the flattening is either lateral, as in the amphipods, or dorso-ventral, as in the isopods and crabs.

In sandy regions, because of the unstable nature of substratum, no such means of attachment as indicated in the foregoing paragraph will suffice to maintain the animals in their almost ceaseless battle with the billows. Most of them must perforce depend on their ability quickly to penetrate into the sand for safety. Some forms endowed with less celerity, such as the sand dollars, are so constructed that their bodies offer no more resistance to wave impact than does a flat pebble.

Temperature, also, is a not inconsiderable factor among those physical forces constantly operating to produce a diversity of forms among seashore animals. At a comparatively shallow depth in the sea, there is small fluctuation of temperatures; and life there exists in surroundings of serene stability, but as the shore is approached, the influence of the sun becomes more and more manifest and the variation is greater. This variation becomes greatest between the tide marks where, because of the very shallow depths and the fresh water from the land, this area is subjected to wide changes in both temperature and salinity.

Nor is a highly competitive mode of life without its bearing on structure as well as habits. In this phase of their struggle for existence, the animals of both the sea and the shore have become possessed of weapons for offense and defense that are correspondingly varied.

Although the life in the sea has been generally considered and treated as separate and distinct from the more familiar life on land, that supposition has no real basis in fact. Life on this planet is one vast unit, depending for its existence chiefly on the same sources of supply. That portion of animal life living in the sea, notwithstanding its strangeness and unfamiliarity, may be consid-

*Reading Passage II (Cont'd)*

ered as but the aquatic fringe of the life on land. It is supported largely by materials washed into the sea, which are no longer available for the support of land animals. Perhaps we have been misled in these considerations of sea life because of the fact that approximately three times as many major types of animals inhabit salt water as live on the land: of the major *types* of animals no fewer than ten are exclusively marine, that is to say, nearly half again as many as land-dwelling types together. A further interesting fact is that despite the greater variety in the form and structure of sea animals about three fourths of all known *kinds* of animals live on the land, while only one fourth lives in the sea. In this connection it is noteworthy that sea life becomes scarcer with increasing distance from land; toward the middle of the oceans it disappears almost completely. For example, the central south Pacific is a region more barren than is any desert area on land. Indeed, no life of any kind has been found in the surface water, and there seems to be none on the bottom.

Sea animals are largest and most abundant on those shores receiving the most copious rainfall. Particularly is this true on the most rugged and colder coasts where it may be assumed that the material from the land finds its way to the sea unaltered and in greater quantities.

12. The best title for this passage might be
    (A) Between the Tides
    (B) Seashore Life
    (C) The Tides
    (D) The Seashore.

13. Of the following adaptations, the one that would enable an organism to live on a sandy beach is
    (A) the ability to move rapidly
    (B) the ability to burrow deeply
    (C) a flattened shape
    (D) spiny extensions of the shell.

14. The absence of living things in mid-ocean might be due to
    (A) lack of rainfall in mid-ocean
    (B) the distance from material washed into the sea
    (C) larger animals feeding on smaller ones which must live near the land
    (D) insufficient dissolved oxygen.

15. A greater variety of living things exists on a rocky shore than on a sandy beach because
    (A) rocks offer a better foothold than sand
    (B) sandy areas are continually being washed by the surf
    (C) temperature changes are less drastic in rocky areas
    (D) the water in rock pools is less salty.

16. Organisms found living at the high-tide mark are adapted to
    (A) maintain themselves in the air for a long time
    (B) offer no resistance to wave impact
    (C) remain permanently fixed to the substratum
    (D) burrow in the ground.

17. The author holds that living things in the sea represent the aquatic fringe of life on land. This is so because
    (A) there are relatively fewer marine forms of animals than there are land-living forms
    (B) there is greater variety among land-living forms
    (C) marine animals ultimately depend upon material from the land
    (D) there are three times as many kinds of animals on land than there are in the sea.

18. A biologist walking along the shore at the low-tide line would not easily find many live animals since
    (A) their flattened shapes make them indistinguishable
    (B) they are washed back and forth by the waves
    (C) they burrow deeply
    (D) they move rapidly.

19. The intent of the author in the last paragraph is to show that
    (A) the temperature and salinity of the sea determine the variety among shore animals
    (B) marine animals are vastly different from terrestrial organisms
    (C) colder areas can support more living things than warm areas
    (D) marine forms have the same problems as terrestrial animals.

20. A scientist wishing to study a great variety of living things would do well to hunt for them
    (A) in shallow waters
    (B) on a rocky seashore
    (C) on a sandy seashore
    (D) on any shore between the tide lines.

21. The most primitive forms of living things in the evolutionary scale are to be found in the sea because
    (A) the influence of the sea is found in land animals
    (B) the sea is relatively stable
    (C) many forms have become extinct on land
    (D) land animals are supposed to have evolved from sea organisms.

22. The author suggests that any area on the shore bounded by the high and low tide lines
    (A) has a greater variety of physical factors than area of similar size any other place
    (B) has a greater variety of living things than any other area of similar size
    (C) can be used to explain the great variations among living things
    (D) can be used to explain the adaptations that are found among living things.

23. Some organisms can withstand wave shock by
    (A) periodic exposures to air
    (B) hiding under stones
    (C) moving out to deep water
    (D) forming new attachments to the substratum.

24. Commercial fishing vessels would find their greatest catch in
    (A) mid-ocean
    (B) off cold land areas
    (C) off warm, moist land areas
    (D) off areas with great rainfall.

25. The greatest variations among shore animals are adaptations to
    (A) changing temperatures
    (B) variations in sub-stratum
    (C) minimize friction
    (D) alterations in salinity.

26. The fact that there is a greater number of kinds of animals living on land than in the sea might be related to the fact that
    (A) water does not show as great extremes in temperature as land does
    (B) evolution has proceeded at a faster pace on land than on the sea
    (C) aquatic animals depend for food upon that which is no longer needed by land animals
    (D) land animals live in a great variety of environments.

27. Live barnacles might be found on the bottom of a rowboat beached for some time just above the low-tide line since
    (A) they require alternate periods of immersion in the sea
    (B) they are protected from the impact of the waves
    (C) they require extremes of temperatures afforded by the beach
    (D) they are incapable of forming new attachments.

# TEST III. VOCABULARY

## TIME: 20 Minutes

*DIRECTIONS: In each of the following questions, one word . . . a numbered word . . . is followed by four or five lettered words or expressions. Choose the lettered word or expression that has most nearly the opposite meaning of the numbered word. Mark the letter preceding that word as the answer to the question.*

1. piquant
   - (A) factitious
   - (B) vain
   - (C) insipid
   - (D) vulture
   - (E) chromatic.

2. opportune
   - (A) dialectical
   - (B) mutable
   - (C) unplanned
   - (D) weird
   - (E) inexpedient.

3. petulant
   - (A) irascible
   - (B) cheerful
   - (C) uncouth
   - (D) abnormal
   - (E) ambulant.

4. savory
   - (A) apathetic
   - (B) clandestine
   - (C) pliant
   - (D) unpalatable
   - (E) capillary.

5. satiated
   - (A) satirical
   - (B) centaur
   - (C) gorgeous
   - (D) delectable
   - (E) hungry.

6. reclusive
   - (A) empyreal
   - (B) obscure
   - (C) gregarious
   - (D) rustic
   - (E) chilblain.

7. courteous
   - (A) flaccid
   - (B) emolient
   - (C) insolent
   - (D) scrupulous
   - (E) flinching.

8. usurp
   - (A) succor
   - (B) predict
   - (C) pacify
   - (D) declaim
   - (E) donate.

9. acrimonious
   - (A) alluvial
   - (B) apocalyptic
   - (C) cursive
   - (D) harmonious
   - (E) flippant.

10. skeptical
    - (A) cryptic
    - (B) credulous
    - (C) discursive
    - (D) eminent
    - (E) caricatured.

11. recondite
    - (A) miniature
    - (B) ceramic
    - (C) arable
    - (D) caraway
    - (E) obvious.

12. redundant
    - (A) dilatory
    - (B) apocryphal
    - (C) astute
    - (D) insufficient
    - (E) calumnious.

13. indubitable
    - (A) fetid
    - (B) aesthetic
    - (C) unmitigated
    - (D) questionable
    - (E) belabored.

14. restitution
    - (A) inflation
    - (B) cataclysm
    - (C) deprivation
    - (D) misogyny
    - (E) changeling.

15. rotundity
    - (A) clemency
    - (B) ebullience
    - (C) angularity
    - (D) contumely
    - (E) chicory.

16. sagacious
    - (A) derelict
    - (B) hazardous
    - (C) articulate
    - (D) verbose
    - (E) ignorant.

17. sanguinary
    - (A) pacific
    - (B) sanctified
    - (C) gastronomical
    - (D) turgid
    - (E) embittered.

18. parsimony
    - (A) miasma
    - (B) antimony
    - (C) clinch
    - (D) fustian
    - (E) prodigality.

19. perspicuity
    (A) cupidity
    (B) salubriousness
    (C) ambiguity
    (D) discrimination
    (E) chrysolite.

20. preposterous
    (A) complaisant
    (B) conceited
    (C) apologetic
    (D) rational
    (E) castellated.

21. placid
    (A) redundant
    (B) poignant
    (C) turbid
    (D) saturnine
    (E) sardonic.

22. blasphemy
    (A) gynecologist
    (B) benediction
    (C) podium
    (D) panacea
    (E) miscegenation.

23. contumacious
    (A) punctilious
    (B) plenteous
    (C) meditative
    (D) obedient
    (E) plebeian.

24. antecedent
    (A) apothegm
    (B) quandary
    (C) auxiliary
    (D) posterior
    (E) orthodontist.

25. tranquility
    (A) complacency
    (B) tumult
    (C) plagiary
    (D) prophecy
    (E) philately.

26. apposite
    (A) incongruous
    (B) diaphanous
    (C) vitriolic
    (D) truculent
    (E) unique.

## TEST IV. VERBAL ANALOGIES

### TIME: 15 Minutes

*DIRECTIONS: In these test questions each of the two CAPI-TALIZED words have a certain relationship to each other. Following the capitalized words are other pairs of words, each designated by a letter. Select the lettered pair wherein the words are related in the same way as the two CAPITALIZED words are related to each other.*

## EXPLANATIONS OF KEY POINTS BEHIND THESE QUESTIONS ARE GIVEN WITH THE ANSWERS

1. CROWN : ROYAL ::

   (A) helmet : military
   (B) cola : sweet
   (C) crucifix : religious
   (D) wrap : ermine
   (E) throne : regal

2. LARGE : BIG ::

   (A) small : tiny
   (B) small : petite
   (C) small : little
   (D) small : diminutive
   (E) small : puny

3. TOCSIN : BITE ::

   (A) taxi : tooth
   (B) tepee : Indian
   (C) bell : animal
   (D) poison : bay
   (E) immorality : mastication

4. REPUGNANCE : ABHORRENCE ::

   (A) cooperation : concurrence
   (B) cowardice : fear
   (C) hate : love
   (D) indifference : admiration
   (E) apathy : laziness

5. RETINUE : MONARCH ::

   (A) cortege : escort
   (B) princess : queen
   (C) return : throne
   (D) second : first
   (E) moon : earth

6. WOOD : MILK ::

   (A) tree : pasture
   (B) nature : industry
   (C) cord : quart
   (D) leaf : cow
   (E) wagon : pail

7. MINARET : MOSQUE ::

   (A) Christian : Moslem
   (B) steeple : church
   (C) dainty : grotesque
   (D) modern : classic
   (E) Romanesque : Gothic

8. WHEAT : CHAFF

   (A) wine : dregs
   (B) bread : roll
   (C) laughter : raillery
   (D) oat : oatmeal
   (E) crop : corn

9. DRAMA : DIRECTOR ::

   (A) class : principal
   (B) movie : scenario
   (C) actor : playwright
   (D) tragedy : Sophocles
   (E) magazine : editor

10. COMMONPLACE : CLICHÉ ::

   (A) serious : play
   (B) annoying : pun
   (C) appreciated : gift
   (D) terse : maxim
   (E) poisonous : snake

11. AFFLUENT : LUCK ::

   (A) charitable : stinginess
   (B) greedy : cruelty
   (C) free-flowing : barrier
   (D) impoverished : laziness
   (E) fluent : hesitance

12. PICCOLO : TUBA ::

   (A) orchestra : band
   (B) concert : opera
   (C) trumpet : trombone
   (D) sweet : sour
   (E) violin : bass

13. BREAD : CAKE::

   (A) shirt : tie
   (B) poverty : riches
   (C) baker : chef
   (D) wheat : flour
   (E) pot : pan

14. MORALITY : LEGALITY ::

   (A) home : court
   (B) man : law
   (C) mayoralty : gubernatorial
   (D) priest : attorney
   (E) sin : crime

15. ELLIPSE : CURVE ::

   (A) ellipsis : speech
   (B) square : circle
   (C) rotation : revolution
   (D) curve : pitch
   (E) earth : sun

16. SUGAR : SACCHARIN ::

   (A) candy : cake
   (B) hog : lard
   (C) cane : stalk
   (D) spice : pepper
   (E) butter : margarine

17. REQUEST : DEMAND ::

   (A) reply : respond
   (B) regard : reject
   (C) inquire : require
   (D) wish : crave
   (E) seek : hide

18. WATER : FAUCET ::

   (A) fuel : throttle
   (B) $H_2O$ : O
   (C) kitchen : sink
   (D) steam : solid
   (E) leak : plumber

19. FLASK : BOTTLE ::

   (A) whiskey : milk
   (B) metal : glass
   (C) powder : liquid
   (D) quart : pint
   (E) brochure : tome

20. MONEY : GREED ::

   (A) finance : creed
   (B) property : desire
   (C) dollar sign : capitalism
   (D) food : voracity
   (E) work : slavery

# TEST V. SENTENCE COMPLETIONS

## TIME: 15 Minutes

*DIRECTIONS: Each of the completion questions in this test consists of an incomplete sentence. Each sentence is followed by a series of lettered words, one of which best completes the sentence. Select the word that best completes the meaning of each sentence, and mark the letter of that word opposite that sentence.*

1. Even when his reputation was in _____, almost everyone was willing to admit that he had genius.

    (A) dialogue
    (B) retaliation
    (C) eclipse
    (D) differentiation
    (E) rebuttal

2. How many of the books published each year in the United States make a(n) _____ contribution toward improving men's _____ with each other?

    (A) conservational . . . reservations
    (B) standardized . . . customs
    (C) referential . . . rudeness
    (D) squalid . . . generalities
    (E) significant . . . relationships

3. No one can say for sure how _____ the awards have been.

    (A) determined
    (B) effective
    (C) reducible
    (D) effervescent
    (E) inborn

4. For fifty years, only such women and the few intellectuals who shared his _____ scorn read Stendhal.

    (A) reverberating
    (B) explicit
    (C) sensational
    (D) sensuous
    (E) retreating

5. The _____ of the chronic balance of payments deficits which have _____ the U.S. Treasury Department under three Presidents is very real.

    (A) temptation . . . reviled
    (B) understanding . . . menaced
    (C) impact . . . underestimated
    (D) dilemma . . . plagued
    (E) strengthening . . . deceived

6. The fact that a business has _____ does not create an _____ on it to give away its prosperity.

    (A) prospered . . . imperative
    (B) halted . . . insensitivity
    (C) incorporated . . . indecision
    (D) supplemented . . . obligation
    (E) accumulated . . . aspect

7. When I watch drivers slam their cars to a halt, take corners _____ on two wheels, and blunder wildly over construction potholes and railroad crossings, I consider it a _____ to automotive design that cars don't shake apart far sooner.

    (A) gradually . . . curiosity
    (B) sensibly . . . blessing
    (C) gracefully . . . misfortune
    (D) habitually . . . tribute
    (E) religiously . . . verdict

8. On the ground, liquid hydrogen must be stored in large stainless steel tanks with double walls filled with _____ and evacuated to a high vacuum.

    (A) velocity          (B) visibility
    (C) sufficiency       (D) elasticity
           (E) insulation

9. The second act, which jumps forward to the late 1930's, a much less interesting period to _____, is nevertheless the more effective of the two.
   (A) caricature
   (B) instigate
   (C) stem
   (D) concentrate
   (E) validate

10. It is true that some of the most interesting novels of our age are in many ways closer to poetry than they are to old-fashioned _____, and the examination of _____ and imagery is by now a standard academic approach to fiction.
    (A) expression . . . styles
    (B) realism . . . symbolism
    (C) romances . . . character
    (D) manners . . . truth
    (E) prose . . . images

11. Britain, for the present, is deeply _____ in economic troubles, and the economic future, heavily _____, looks uncertain.
    (A) engrossed . . . responsive
    (B) ingrained . . . skeptical
    (C) saturated . . . enveloped
    (D) mired . . . mortgaged
    (E) perplexed . . . obligated

12. Ontology is the word now used in place of metaphysics, on the grounds that it is less _____ and supernatural.
    (A) theological
    (B) applicable
    (C) reliable
    (D) philosophical
    (E) approximate

13. The "loop" is a cheap, highly effective _____ device perfected in America and widely distributed throughout India.
    (A) validating
    (B) restraining
    (C) participating
    (D) contraceptive
    (E) reactionary

14. Our Constitution was based on the belief that the free _____ of ideas, peoples, and cultures is essential to the _____ of a democratic society.
    (A) selection . . . concurrence
    (B) interchange . . . preservation
    (C) reversal . . . upholding
    (D) dissemination . . . congruence
    (E) blasphemy . . . status

15. Sometimes the single building is not particularly historic, but in _____ with other buildings it takes on meaning.
    (A) distinction
    (B) correlation
    (C) design
    (D) detail
    (E) conjunction

16. As this country has become more _____, industrialized, and internationalized, it has —like all Western democracies—experienced a necessary increase in the _____ of the executive.
    (A) civilized . . . convenience
    (B) urbanized . . . role
    (C) objective . . . wealth
    (D) synthesized . . . efficiency
    (E) callous . . . selfishness

17. The sea air was _____ through the nine-foot windows, and one could stand in the breeze and look across the tennis courts to the herring boats, with their drooping nets _____ offshore.
    (A) swishing . . . floating
    (B) rampaging . . . waving
    (C) skipping . . . wilting
    (D) billowing . . . bobbing
    (E) drifting . . . flopping

18. The interior of the concert hall is a _____ feast, with a modern stateliness of line and color reigning throughout.
    (A) veritable
    (B) remarkable
    (C) visual
    (D) glowing
    (E) delicious

19. Education is enjoying a new and unaccustomed _____ to which it has not yet _____ and it is being widely hailed as the nation's "major growth industry."
    (A) resurgence . . . settled
    (B) improvement . . . accepted
    (C) impetus . . . related
    (D) refinement . . . responded
    (E) affluence . . . adjusted

20. Spectacle films seldom cause much interest among cinematic purists, mainly because their stories are so often on the _____ side, their sound-tracks more thunderous than _____, and their aim to fill the screen with physical action.
    (A) blasphemous . . . silent
    (B) dubious . . . simple
    (C) primitive . . . literate
    (D) sympathetic . . . violent
    (E) earthy . . . professional

# TEST VI. QUANTITATIVE ABILITY

## TIME: 60 Minutes

*DIRECTIONS: For each of the following questions, select the choice which best answers the question or completes the statement.*

### EXPLANATIONS ARE GIVEN WITH THE ANSWERS

1. Which of the following fractions is more than ¾?

   (A) $^{35}/_{71}$  (B) $^{13}/_{20}$
   (C) $^{71}/_{101}$  (D) $^{19}/_{24}$
   (E) $^{15}/_{20}$

**DO YOUR FIGURING HERE**

2. If $820 + R + S - 610 = 342$, and if $R = 2S$, Then
   $S =$

   (A) 44
   (B) 48
   (C) 132
   (D) 184
   (E) 192

3. What is the cost, in dollars, to carpet a room x yards long and y yards wide, if the carpet costs two dollars per square foot?

   (A) xy
   (B) 2xy
   (C) 3xy
   (D) 6xy
   (E) 18xy

4. If $7M = 3M - 20$, then $M + 7 =$

   (A) 0
   (B) 2
   (C) 5
   (D) 12
   (E) 17

5. In circle O below, AB is a diameter, angle BOD contains 15° and angle EOA contains 85°. Find the number of degrees in angle ECA.

   (A) 15
   (B) 35
   (C) 50
   (D) 70
   (E) 85

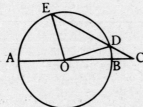

6. The diagonal of a rectangle is 10. The area of the rectangle
   (A) must be 24
   (B) must be 48
   (C) must be 50
   (D) must be 100
   (E) cannot be determined from the data given

7. In triangle PQR in the figure below, angle P is greater than angle Q and the bisectors of angle P and angle Q meet in S. Then

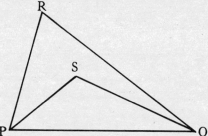

   (A) SQ > SP
   (B) SQ = SP
   (C) SQ < SP
   (D) SQ ≥ SP
   (E) no conclusion concerning the relative lengths of SQ and SP can be drawn from the data given

8. The coordinates of vertices X and Y of an equilateral triangle XYZ are (−4, 0) and (4, 0), respectively. The coordinates of Z may be
   (A) $(0, 2\sqrt{3})$
   (B) $(0, 4\sqrt{3})$
   (C) $(4, 4\sqrt{3})$
   (D) (0, 4)
   (E) $(4\sqrt{3}, 0)$

9. Given: All men are mortal. Which statement expresses a conclusion that logically follows from the given statement?
   (A) All mortals are men.
   (B) If X is a mortal, then X is a man.
   (C) If X is not a mortal, then X is not a man.
   (D) If X is not a man, then X is not a mortal.
   (E) Some mortals are not men.

10. In the accompanying figure, ACB is a straight angle and DC is perpendicular to CE. If the number of degrees in angle ACD is represented by x, the number of degrees in angle BCE is represented by
    (A) 90 − x
    (B) x − 90
    (C) 90 + x
    (D) 180 − x
    (E) 45 + x

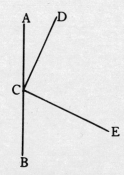

11. What is the smallest positive number which, when it is divided by 3, 4, or 5, will leave a remainder of 2?

    (A) 22
    (B) 42
    (C) 62
    (D) 122
    (E) 182

12. A taxi charges 20 cents for the first quarter of a mile and 5 cents for each additional quarter of a mile. The charge, in cents, for a trip of d miles is

    (A) $20 + 5d$
    (B) $20 + 5 (4d - 1)$
    (C) $20 + 20d$
    (D) $20 + 4 (d - 1)$
    (E) $20 + 20 (d - 1)$

13. In a certain army post, 30% of the men are from New York State, and 10% of these are from New York City. What percent of the men in the post are from New York City?

    (A) 3
    (B) .3
    (C) .03
    (D) 13
    (E) 20

14. From 9 A.M. to 2 P.M., the temperature rose at a constant rate from $-14°F$ to $+36°F$. What was the temperature at noon?

    (A) $-4°$
    (B) $+6°$
    (C) $+16°$
    (D) $+26°$
    (E) $+31°$

15. There are just two ways in which 5 may be expressed as the sum of two different positive (non-zero) integers; namely, $5 = 4 + 1 = 3 + 2$. In how many ways may 9 be expressed as the sum of two different positive (non-zero) integers?

    (A) 3
    (B) 4
    (C) 5
    (D) 6
    (E) 7

16. A board 7 feet 9 inches long is divided into three equal parts. What is the length of each part?

    (A) 2 ft. 7 in.
    (B) 2 ft. 6⅓ in.
    (C) 2 ft. 8⅓ in.
    (D) 2 ft. 8 in.
    (E) 2 ft. 9 in.

**DO YOUR FIGURING HERE**

17. In the figure below, the largest possible circle is cut out of a square piece of tin. The area of the remaining piece of tin is approximately (in square inches)

    (A) .75
    (B) 3.14
    (C) .14
    (D) .86
    (E) 1.0

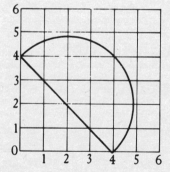

**DO YOUR FIGURING HERE**

18. Which of the following is equal to 3.14 x 10⁶?

    (A) 314
    (B) 3,140
    (C) 31,400
    (D) 314.000
    (E) 3,140,000

19.

$$\frac{36}{29 - \frac{4}{0.2}} =$$

    (A) ⅓
    (B) 2
    (C) 4
    (D) ¾
    (E) 18

20. In terms of the square units in the figure below, what is the area of the semicircle?

    (A) 32π
    (B) 16π
    (C) 8π
    (D) 4π
    (E) 2π

21. The sum of three consecutive odd numbers is always divisible by I. 2 II. 3 III. 5 IV. 6

    (A) only I
    (B) only IV
    (C) only I and II
    (D) only I and III
    (E) only II and IV

22. In the diagram, triangle ABC is inscribed in a circle and CD is tangent to the circle. If angle BCD is 40° how many degrees are there in angle A?

    (A) 20
    (B) 30
    (C) 40
    (D) 50
    (E) 60

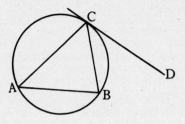

23. If a discount of 20% off the marked price of a suit saves a man $15, how much did he pay for the suit?

    (A) $35
    (B) $60
    (C) $75
    (D) $150
    (E) $300

24. The ice compartment in a refrigerator is 8 inches deep, 5 inches high, and 4 inches wide. How many ice cubes will it hold, if each cube is 2 inches on a side?

    (A) 16
    (B) 20
    (C) 40
    (D) 80
    (E) 160

25. Find the last number in the series:
    8 , 4 , 12 , 6 , 18 , 9 , ?

    (A) 19
    (B) 20
    (C) 22
    (D) 24
    (E) 27

26. A 15–gallon mixture of 20% alcohol has 5 gallons of water added to it. The strength of the mixture, as a percent, is near

    (A) 15
    (B) 13⅓
    (C) 16⅔
    (D) 12½
    (E) 20

27. In the figure below, QXRS is a parallelogram and P is any point on side QS. What is the ratio of the area of triangle PXR to the area of QXRS?

    (A) 1 : 4
    (B) 1 : 3
    (C) 2 : 3
    (D) 3 : 4
    (E) 1 : 2

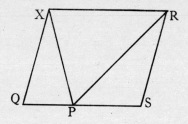

28. If x (p + 1) = M, then p =

    (A) M — 1
    (B) M
    (C) $\dfrac{M-1}{x}$
    (D) M — x — 1
    (E) $\dfrac{M}{x} - 1$

29. If T tons of snow fall in 1 second, how many tons fall in M minutes?

    (A) 60 MT
    (B) MT + 60
    (C) MT
    (D) $\dfrac{60\,M}{T}$
    (E) $\dfrac{MT}{60}$

30. If $\dfrac{P}{Q} = \dfrac{4}{5}$, what is the value of 2 P + Q ?

    (A) 14
    (B) 13
    (C) — 1
    (D) 3
    (E) cannot be determined from the information given

31. The figure shows one square inside another and a rectangle of diagonal T. The best approximation to the value of T, in inches, is given by which of the following inequalities?

    (A) 6 < T < 9
    (B) 11 < T < 12
    (C) 12 < T < 13
    (D) 9 < T < 11
    (E) 10 < T < 11

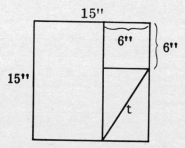

32. What is the smallest positive integer $K > 1$ Such that $R^2 = S^3 = K$, for some integers R and S?

    (A) 4
    (B) 8
    (C) 27
    (D) 64
    (E) 81

DO YOUR FIGURING HERE

33. The number of square units in the area of triangle RST is

    (A) 10
    (B) 12.5
    (C) 15.5
    (D) 17.5
    (E) 20

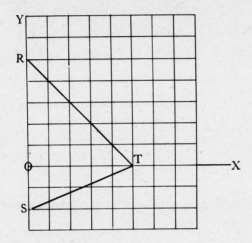

34. In the figure, PQR is an equilateral triangle of side 10 inches. At each vertex, a small equilateral $\triangle$ of side X is cut off to form a regular hexagon. What is the length of X, in inches?

    (A) 3
    (B) 3⅓
    (C) 3½
    (D) 4
    (E) 4½

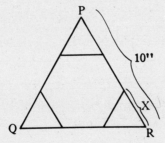

35. Which of the following has the same value as $\dfrac{P}{Q}$ ?

    (A) $\dfrac{P-2}{Q-2}$
    (B) $\dfrac{1+P}{1+Q}$
    (C) $\dfrac{P^2}{Q^2}$
    (D) $\dfrac{3P}{3Q}$
    (E) $\dfrac{P+3}{Q+3}$

# TEST VII. PERCEPTUAL MOTOR ABILITY

## TIME: 20 Minutes

DIRECTIONS: *Each question in this test consists of a numbered picture showing a piece of cardboard that is to be folded. The dotted lines show where folds are to be made. The problem is to choose the lettered picture, A, B, C, or D which would be made by folding the cardboard in the numbered picture. For each question blacken the space on your answer sheet corresponding to the letter of the best answer.*

*Correct key answers to all these test questions will be found at the end of the test.*

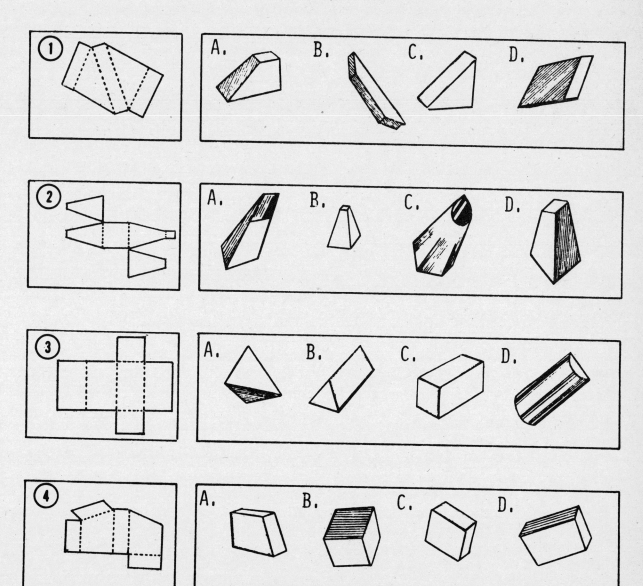

S2044

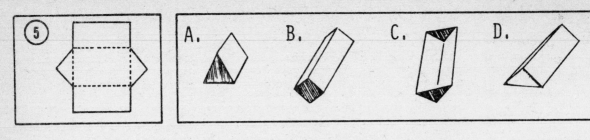

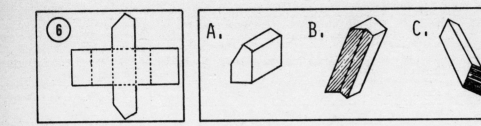

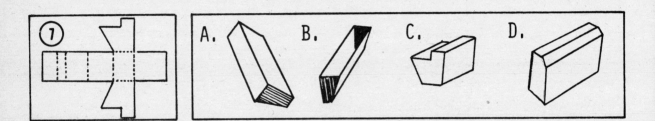

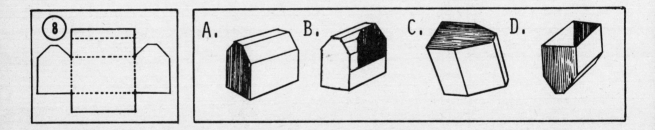

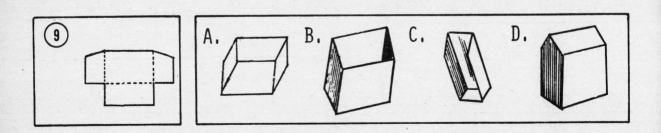

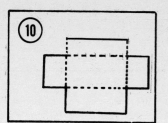
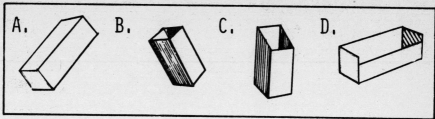

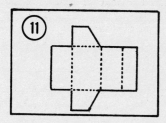
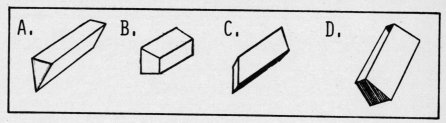

# CORRECT ANSWERS FOR PREDICTIVE EXAMINATION III.

*(Please make every effort to answer the questions on your own before look-ing at these answers. You'll make faster progress by following this rule.)*

## TEST I. BIOMEDICAL SCIENCE

| | | | | | | | |
|---|---|---|---|---|---|---|---|
| 1. 2 | 7. 2 | 13. 4 | 19. 3 | 25. 1 | 31. 3 | 36. 4 | 41. 3 |
| 2. 2 | 8. 3 | 14. 4 | 20. 1 | 26. 2 | 32. 1 | 37. 3 | 42. 3 |
| 3. 4 | 9. 1 | 15. 1 | 21. 4 | 27. 4 | 33. 1 | 38. 1 | 43. 4 |
| 4. 1 | 10. 2 | 16. 2 | 22. 4 | 28. 2 | 34. 1 | 39. 1 | 44. 3 |
| 5. 1 | 11. 3 | 17. 4 | 23. 3 | 29. 2 | 35. 4 | 40. 1 | 45. 3 |
| 6. 3 | 12. 4 | 18. 4 | 24. 1 | 30. 1 | | | |

## TEST II. INTERPRETATION OF SCIENCE READINGS

| | | | | | | | |
|---|---|---|---|---|---|---|---|
| 1. C | 5. D | 9. D | 13. A | 16. A | 19. D | 22. A | 25. C |
| 2. C | 6. D | 10. A | 14. B | 17. C | 20. D | 23. A | 26. B |
| 3. A | 7. B | 11. C | 15. B | 18. D | 21. B | 24. D | 27. A |
| 4. B | 8. D | 12. B | | | | | |

## TEST III. VOCABULARY

| | | | | | | | |
|---|---|---|---|---|---|---|---|
| 1. C | 5. E | 9. D | 12. D | 15. C | 18. E | 21. C | 24. D |
| 2. E | 6. C | 10. B | 13. D | 16. E | 19. C | 22. B | 25. B |
| 3. B | 7. C | 11. E | 14. C | 17. A | 20. D | 23. D | 26. A |
| 4. D | 8. E | | | | | | |

## TEST IV. VERBAL ANALOGIES

| | | | | | | | |
|---|---|---|---|---|---|---|---|
| 1. C | 4. E | 7. B | 10. D | 13. A | 15. D | 17. D | 19. E |
| 2. C | 5. E | 8. A | 11. D | 14. E | 16. E | 18. A | 20. D |
| 3. D | 6. C | 9. E | 12. E | | | | |

## TEST IV. EXPLANATORY ANSWERS

1. **(C)** A crown (when worn) indicates a royal state; a crucifix (when worn) indicates a religious attachment. Note that a throne also has a regal association, but the throne is not worn.

2. **(C)** A general synonym for large is big; a general synonym for small is little. The words tiny, petite, diminutive, and puny have special connotations.

3. **(D)** The homophone of tocsin is toxin; the homophone of bite is bight. Toxin means poison—bight means bay.

4. **(E)** Abhorrence is an extreme form of repugnance; laziness is an extreme form of apathy.

5. **(E)** A retinue attends a person of rank such as a monarch; the moon is a satellite (smaller body attending upon a larger one) attending upon and revolving round the earth.

6. **(C)** A cord is a wood unit of measurement; a quart is a milk unit of measurement.

7. **(B)** A minaret is a high tower attached to a mosque; a steeple is a high structure rising above a church.

8. **(A)** Chaff is that worthless part of the grain left over after threshing; dregs constitute the worthless residue in the process of making wine.

9. **(E)** A director is responsible for the production of the drama; an editor is responsible for the publication of the magazine.

10. **(D)** A cliché is commonplace; a maxim is terse.

11. **(D)** A person frequently becomes affluent because of luck; a person frequently becomes impoverished because of laziness.

12. **(E)** A piccolo is a wind instrument pitched an octave higher than an ordinary flute, whereas a tuba is a much larger and lower-pitched wind instrument; a violin, in comparison with a bass, is smaller and higher-pitched.

13. **(A)** Bread is a necessity, cake is not; a shirt is a necessity, a tie is not.

14. **(E)** A sin is immoral; a crime is illegal.

15. **(D)** An ellipse is a type of curve (plane curve); a curve is a type of baseball pitch.

16. **(E)** Saccharin is a chemical compound used as a substitute for sugar; margarine, made from vegetable oils and milk, is a substitute for butter.

17. **(D)** To demand is to request in a strong manner; to crave is to wish in a strong manner.

18. **(A)** A faucet controls the flow of water; a throttle controls the flow of fuel.

19. **(E)** A flask is a smaller version of a bottle; a brochure is a smaller version of a tome.

20. **(D)** Some people have an insatiable desire (greed) for money; some have an insatiable desire (voracity) for food.

## TEST V. SENTENCE COMPLETIONS

| | | | | | | | |
|---|---|---|---|---|---|---|---|
| 1. C | 4. D | 7. D | 10. B | 13. D | 15. E | 17. D | 19. E |
| 2. E | 5. D | 8. E | 11. D | 14. B | 16. B | 18. C | 20. C |
| 3. B | 6. A | 9. A | 12. A | | | | |

## TEST VI. QUANTITATIVE ABILITY

| | | | | | | | |
|---|---|---|---|---|---|---|---|
| 1. D | 6. E | 11. C | 16. A | 20. D | 24. A | 28. E | 32. D |
| 2. A | 7. A | 12. B | 17. D | 21. B | 25. E | 29. A | 33. D |
| 3. E | 8. B | 13. A | 18. E | 22. C | 26. A | 30. E | 34. B |
| 4. B | 9. C | 14. C | 19. C | 23. B | 27. E | 31. E | 35. D |
| 5. B | 10. A | 15. B | | | | | |

## TEST VII. PERCEPTUAL MOTOR ABILITY

| | | | | | | | |
|---|---|---|---|---|---|---|---|
| 1. C | 3. C | 5. D | 7. C | 8. B | 9. A | 10. D | 11. B |
| 2. B | 4. A | 6. A | | | | | |

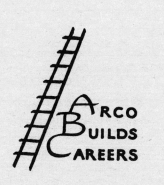

2

# PART TWO

## *Pinpoint Practice To Raise Your Mark*

### *Biomedical Science*
### *Reading Interpretation in Science*

# DIRECTIONS FOR ANSWERING QUESTIONS

*DIRECTIONS: For each question read all the choices carefully. Then select that answer which you consider correct or most nearly correct. Write the letter preceding your best choice next to the question. Should you want to answer on the kind of answer sheet used on machine-scored examinations, we have provided several such facsimiles. On some machine-scored exams you are instructed to "place no marks whatever on the test booklet." In other examinations you may be instructed to mark your answers in the test booklet. In such cases you should be careful that no other marks interfere with the legibility of your answers. It is always best NOT to mark your booklet unless you are sure that it is permitted. It is most important that you learn to mark your answers clearly and in the right place.*

*FOR THE SAMPLE QUESTION that follows, select the appropriate letter preceding the word which is most nearly the same in meaning as the capitalized word:*

1. DISSENT:     (A) approve     (B) depart
                (C) disagree    (D) enjoy

*DISSENT is most nearly the same as (C), disagree, so that the acceptable answer is shown thus on your answer sheet:*

```
  A   B   C   D
  ::  ::  I   ::
```

# Practice Using Answer Sheets

**Alter numbers to match the practice and drill questions in each part of the book.
Make only ONE mark for each answer. Additional and stray marks may be counted as mistakes.
In making corrections, erase errors COMPLETELY. Make glossy black marks.....**

# SCIENCE AS A FIELD

*Most people, like yourself, who take exams are busy people. They cannot afford to waste time; that is why you bought this book, to help provide you with the best preparation possible. This chapter material will help do just that. It is a workable plan for broadening your background in a subject likely to occur on your exam.*

## SCIENCE TEST ONE

### TIME: 20 Minutes

*The following are representative examination type questions. They should be carefully studied and completely understood. The actual test questions will probably not be quite as difficult as these.*

*DIRECTIONS: For each of the following questions, select the choice which best answers the question or completes the statement.*

## A FAIR SAMPLING OF THE QUESTIONS YOU'LL BE ASKED

1. The normal height of a mercury barometer at sea level is
   (A) 15 inches
   (B) 30 inches
   (C) 32 feet
   (D) 34 feet.

2. Of the following phases of the moon, the invisible one is called
   (A) crescent
   (B) full moon
   (C) new moon
   (D) waxing and waning.

3. Of the following, the statement that best describes a "high" on a weather map is
   (A) the air extends farther up than normal
   (B) the air pressure is greater than normal
   (C) the air temperature is higher than normal
   (D) the air moves faster than normal.

4. The nerve endings for the sense of sight are located in the part of the eye called the
   (A) cornea
   (B) sclera
   (C) iris
   (D) retina.

5. Of the following, the one which causes malaria is
   (A) a bacterium
   (B) a mosquito
   (C) a protozoan
   (D) bad air.

6. A 1000-ton ship must displace a weight of water equal to
   (A) 500 tons
   (B) 1000 tons
   (C) 1500 tons
   (D) 2000 tons.

7. Of the following instruments, the one that can convert light into an electric current is the
   (A) radiometer
   (B) dry cell
   (C) electroylsis apparatus
   (D) photo-electric cell.

8. On the film in a camera, the lens forms an image which, by comparison with the original subject, is
   (A) right side up and reversed from left to right
   (B) upside down and reversed from left to right
   (C) right side up and not reversed from left to right
   (D) upside down and not reversed from left to right.

9. Of the following, the plant whose seeds are *not* spread by wind is the
   (A) cocklebur          (B) maple
   (C) dandelion          (D) milkweed.

10. Of the following, the insect which is harmful to man's food supply is the
   (A) dragonfly          (B) grasshopper
   (C) ladybug            (D) praying mantis.

11. Of the following, the one which is fall-blooming generally is the
   (A) azalea             (B) hickory
   (C) tulip              (D) witch hazel.

12. At the beginning of a community succession, the first of the following living things to get a foothold on bare rocks, other things being equal, are
   (A) mosses             (B) ferns
   (C) algae              (D) lichens.

13. Ciliated male gametes may be found in the cells of

   (A) bread mold         (B) gingko
   (C) protococcus        (D) slime mold.

14. The shape of which of the following does the vibrio shape of certain bacteria most closely resemble?
   (A) bacilli            (B) spirilla
   (C) cocci              (D) Rickettsia.

15. Nutrition in mushrooms is
   (A) symbiotic          (B) saprophytic
   (C) parasitic          (D) holophytic.

16. In a demonstration in class of a test for vitamin C, one might effectively use
   (A) acetic acid        (B) brom thymol blue
   (C) congo red          (D) indophenol.

17. Rod-shaped bacteria are classified as
   (A) bacilli            (B) cocci
   (C) vibrios            (D) spirilla.

18. A stain used in classifying pathogenic bacteria is
   (A) Gram's             (B) Wright's
   (C) Loeffler's         (D) Giemsa.

19. Bacteriophage is a type of
   (A) enzyme             (B) toxin
   (C) bacterium          (D) virus.

20. Coral is formed by
   (A) marine algae
   (B) a mollusc found in the Caribbean
   (C) an animal related to the sea anemone
   (D) a seed plant.

## CONSOLIDATE YOUR KEY ANSWERS HERE

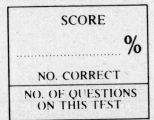

### Answers: Test 1.

| | | | |
|---|---|---|---|
| 1. B | 6. B | 11. D | 16. D |
| 2. C | 7. D | 12. D | 17. A |
| 3. B | 8. B | 13. B | 18. A |
| 4. D | 9. A | 14. B | 19. D |
| 5. C | 10. B | 15. B | 20. C |

| SCORE |
|---|
| % |
| ............................ |
| NO. CORRECT |
| NO. OF QUESTIONS ON THIS TEST |

# SCIENCE TEST TWO

TIME: 10 Minutes

*DIRECTIONS: For each of the following questions, select the choice which best answers the question or completes the statement.*

## A FAIR SAMPLING OF THE QUESTIONS YOU'LL BE ASKED

1. One-celled animals belong to the group of living things known as
   - (A) protozoa
   - (B) porifera
   - (C) annelida
   - (D) arthropoda.

2. Spiders can be distinguished from insects by the fact that spiders have
   - (A hard outer coverings
   - (B) large abdomens
   - (C) four pairs of legs
   - (D) biting mouth parts.

3. An important ore of uranium is called
   - (A) hematite
   - (B) bauxite
   - (C) chalcopyrite
   - (D) pitchblende.

4. Of the following, the lightest element known on earth is
   - (A) hydrogen
   - (B) helium
   - (C) oxygen
   - (D) air.

5. Of the following gases in the air, the most plentiful is
   - (A) argon
   - (B) nitrogen
   - (C) oxygen
   - (D) carbon dioxide.

6. The time it takes for light from the sun to reach the earth is approximately
   - (A) four years
   - (B) four months
   - (C) eight minutes
   - (D) sixteen years.

7. Of the following types of clouds, the ones which occur at the greatest height are called
   - (A) cirrus
   - (B) cumulus
   - (C) nimbus
   - (D) stratus.

8. The time that it takes for the earth to rotate 45° is
   - (A) one hour
   - (B) three hours
   - (C) four hours
   - (D) ten hours.

9. Of the following glands, the one which regulates the metabolic rate is the
   - (A) adrenal
   - (B) salivary
   - (C) thyroid
   - (D) thymus.

10. All of the following are Amphibia *except* the
    - (A) salamander
    - (B) lizard
    - (C) frog
    - (D) toad.

## CONSOLIDATE YOUR KEY ANSWERS HERE

**Answer Sheet**

|   | A | B | C | D | E |
|---|---|---|---|---|---|
| 1 | ‖ | ‖ | ‖ | ‖ | ‖ |
| 2 | ‖ | ‖ | ‖ | ‖ | ‖ |
| 3 | ‖ | ‖ | ‖ | ‖ | ‖ |
| 4 | ‖ | ‖ | ‖ | ‖ | ‖ |
| 5 | ‖ | ‖ | ‖ | ‖ | ‖ |

**Answer Sheet**

|   | A | B | C | D | E |
|---|---|---|---|---|---|
| 6 | ‖ | ‖ | ‖ | ‖ | ‖ |
| 7 | ‖ | ‖ | ‖ | ‖ | ‖ |
| 8 | ‖ | ‖ | ‖ | ‖ | ‖ |
| 9 | ‖ | ‖ | ‖ | ‖ | ‖ |
| 10 | ‖ | ‖ | ‖ | ‖ | ‖ |

## Answers: Test 2.

*(You'll learn more by writing your own answers before comparing them with these.)*

| 1. A | 4. A | 6. C | 8. B |
|------|------|------|------|
| 2. C | 5. B | 7. A | 9. C |
| 3. D |      |      | 10. B |

| SCORE | .............................. % |
|---|---|
| NO. CORRECT ÷ | |
| NO. OF QUESTIONS ON THIS TEST | |

S1627

# ACHIEVEMENT TEST IN BIOLOGY

*For each question read all the choices carefully. Then select
that answer which you consider correct or most nearly correct.
Write the letter preceding your best choice next to the question.*

1. The idea of spontaneous reproduction was attacked by the experiments of
   (A) Aristotle      (B) Galen
   (C) Redi          (D) Schleiden.

2. The scientist who first synthesized DNA was
   (A) Kornberg      (B) Ochoa
   (C) Sanger        (D) du Vigneaud.

3. The ideas of Lysenko in the field of genetics are most similar to those of which one of the following?
   (A) Darwin        (B) Lamarck
   (C) Morgan        (D) Weismann.

4. Tissue culture has been extensively used as a research method in all of the following fields of biological investigation *except*
   (A) photosynthesis
   (B) virology
   (C) development of nerve cells
   (D) experimental embryology.

5. Of the following, the highest bactericidal activity of light occurs at a wave length in Angstrom units of
   (A) 2536          (B) 3256
   (C) 5236          (D) 6532.

6. After each transfer of a culture of bacteria, the wire loop should be
   (A) dipped into alcohol
   (B) held in a flame
   (C) dipped into liquid soap
   (D) washed repeatedly in water.

7. For the extraction in the classroom of chlorophyll from green leaves, the alcohol is most safely heated by
   (A) a Bunsen burner
   (B) an electric hot plate
   (C) a wing-top burner
   (D) a gas hot plate.

8. To demonstrate the action of ptyalin on starch, which one of the following should be used?
   (A) Robert's solution
   (B) Benedict's solution
   (C) Lugol's solution
   (D) Wright's stain.

9. In making artificial gastric juice, hydrochloric acid is added to a solution of
   (A) rennin         (B) pancreatin
   (C) ox-gall        (D) pepsin.

10. When inserting a thistle tube through a rubber stopper, one should grasp
    (A) the bowl firmly
    (B) the tubing near the bowl
    (C) the tubing near its middle
    (D) the tubing near the stopper.

11. In the bell-jar model used to demonstrate breathing, the Y tube represents the
    (A) diaphragm and trachea
    (B) trachea and bronchi
    (C) diaphragm and bronchi
    (D) bronchi and lungs.

12. Transduction is a term applied to a method of
    (A) liquid transfer in vascular plants
    (B) electrolyte diffusion through a cell membrane
    (C) oxygen absorption of a red corpuscle
    (D) genetic transmission in bacteria.

13. In which one of the following ways does combustion differ from cellular respiration?
    (A) it produces more heat
    (B) it wastes more energy
    (C) it is less rapid
    (D) it occurs at a higher temperature.

14. Of the following processes, the one carried on exclusively by bacteria is
    (A) maturing of cheese
    (B) synthesis of antibiotics
    (C) formation of humus
    (D) synthesis of Vitamin K in the intestine.

15. The basic mechanism of hereditary transmission is
    (A) sexual reproduction
    (B) polyploidy
    (C) splitting of chromosomes
    (D) the mitotic mechanism.

16. Of the following, an enzyme responsible for the digestion of proteins is
    (A) maltase
    (B) trypsin
    (C) ptyalin
    (D) steapsin.

17. Failure of blood to clot readily when exposed to air may be due to
    (A) an oversupply of erythrocytes
    (B) a deficiency of leucocytes
    (C) an overabundance of fibrin
    (D) an inadequacy of thrombokinase

18. The tissue to which gland cells belong is
    (A) connective
    (B) epithelial
    (C) secretory
    (D) nerve.

19. Cone cells are most closely associated with the function of
    (A) digestion
    (B) absorption
    (C) vision
    (D) secretion.

20. Semicircular canals are thought to be most sensitive to which one of the following?
    (A) light
    (B) odor
    (C) gravity
    (D) sound.

21. Most of the carbon dioxide in the blood is carried in the
    (A) liquid portion
    (B) leucocytes
    (C) erythrocytes
    (D) platelets.

22. A synaptic phenomenon involved in learning is
    (A) accumulation
    (B) summation
    (C) facilitation
    (D) association.

23. Increased blood pressure may be brought about by excess secretion of
    (A) thyroxin
    (B) insulin
    (C) ACTH
    (D) adrenalin.

24. Acromegaly is directly caused by malfunction of the
    (A) thyroid
    (B) pituitary
    (C) parathyroid
    (D) adrenal.

25. Of the following, the plant hormone concerned with growth is
    (A) auxin
    (B) estrogen
    (C) testosterone
    (D) ATP.

26. Bread mold resembles ferns in that both develop
    (A) mycelia
    (B) hyphae
    (C) pinnules
    (D) spores.

27. An American tree which disease has rendered almost extinct in the United States is the
    (A) tulip tree
    (B) chestnut
    (C) elm
    (D) horse chestnut.

28. Of the following, the plant which does *not* belong to the family Compositae is
    (A) dandelion
    (B) snapdragon
    (C) daisy
    (D) goldenrod.

29. Sap rises in woody stems because of root pressure and
    (A) transpiration pull
    (B) enzyme action
    (C) molecular adhesion
    (D) photosynthesis.

30. Vascular plants contain vessels called xylem and
    (A) cambium
    (B) phloem
    (C) meristem
    (D) lenticels.

31. The specific function of light energy in the process of photosynthesis is to
    (A) activate chlorophyll
    (B) split water
    (C) reduce carbon dioxide
    (D) synthesize glucose.

32. Stored food for the embryo of a bean seed is found in the
    (A) plumule
    (B) hypocotyl
    (C) cotyledons
    (D) testa.

33. Of the following, an example of carnivorous plants is the
    (A) sundew
    (B) mandrake
    (C) cowslip
    (D) jewelweed.

34. In the structure of a flower, the stigma is most closely associated with the
    (A) style
    (B) ovary
    (C) sepal
    (D) ovule.

35. Of the following animal phyla, the one which is probably more varied and abundant now than in previous geological periods is the
    (A) Protozoa
    (B) Bryozoa
    (C) Brachiopoda
    (D) Echinodermata.

36. Of the following, one difference between frog and man is that the frog has no
    (A) salivary glands
    (B) thyroid gland
    (C) pancreas
    (D) adrenal gland.

37. Of the following organisms, the one that is *not* in the same taxonomic class as the others is the
    (A) salamander
    (B) mud puppy
    (C) newt
    (D) lizard.

38. The vocal organ of birds is the
    (A) trachea
    (B) larynx
    (C) syrinx
    (D) air sac.

39. Of the following, the marsupial native to the United States is the
    (A) raccoon
    (B) wombat
    (C) opossum
    (D) armadillo.

40. Of the following, a structure found in mammals but *not* in reptiles is the
    (A) lung
    (B) brain
    (C) diaphragm
    (D) ventricle.

41. The first fully terrestrial vertebrates were the
    (A) amphibia
    (B) reptiles
    (C) birds
    (D) mammals.

42. A cartilaginous vertebrate that parasitizes fishes is the
    (A) pilot fish
    (B) lamprey
    (C) barracuda
    (D) moray eel.

43. Of the following, the one to which the horse-shoe crab is most closely related is the
    (A) blue crab
    (B) lobster
    (C) garden spider
    (D) chambered nautilus.

44. The titanotheres were a group of fossil
    (A) fish
    (B) amphibians
    (C) reptiles
    (D) mammals.

45. Of the following, a crustacean that lives on land is the
    (A) centipede
    (B) millipede
    (C) sow bug
    (D) tick.

46. Of the following, the one that is not an animal is the
    (A) sea lily
    (B) sea cucumber
    (C) sand dollar
    (D) diatom.

47. Of the following, the hydra is most closely related to the
    (A) coral
    (B) flatworm
    (C) sponge
    (D) roundworm.

48. A probably unforeseen result of the widespread use of DDT is
    (A) the control of mosquitoes
    (B) the development of insects immune to DDT
    (C) the development of fishes immune to DDT
    (D) the destruction of harmful birds.

49. Oxygen enters protozoa chiefly through the
    (A) surface protoplasm
    (B) vacuoles
    (C) oral grooves
    (D) pseudopodia.

50. Air passes into and out of the insect body by way of
    (A) gills
    (B) lungs
    (C) skin
    (D) tracheae.

51. The best basis for choosing a bull to sire a productive dairy herd is
    (A) milk production by the bull's female ancestors
    (B) milk production by the bull's sisters
    (C) milk production by the bull's daughters
    (D) the physical characteristics of the bull itself.

52. The result of the loss of a retina in an eye is
    (A) near-sightedness
    (B) far-sightedness
    (C) astigmatism
    (D) lack of vision in the affected eye.

53. The largest percentage of the salt excreted from the body normally passes out through the
    (A) kidneys
    (B) skin
    (C) large intestine
    (D) lachrymal glands.

54. Of the following, a condition *not* usually considered to be associated with heavy cigarette smoking is
    (A) shorter life span
    (B) slowing of the heartbeat
    (C) cancer of the lung
    (D) heart disease.

55. Damage to the cerebellum would interfere mainly with which one of the following?
    (A) memory
    (B) voluntary acts
    (C) sensation
    (D) equilibrium.

56. The number of "senses" in man is
    (A) less than five
    (B) five
    (C) seven
    (D) more than seven.

57. The center which maintains the rhythm of breathing is located in the
    (A) cerebellum
    (B) medulla
    (C) cerebrum
    (D) spinal cord.

58. The major function of bile is
    (A) digestion
    (B) emulsification
    (C) absorption
    (D) lubrication.

59. The surgical removal of the stomach would interfere mainly with the functioning in the body of which one of the following?
    (A) enzyme secretion
    (B) fat digestion
    (C) food storage
    (D) protein absorption.

60. The liquid portion of whole blood is called
    (A) serum
    (B) lymph
    (C) plasma
    (D) water.

61. Failure of lymph to circulate would most directly affect which one of the following?
    (A) fat digestion
    (B) transport between the body cells and blood
    (C) production of red blood cells
    (D) circulation of blood platelets.

62. If in a given sample of blood, clumping occurred with both A serum and B serum, the blood type was
    (A) A          (B) B
    (C) AB         (D) O

63. Recent work indicates that the commonest normal human diploid chromosome number is
    (A) 45         (B) 46
    (C) 47         (D) 48

64. The glomeruli are most closely related to the system involved in
    (A) reproduction
    (B) support and movement
    (C) digestion
    (D) excretion.

65. Of the following, the area in whose functions the effects of alcohol are first observed is the
    (A) cerebrum      (B) cerebellum
    (C) medulla       (D) spinal cord.

66. Inhalation in man is caused by
    (A) lowering the ribs and raising the diaphragm
    (B) raising the ribs and raising the diaphragm
    (C) lowering the ribs and the diaphragm
    (D) raising the ribs and lowering the diaphragm.

67. In man, diffusion of carbon dioxide and oxygen occurs mainly in the
    (A) pharynx       (B) alveoli
    (C) bronchi       (D) glottis.

68. Of the following, a structure which normally serves as a common passageway for both food and air is the
    (A) glottis       (B) pharynx
    (C) trachea       (D) glottis.

69. The kidney is to renal corpuscles as the skin is to
    (A) oil glands    (B) sweat glands
    (C) pores         (D) epidermis.

70. Deamination of proteins occurs mainly in the
    (A) small intestine  (B) spleen
    (C) pancreas         (D) liver.

71. Of the following, the one which is a final waste product of protein metabolism is
    (A) pepsinogen    (B) amino acid
    (C) urea          (D) urine.

72. The lowest concentration of nitrogenous waste may be found in blood passing through the
    (A) pulmonary artery  (B) renal artery
    (C) hepatic vein      (D) renal vein.

73. The liquid which collects in the cavity of Bowman's capsule is
    (A) urine in concentrated form
    (B) blood plasma minus plasma proteins
    (C) freshly aerated blood
    (D) used bile ready for excretion.

74. Of the following, which one most closely indicates the approximate number of calories required by an average man who does office work?
    (A) 1500-1800     (B) 2000-2200
    (C) 2400-2700     (D) 3000-3300.

75. Of the following vitamins, the one which can most readily be manufactured in our bodies is
    (A) A             (B) B1
    (C) C             (D) D

76. The chief function of roughage is to
    (A) build muscle tissue
    (B) provide quick energy
    (C) provide certain vitamins
    (D) stimulate peristalsis.

77. The passage of food into the larynx is normally prevented by the
    (A) pharynx       (B) trachea
    (C) epiglottis    (D) hard palate.

78. If an organism has 2n chromosomes in each of its body cells, the mature sperm will contain the number of chromosomes represented by
    (A) 2n            (B) n
    (C) n/2           (D) 4n.

79. Genetical experiments with Neurospora have shown that
    (A) heterosis is based upon enzymes
    (B) pure line selection minimizes variations
    (C) inbreeding is generally harmful
    (D) genes control the production of many enzymes.

80. Severing the vagus nerve
    (A) augments the flow of gastric juice
    (B) completely stops the flow of gastric juice
    (C) reduces the flow of gastric juice
    (D) stops the production of gastrin.

81. From the ovary, the egg of the mammal next goes into the
    (A) follicle
    (B) abdominal cavity
    (C) oviduct
    (D) uterus.

82. All of the following may be caused by a virus *except*
    (A) poliomyelitis
    (B) influenza
    (C) malaria
    (D) smallpox.

83. The female drosophila can be distinguished from the male by noting that
    (A) the female possesses a fringe of black bristles in the uppermost joint of the first pair of legs
    (B) the tip of the abdomen in the female is elongated and more rounded
    (C) the first pair of legs in the male is longer than in the female
    (D) the female has dark bristles in the third pair of legs.

84. Lichens are composites, consisting of fungi and
    (A) bacteria
    (B) algae
    (C) mosses
    (D) protozoa.

85. The main tissue in the pyloric sphincter is
    (A) muscle
    (B) epithelium
    (C) connective
    (D) nerve.

86. The crayfish is a member of the class
    (A) chilopoda
    (B) arachinda
    (C) arthropoda
    (D) crustacea.

87. The structure in a mammal that carries sperm cells from the testes to the urethra is the organ called the
    (A) seminiferous tubule
    (B) urachis
    (C) ureter
    (D) vas deferens.

88. The tubercle bacillus is best stained with
    (A) hematoxylin
    (B) acid fast stain
    (C) chromic acid
    (D) glacial acetic acid.

89. Stock cultures of drosophila should be kept in rooms which have no greater range in temperature than from
    (A) 15-20 degrees C.
    (B) 20-25 degrees C.
    (C) 25-30 degrees C.
    (D) 35-40 degrees C.

90. The flagella of collar cells waft small particles of food into the collars whence the food passes into gastric vacuoles in the individual cells of the
    (A) hydra
    (B) planaria
    (C) starfish
    (D) sponge.

91. Of the following, the one *never* found in invertebrates is
    (A) coelom
    (B) triploblastic embryo
    (C) dorsal nerve cord
    (D) red blood corpuscles.

92. Enzymes can best be classified as which one of the following?
    (A) carbohydrates
    (B) inorganic trace elements
    (C) proteins
    (D) phospholipid - nucleic acids.

93. Autocatalysis in cytology refers to
    (A) protein digestion
    (B) hormonal activity
    (C) bacterial disintegration
    (D) gene duplication.

94. In passing to the lungs, air passes in order through the
    (A) larynx, pharynx, bronchioles and bronchi
    (B) pharynx, larynx, bronchi and bronchioles
    (C) pharynx, larynx, bronchioles and bronchi
    (D) larynx, pharynx, bronchi and bronchioles.

95. Of the following larvae, the one which may pass through snail and fish before entering the human body are those of the
    (A) Chinese liver fluke
    (B) trichina
    (C) hookworm
    (D) tapeworm.

96. Bread mold illustrates the type of nutrition which is
    (A) holophytic
    (B) parasitic
    (C) xerophytic
    (D) saprophytic.

97. The ciliary muscle is used for the process of
    (A) locomotion
    (B) food transportation
    (C) accommodation
    (D) dust removal.

98. Infection may be spread rapidly in the mastoid bone because of which one of the following characteristics?
    (A) spongy in texture
    (B) close to the cerebrum
    (C) unable to circulate antibodies
    (D) essentially non-living in composition.

99. Haversian systems are found in
    (A) fibrous cartilage
    (B) elastic cartilage
    (C) bone
    (D) areolar tissue.

100. Of the following, an example of evolutionary stagnation is (are)
    (A) Crossopterygians
    (B) lungfish
    (C) archaeopteryx
    (D) Cro-Magnon man

101. In the chemical expression, A $\sim$ P, the symbol $\sim$ represents
    (A) release of gases
    (B) precipitation
    (C) high energy bond
    (D) low energy bond.

102. Phage is parasitic on
 (A) bacteria      (B) virus
 (C) molds      (D) rickettsia.

103. Pasteur's famous experiment with two groups of sheep and other cattle demonstrated the success of his vaccine against
 (A) rabies      (B) cholera
 (C) tuberculosis      (D) anthrax.

104. The blood constituent most likely to provide antibodies is
 (A) albumin      (B) fibrinogen
 (C) globulin      (D) heparin.

105. The tricuspid valve is between the
 (A) left auricle and left ventricle
 (B) right auricle and right ventricle
 (C) right ventricle and pulmonary artery
 (D) aorta and left ventricle.

106. The ability to taste PTC paper is
 (A) acquired
 (B) inherited as a recessive trait
 (C) inherited as a dominant trait
 (D) sex-linked among the Mongoloids.

107. The body obtains important coenzymes from foods containing which one of the following?
 (A) vitamins      (B) lipoids
 (C) steroids      (D) amino acids.

108. A micron is equal to
 (A) .1 mm.      (B) .01 mm.
 (C) .001 mm.      (D) .0001 mm.

109. The cells that are mainly responsible for regeneration in the hydra are
 (A) endodermal      (B) neuromuscular
 (C) mesenchymal      (D) epidermal.

110. A sphygmomanometer is used to measure
 (A) basal metabolism
 (B) sedimentation rate
 (C) clotting time
 (D) blood pressure.

111. Of the following systems, the one to which the tonsils belong is the
 (A) respiratory      (B) lymphatic
 (C) digestive      (D) circulatory.

112. The skeleton of a shark is made of
 (A) bone      (B) chitin
 (C) cartilage      (D) calcareous plates.

113. Of the following organisms, the two which probably existed during the same period are
 (A) Polycosaurs and flowering plants
 (B) Pterosaurs and giant dragon flies
 (C) Cycads and Gingkos
 (D) Australopithecines and Trilobites

114. Viruses and chloroplasts behave alike in that they
 (A) replicate in living cells only
 (B) are essentially made up of DNA
 (C) are saprophytic
 (D) reproduce in a cell-free medium.

115. Liverworts are most closely related to which one of the following?
 (A) ferns      (B) algae
 (C) lichens      (D) mosses.

116. Studies in which one of the following fields led most directly to the conception that ontogeny recapitulates phylogeny?
 (A) paleontology
 (B) embryology
 (C) comparative anatomy
 (D) taxonomy.

117. The relationship between termites and ciliates is known as
 (A) mutualism      (B) parasitism
 (C) commensalism      (D) holophytism.

118. To insure a satisfactory classroom demonstration of the "scratch" reflex in a frog, the teacher should destroy the frog's
 (A) brain
 (B) spinal cord
 (C) brain and spinal cord
 (D) sciatic nerve.

119. The hammer, anvil, and stirrup bones lie in the
 (A) outer ear      (B) middle ear
 (C) inner ear      (D) semicircular canals.

120. The cellular structure that helps to regulate turgor is the
 (A) Goli apparatus      (B) reticular apparatus
 (C) tonoplast      (D) mitochondrion.

121. Clams, snails, and octopi are similar in that they possess
 (A) conspicuous shell and foot
 (B) conspicuous shell and mantle
 (C) gills and foot
 (D) gills and mantle.

122. The phylum to which the leech belongs is the
 (A) platyhelmenthes      (B) nematoda
 (C) arthropoda      (D) annelida.

123. The Salk polio vaccine is produced from viruses grown in tissue from which one of the following?
 (A) rabbits      (B) sheep
 (C) monkeys      (D) guinea pigs.

124. Which one of the following is not found in the skull?
(A) turbinals
(B) hyoid
(C) mastoid
(D) parietal.

125. In vascular plants, the stele is surrounded by
(A) collenchyma
(B) meristem
(C) endodermis
(D) phellogen.

126. Which one of the following is *not* associated with the others in the performance of a related function?
(A) calcium ion
(B) fibrinogen
(C) monocytes
(D) platelets.

127. Erythroblasts are found normally only in the
(A) blood
(B) spleen
(C) liver
(D) bone marrow.

128. Which one of the following genuses was the result of a hoax?
(A) Eoanthropus
(B) Pithecanthropus
(C) Dryopithecus
(D) Sinanthropus.

129. Enucleate erythrocytes are characteristic of which one of the following?
(A) reptiles
(B) fish
(C) amphibians
(D) mammals.

130. Beta particles are
(A) protons
(B) neutrons
(C) electrons
(D) neutrons and protons.

131. Hiccups are a result of spasmodic, involuntary contractions of the
(A) stomach muscles
(B) diaphragm
(C) abdominal muscles
(D) rib muscles.

132. Genes are composed principally of
(A) DNA
(B) ATP
(C) 2-4D
(D) hormones.

133. The type of kidney found in fully matured reptiles, birds and mammals is the
(A) mesonephros
(B) ananephros
(C) metanephros
(D) pronephros.

134. The taiga is practically absent in the
(A) Southern Hemisphere
(B) northern part of Siberia
(C) mountains of India
(D) Burmese jungle.

135. Variations in the colors of wheat kernels is best ascribed to the effects of
(A) xenia
(B) maternal inheritance
(C) multiple alleles
(D) photoperiodism.

136. The actual incidence of hemophilia is less than the theoretically predictable level because
(A) hemophilia is sex-linked
(B) of adverse marriage selection pressure against hemophiliacs
(C) the gene for hemophilia is recessive
(D) homozygosity is seldom found in the female.

137. The frequency of crossing-over of genes tends to vary
(A) inversely with the distance between genes in allelic chromosomes
(B) inversely with the number of genes near the centromere
(C) directly with the character of the gene
(D) inversely with the increasing complexity of the organism.

138. Certain ultraviolet radiations are an effective agent for mutations principally because
(A) they produce thermal effects
(B) they can be easily administered
(C) nucleoproteins absorb some ultraviolet radiations
(D) they may produce hemolysis

139. Of the following diseases, the one that is seriously affecting the rabbit population is
(A) glanders
(B) malta fever
(C) elephantiasis
(D) myxomatosis.

140. The human embryo's placenta is derived from the
(A) decidua vera
(B) chorion
(C) amnion
(D) corpus luteum.

141. The structures that produce sex cells in the prothallium are
(A) anthers and archegonia
(B) ovaries and anthers
(C) testes and archegonia
(D) antheridia and archegonia.

142. The thyrotrophic hormone is produced by the
(A) thyroid
(B) thymus
(C) pituitary
(D) adrenal.

143. Smooth muscle cells are innervated by the
(A) peripheral nervous system
(B) central nervous system
(C) parasympathetic nerves
(D) autonomic nervous system.

144. Of the following, the one which is a hormone which acts to produce secondary sex characteristics of the male is
(A) pitocin
(B) gonadotrophin II
(C) androsterone
(D) estradiol.

145. Meiosis occurs in the spirogyra
 (A) as the zygospore germinates
 (B) in preparation for conjugation
 (C) during the vegetative stage
 (D) as the protoplasmic bridges form.

146. Egestion in planaria takes place through the
 (A) anus          (B) flame cells
 (C) mouth         (D) collar cells.

147. Experimental evidence shows that the replication of DNA molecules occurs essentially during the
 (A) interphase    (B) late prophase
 (C) metaphase     (D) early anaphase.

148. Striated muscle tissue is called a syncytium because the fibers contain many
 (A) myofibrils
 (B) light and dark bands
 (C) transverse stripes
 (D) nuclei.

149. The basic chemical formula for starch is
 (A) $(C_6H_{10}O_5)n$      (B) $(C_6H_{12}O_6)n$
 (C) $C_{12}H_{22}O_{11}$   (D) $C_6H_{12}O_6$

150. Of the following, an animal with an evertible alimentary structure is the
 (A) hydra          (B) dogfish
 (C) amphioxus      (D) molgula.

151. The branched type of gastrovascular cavity is well exemplified by a
 (A) planaria       (B) hydra
 (C) sponge         (D) tapeworm.

152. The sexual generation of obelia is the
 (A) zooid          (B) planula
 (C) hydrotheca     (D) medusa.

153. Most scientific names of plants and animals have two parts of which the second is the
 (A) variety        (B) genus
 (C) species        (D) family

154. A working muscle under anaerobic conditions does not
 (A) use up glycogen reserves rapidly
 (B) accumulate lactic acid rapidly
 (C) accumulate inorganic phosphates
 (D) convert lactic acid into glycogen.

155. Somatotrophin is the hormone of the pituitary gland which influences
 (A) use of sugar by cells
 (B) growth of the skeleton
 (C) maturing of the gonads
 (D) water content of the skeleton.

156. Chordate animals display three unique features at some stage in their development—a notochord, a dorsal nerve cord and
 (A) gill clefts
 (B) a diaphragm
 (C) a closed circulatory system
 (D) a dorsally situated heart.

157. The excretory organs (green glands) of the crayfish are located closest to which one of the following?
 (A) midgut         (B) heart
 (C) eyes           (D) gonads.

158. The relationship which exists between the shark and remora is
 (A) symbiosis      (B) commensalism
 (C) parasitism     (D) mutualism.

159. Which one of the following is deposited in the cell wall of diatoms?
 (A) silicon        (B) lime
 (C) chitin         (D) gelatin.

160. Peyer's patches are located in the
 (A) pancreas       (B) nasopharynx
 (C) ileum          (D) hypothalamus.

161. Secretin is produced by cells of the
 (A) liver          (B) ileum
 (C) jejunum        (D) duodenum.

162. A cephalothorax is characteristic of which one of the following?
 (A) grasshopper    (B) crayfish
 (C) scorpion       (D) centipede.

163. Grana are constituents of
 (A) cytoplasmic granules
 (B) chromatin granules
 (C) reticulocytes
 (D) chloroplasts.

164. Sucrose, during digestion, is broken down into
 (A) glucose and fructose
 (B) galactose and glucose
 (C) galactose and fructose
 (D) maltose and glucose.

$$COOH$$
$$H_2N - C - H$$
$$R$$

165. The structural formula above represents a (an)
 (A) lipoid         (B) coenzyme
 (C) protein        (D) amino acid.

166. Cell turgor is increased when the external medium is
 (A) hypertonic
 (B) isotonic
 (C) hypotonic
 (D) isoelectrically equivalent.

167. Which one of the following is an evolutionary link between reptiles and birds?
(A) chondricthyes        (B) archaeopteryx
(C) pterodactyl          (D) didelphys.

168. A hormone which regulates the use of calcium by bones is produced by the
(A) thymus               (B) parathyroid
(C) thyroid              (D) pituitary.

169. A Sonoran habitat would most likely be found at which one of the following?
(A) seashore
(B) mouth of a river
(C) base of mountains
(D) peaks of foothills or on mountains.

170. Among vertebrates the embryonic ectoderm gives rise to which one of the following?
(A) nervous system    (B) digestive system
(C) skeletal system   (D) respiratory system.

171. A diet inadequate with respect to iodine will probably result in
(A) exophthalmic goiter
(B) Basedow's disease
(C) endemic goiter
(D) Graves's disease.

172. The main extensor muscle of the arm is the
(A) pectoralis major   (B) triceps
(C) biceps             (D) gastrocnemius.

173. Pioneer studies on the effects of deuterium on intermediary metabolism were performed by
(A) Schoenheimer       (B) Urey
(C) Fermi              (D) Oppenheimer.

174. The vegetation of dry plains, semideserts, and true deserts is composed of
(A) hydrophytes        (B) parasites
(C) saprophytes        (D) xerophytes.

175. The color of certain Hydrangea flowers may be changed to blue by the addition to the soil of
(A) $SO_2$             (B) Al
(C) CO                 (D) CaO.

176. The *incorrect* sequence in the following groups of food chains is
(A) insect-spider-frog-fish-otter
(B) algae-protozoa-aquatic insect-black bass-pickerel
(C) grass-cricket-frog-snake-hawk
(D) protozoa-aquatic insect larvae-diatoms-copepods-bass-raccoon.

177. A successful graft of an apple scion on a pear stock would result in
(A) genetic resistance
(B) clonal selection
(C) growth of apples on the scion
(D) growth of pears on the scion.

178. A cloaca is *not* found in which one of the following?
(A) reptiles           (B) salamanders
(C) rays               (D) sunfish.

179. Of the following scientists, the one *least* associated with studies in the field of evolution is
(A) Goldschmidt        (B) Buffon
(C) Simpson            (D) Bonner.

180. Hexokinase acts upon which one of the following?
(A) fructose
(B) glucose
(C) phosphoglyceraldehyde
(D) glycogen.

181. Of the following, the one which is a link between the annelids and the arthropods is the
(A) nautilus           (B) trilobite
(C) limulus            (D) peripatus.

182. Addison's disease is due to the malfunctioning of
(A) hypophysis         (B) epiphysis
(C) adrenals           (D) epididymis.

183. Bast fibers in a woody stem lie in the
(A) cork               (B) phloem
(C) cortex             (D) xylem.

184. Cattle may develop the condition known as "blind staggers" after ingesting feed containing
(A) selenium           (B) cobalt
(C) manganese          (D) thorium.

185. Of the following, one of the foremost contributors to our knowledge of the cytochrome system is
(A) Rittenberg         (B) Iwanowsky
(C) Beadle             (D) Warburg.

186. Book lungs may be found in dissections of which one of the following?
(A) aphids             (B) spiders
(C) silverfish         (D) finches.

187. Balanced lethals are used in drosophila crosses to
(A) determine on which chromosome a recessive mutant gene is located
(B) show the effect of hypostatic alleles
(C) prove that a fly is heterozygous for a selected trait
(D) test for sex-linkage.

188. The nerve endings for the sense of sight are located in the part of the eye called the
(A) cornea
(B) sclera
(C) iris
(D) retina.

189. Of the following, the one which causes malaria is
(A) a bacterium
(B) a mosquito
(C) a protozoan
(D) bad air.

190. Of the following, the plant whose seeds are *not* spread by wind is the
(A) cocklebur
(B) maple
(C) dandelion
(D) milkweed.

191. Of the following, the insect which is harmful to men's food supply is the
(A) dragonfly
(B) grasshopper
(C) ladybug
(D) praying mantis.

192. One-celled animals belong to the group of living things known as
(A) protozoa
(B) porifera
(C) annelida
(D) arthropoda.

193. Spiders can be distinguished from insects by the fact that spiders have
(A) hard outer coverings
(B) large abdomens
(C) four pairs of legs
(D) biting mouth parts.

194. Of the following glands, the one which regulates the metabolic rate is the
(A) adrenal
(B) salivary
(C) thyroid
(D) thymus.

195. All of the following are Amphibia *except* the
(A) salamander
(B) lizard
(C) frog
(D) toad.

196. Of the following, the scientist who originated and developed the system of classifying the plants and animals of the earth was
(A) Linnaeus
(B) Darwin
(C) Mendel
(D) Agassiz.

197. Protoplasmic streaming may best be observed in
(A) ameba
(B) cheek cells
(C) onion skin cells
(D) striated muscle.

198. A plant structure which consists of a single cell is a
(A) lenticel
(B) root hair
(C) stomate
(D) terminal bud.

199. A monocotyledonous plant that is used for food by man is the
(A) bean
(B) carrot
(C) corn
(D) radish.

200. The largest number of species of any group in the animal kingdom is found in the class
(A) Crustacea
(B) Insecta
(C) Mammalia
(D) Myriapoda.

## Test In Biology

## Correct Answers

*(You'll learn more by writing your own answers before comparing them with these.)*

| | | | | |
|---|---|---|---|---|
| 1. C | 41. B | 81. C | 121. C | 161. D |
| 2. A | 42. B | 82. C | 122. D | 162. B |
| 3. B | 43. C | 83. B | 123. C | 163. D |
| 4. A | 44. D | 84. B | 124. B | 164. A |
| 5. A | 45. C | 85. A | 125. C | 165. D |
| 6. B | 46. D | 86. D | 126. C | 166. C |
| 7. B | 47. A | 87. D | 127. D | 167. B |
| 8. C | 48. B | 88. B | 128. A | 168. B |
| 9. D | 49. A | 89. B | 129. D | 169. A |
| 10. D | 50. D | 90. D | 130. C | 170. A |
| 11. B | 51. C | 91. C | 131. B | 171. C |
| 12. D | 52. D | 92. C | 132. A | 172. B |
| 13. B | 53. A | 93. D | 133. C | 173. A |
| 14. D | 54. B | 94. B | 134. A | 174. D |
| 15. C | 55. D | 95. A | 135. D | 175. D |
| 16. B | 56. D | 96. D | 136. B | 176. D |
| 17. D | 57. B | 97. C | 137. B | 177. C |
| 18. B | 58. B | 98. A | 138. C | 178. D |
| 19. C | 59. A | 99. C | 139. D | 179. D |
| 20. C | 60. C | 100. B | 140. B | 180. B |
| 21. A | 61. A | 101. C | 141. D | 181. D |
| 22. C | 62. D | 102. A | 142. C | 182. C |
| 23. D | 63. B | 103. D | 143. D | 183. B |
| 24. B | 64. D | 104. C | 144. C | 184. A |
| 25. A | 65. D | 105. B | 145. A | 185. D |
| 26. D | 66. D | 106. B | 146. C | 186. B |
| 27. B | 67. B | 107. A | 147. A | 187. C |
| 28. B | 68. B | 108. C | 148. D | 188. D |
| 29. A | 69. B | 109. C | 149. A | 189. C |
| 30. B | 70. D | 110. D | 150. A | 190. A |
| 31. B | 71. C | 111. B | 151. A | 191. B |
| 32. C | 72. D | 112. C | 152. D | 192. A |
| 33. A | 73. B | 113. C | 153. C | 193. C |
| 34. A | 74. C | 114. A | 154. D | 194. D |
| 35. A | 75. D | 115. D | 155. B | 195. A |
| 36. A | 76. D | 116. B | 156. A | 196. B |
| 37. D | 77. C | 117. A | 157. C | 197. A |
| 38. C | 78. B | 118. A | 158. B | 198. B |
| 39. C | 79. D | 119. B | 159. A | 199. C |
| 40. C | 80. A | 120. C | 160. C | 200. B |

# ADVANCED BIOLOGY EXAMINATION

*Directions:* Select from the lettered choices that choice which best completes the statement or answers the question. Indicate the letter of your choice on the answer sheet.

## A FAIR SAMPLING OF THE QUESTIONS YOU'LL BE ASKED

1. Pollination characteristically occurs among which one of the following pairs?

 (A) angiosperms and psilopsids
 (B) angiosperms and gymnosperms
 (C) pteridophytes and bryophytes
 (D) bryophytes and angiosperms
 (E) angiosperms and fungi

2. A nerve impulse results in

 (A) the cessation of an electric current
 (B) a chemical flow throughout the nerve fiber
 (C) synaptic secretion of acetylcholine
 (D) a wave of electrical depolarization
 (E) a wave of electrical polarization

3. Much of the phenomena of tropistic responses of plants to light were first observed by which one of the following?

 (A) Charles Darwin
 (B) Hugo DeVries
 (C) Ivan Pavlov
 (D) Lloyd Morgan
 (E) Jacques Loeb

4. Ferns, conifers, and flowering plants are classified as

 (A) bryophyta
 (B) spermatophyta
 (C) psilophyta
 (D) chlorophyta
 (E) tracheophyta

5. Cellulose is digested in the rumen of cattle by the enzyme cellulase secreted by

 (A) protozoa
 (B) bacteria
 (C) the rumen
 (D) the esophagus
 (E) windpipe

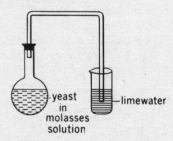

yeast in molasses solution — limewater

6. If the apparatus shown is placed in a moderately warm location, within a few hours the

 (A) molasses solution will flow into the beaker
 (B) molasses solution will turn brown
 (C) limewater will turn milky
 (D) limewater will flow into the flask
 (E) none of these

*Questions 7-8*

Most tissue-culture media contain some type of animal serum as one component. If chicken plasma is wanted, the clotted plasma must be ground with sand as the fibrin in the clot is tough. At one time it was thought necessary to culture cells in serum homologous to that species. However, growth and protective proteins have been proven by recent

S1301

experimentation to be nonspecific. By heating horse serum in a water bath at 56°C for one-half hour many of the specific proteins are denatured to the extent that the serum may be used for all species. Indeed, in some laboratories, horse serum is routinely used for culturing cells from all types of animals. With proper dilution for isotonicity it can be used even for cold-blooded forms. The use of horse serum is also advantageous because it can be stored for long periods at 0° to 5°C, and can be obtained in large quantities. Furthermore it tends to inhibit the liquefaction of the clotted medium caused by some mammalian tumor cells.

7. Which one of the following statements is *least* true?

   (A) Cells of cold-blooded forms do not require media of different isotonic strength.
   (B) Certain proteins in horse serum are not nonspecific.
   (C) Heterologous sera may be used in culturing all types of animal cells.
   (D) Some actions of tumor cells are inhibited by horse serum.
   (E) None of these.

8. Which one of the following statements is *best* supported by the paragraph?

   (A) Formerly it was thought unnecessary to provide homologous sera for culture cells.
   (B) Horse serum inhibits liquefaction of clotted media.
   (C) Protein needed for growth and protection is not different for different species.
   (D) Isotonic horse serum cannot be used for warm-blooded forms.
   (E) None of these.

*Questions 9-11*

In the atoms of heavier elements (whose nuclei have larger electrical charges) the consecutive electron shells are arranged in the same pattern as those in the hydrogen atom, but the diameters of the shells are somewhat smaller. In these atoms the increased electrical attraction of the proton-packed nucleus is not completely balanced by the increased electrical repulsion of the negatively charged electrons, so the electrons are pulled closer to the nucleus. This presents something of a prob-

lem, because heavier nuclei have an increasingly large number of electrons orbiting around them. However, because of the exclusion principle, atoms tend to remain approximately the same in size.

9. Which concept is *best* supported by the paragraph?

   (A) All elements have approximately the same mass.
   (B) An extra electron in an atom causes it to be negatively charged.
   (C) Electron shells of atoms tend to remain at the same distance from the nucleus in all atoms of elements.
   (D) The sizes, rather than the weights or "electron densities" of atoms of elements tend to be constant.
   (E) All compounds have the same size and mass.

10. How does the size of an oxygen atom compare with the size of an uranium atom?

    (A) Oxygen atoms are larger.
    (B) Oxygen atoms are smaller.
    (C) They are approximately equal.
    (D) They cannot be compared, since the two elements exist in different states of matter.
    (E) Uranium atomic size has not as yet been determined.

11. The statement that electrons will not be pushed farther away if the atom's nucleus has more neutrons than protons is

    (A) contradicted by the passage
    (B) implied in the passage
    (C) directly stated in the passage
    (D) suggested by the passage but contradicted by actual evidence
    (E) neither stated nor implied in the passage

12. An organism lacking chlorophyll, but nevertheless able to carry out photosynthesis has been found among which one of the following?

    (A) bacteria
    (B) viruses
    (C) phaeophytes
    (D) zoophytes
    (E) protozoa

13. Of the following, which one best describes phenylketonuria?

   (A) a vitamin deficiency resulting in abnormal metabolism of proteins
   (B) an inherited metabolic disorder resulting in a lack of an enzyme
   (C) a mineral deficiency resulting in abnormal bone formation
   (D) an abnormal shape in red blood cells
   (E) a chronic disease of unknown causes

14. Of the following characteristics, the one relevant to trace elements is that they

   (A) are radioactive and can be located with a Geiger Counter
   (B) exist in minute amounts in protoplasm
   (C) are not readily absorbed into protoplasm
   (D) act as inhibitors of enzymatic reactions
   (E) control the passage of materials through the pores in the cell membrane

15. Solutions of crystal violet, iodine and alcohol are used in a staining procedure known as

   (A) acid-fast stain
   (B) Wright's stain
   (C) Giemsa's stain
   (D) Gram stain
   (E) spore stain

### Questions 16-21

The first representatives of the Osteichthyes appeared in the middle Devonian, soon after the earliest sharks. As the fossils are known, these bony fishes are separated at the outset into the three types of lobe-finned fishes, ray-finned fishes, and lung-fishes, which means that their differentiation from a common ancestry was well advanced. The lobe-fins in turn can be identified as including forms that were forerunners of the first land vertebrates.

Surprising as it may seem, a lung or lungs appear to have been present in many, if not all, of these early bony fishes, perhaps as an adaptation to life in stagnant pools that may have been formed recurrently in the watercourses under the climatic conditions of the Devonian. Apparently the swim bladder of modern bony fishes, which is homologous with the lungs of tetrapod vertebrates is not the organ from which lungs arose but a modification of the primitive lung in the early ancestors of these fishes. After making a beginning of air-breathing it seems that one line, the lobe-finned fishes gave rise to the Amphibia and so to the land vertebrates . . . , while another line, the ray-finned fishes, gave rise to the bony fishes of the present day, in which the primitive lung was transformed into a hydrostatic organ, the swim bladder.

It is significant in this connection that in the most primitive of existing ray-finned fishes, such as the "bichir" of the Nile, *Polypterus,* the lung still persists in its original function; another and independent survival of the primitive lung appears in the three genera of lung-fishes (Dipnoi), *Ceratodus, Protopterus,* and *Lepidosiren.* In North America the sturgeon, *Acipenser,* the paddle fish, *Polyodon,* the gar pike, *Lepisosteus,* and the bow-fin, *Amia,* are ray-fins of primitive type although they do not have lungs as does the more primitive *Polypterus.* The more specialized ray-fins include all the most familiar fishes of fresh and salt water, such as the trout, salmon, carp, bass, perch, catfish, cod, herring, mackerel, and many others that are highly specialized.

16. The word *homologous* as used in the section means

   (A) compatible
   (B) having the same function
   (C) having the same origin
   (D) having the same structure
   (E) incompatible

17. Which one of the following belongs to the most primitive type

   (A) catfish
   (B) codfish
   (C) frog
   (D) toad
   (E) sturgeon

18. The mammals are derived from

   (A) fish with swim bladders
   (B) the Dipnoi
   (C) the lobe-fins
   (D) the ray-fins
   (E) fish without lobe-fins

19. The Devonian is a

   (A) climatic region
   (B) geological period
   (C) region infested with sharks
   (E) oceanic drift area
   (D) sunken continent

20. The *Osteichthyes* are

    (A) algae
    (B) amphibians
    (C) fungi
    (D) sharks
    (E) bony fish

21. The gar pike, found in midwestern U.S.A., is a

    (A) lobe-finned fish
    (B) lung-fish
    (C) ray-finned fish
    (D) tetrapod vertebrate
    (E) amphibian

22. The fossil, Hesperornis, is significant because it

    (A) had claws on its hind limbs
    (B) had feathers and teeth
    (C) was a link between birds and mammals
    (D) was a link between amphibia and reptiles
    (E) was a link between fish and amphibia

23. Colonies of coelenterates with individuals of more than one body form are said to exhibit

    (A) polymorphism
    (B) radial symmetry
    (C) orthogenesis
    (D) divergence
    (E) neotony

24. To which one of the following is the Haversian system related?

    (A) endocrine system
    (B) skeletal system
    (C) reproductive system
    (D) respiratory system
    (E) nervous system

25. A section of the circulatory system which plays an important role in fishes, but which disappears in higher land animals is the

    (A) hepatic portal system
    (B) renal portal system
    (C) renal arteries
    (D) hepatic arteries
    (E) hepatic veins

26. Of the following organisms, the one that has an incomplete, but functional, digestive system is

    (A) lumbricus
    (B) lobster
    (C) clam
    (D) grasshopper
    (E) planaria

*Questions 27-31*

Chemical investigations show that during muscle contraction the store of organic phosphates in the muscle fibers is altered as energy is released. In doing so, the organic phosphates (chiefly adenosine triphosphate and phospho-creatine) are transformed anaerobically to organic compounds plus phosphates. As soon as the organic phosphates begin to break down in muscle contraction, the glycogen in the muscle fibers also transforms into lactic acid plus free energy. This energy the muscle fiber uses to return the organic compounds plus phosphates into high-energy organic phosphates ready for another contraction. In the presence of oxygen, the lactic acid from the glycogen decomposition is changed also. About one-fifth of it is oxidized to form water and carbon dioxide and to yield another supply of energy. This time the energy is used to transform the remaining four-fifths of the lactic acid into glycogen again.

27. The energy for muscle contraction comes directly from the

    (A) breakdown of the organic phosphates
    (B) resynthesis of adenosine triphosphate
    (C) breakdown of glycogen into lactic acid
    (D) oxidation of lactic acid
    (E) breakdown of lactic acid into glycogen

28. Lactic acid does not accumulate in a muscle that

    (A) is in a state of lacking oxygen
    (B) has an ample supply of oxygen
    (C) is in a state of fatigue
    (D) is repeatedly being stimulated
    (E) is in a state of tetanus

29. The energy for the resynthesis of adenosine triphosphate and phospho-creatine comes from

    (A) synthesis of organic phosphates
    (B) oxidation of lactic acid
    (C) change from glycogen to lactic acid
    (D) resynthesis of glycogen
    (E) none of the above

30. The energy for the resynthesis of glycogen comes from the

    (A) breakdown of organic phosphates
    (B) resynthesis of organic phosphates
    (C) change occurring in one-fifth of the lactic acid
    (D) change occurring in four-fifths of the lactic acid
    (E) none of these changes

31. The breakdown of the organic phosphates into organic compounds plus phosphates is an

    (A) anabolic reaction
    (B) aerobic reaction
    (C) endothermic reaction
    (D) anaerobic reaction
    (E) metabolic reaction

32. Sodium citrate is added to bottles of donor blood to prevent clotting because it removes the

    (A) serum          (B) plasma
    (C) calcium        (D) prothrombin
         (E) fibrinogen

33. Protective mimicry is illustrated by

    (A) aphids and ants
    (B) hermit crab and sea anemone
    (C) monarch and viceroy butterflies
    (D) pilot fish and shark
    (E) termite and trichonympha

34. The evolutionary development of the animal kingdom can best be represented as which one of the following?

    (A) ladder        (B) web
    (C) circle        (D) chain
         (E) tree

35. A pupil treated guppies with a hormone and found that the normally dull-colored females developed bright colors. The hormone was most probably

    (A) androgen
    (B) estradiol
    (C) pitocin
    (D) thyroxin
    (E) parathormone

36. The destruction of coyotes because they may prey on sheep often results in the

    (A) large-scale increase in the numbers of sheep
    (B) starvation of sheep in competition with rabbits
    (C) increase in the quality of mutton
    (D) increase in diseases of sheep
    (E) decrease in diseases of all animals in the given environment

37. It is probable that a mammal smaller than a shrew could not exist because it would

    (A) not get sufficient oxygen
    (B) reproduce too rapidly
    (C) have to eat at too tremendous a rate
    (D) not be able to defend itself
    (E) be unable to bear live young

38. The fruit composed of a hard endocarp and usually one seed is classified as which one of the following?

    (A) capsule
    (B) drupe
    (C) achene
    (D) samara
    (E) none of these

39. Of the following, the important fossil that was intermediate between mammals and reptiles is

    (A) Dipterus
    (B) Cynognathus
    (C) Seymouria
    (D) Smilodon
    (E) Amphioxus

# ANSWER KEY TO SAMPLE TEST (1) IN BIOLOGY

*In order to help you pinpoint your weaknesses, the specific area of each question is indicated in parentheses after the answer. Refer to textbooks and other study material wherever you have an incorrect answer.*

| | | |
|---|---|---|
| EVOLUTION AND THE SPECIES CONCEPT | = ESC | ORGANIZATION = O |
| IRRITABILITY AND RESPONSE | = IR | REGULATION AND CONTROL = RC |
| METABOLISM AND ENERGETICS | = ME | SPECIFICITY = S |
| MORPHOGENESIS | = M | |

|  |  |  |  |
|---|---|---|---|
| 1. B(O) | 11. E(S) | 21. C(ESC) | 31. D(IR) |
| 2. D(IR) | 12. A(ME) | 22. B(ESC) | 32. E(ME) |
| 3. E(IR) | 13. B(ME) | 23. A(M) | 33. C(ESC) |
| 4. E(S) | 14. B(M) | 24. B(M) | 34. E(ESC) |
| 5. B(ME) | 15. D(M) | 25. B(M) | 35. A(RC) |
| 6. C(ME) | 16. C(ESC) | 26. E(S) | 36. B(RC) |
| 7. A(S) | 17. E(ESC) | 27. A(IR) | 37. C(S) |
| 8. B(S) | 18. C(ESC) | 28. B(IR) | 38. C(S) |
| 9. D(S) | 19. B(ESC) | 29. C(IR) | 39. B(ESC) |
| 10. C(S) | 20. E(ESC) | 30. C(IR) | |

| SCORE 1 |
|---|
| .......................... % |
| NO. CORRECT ÷ |
| NO. OF QUESTIONS ON THIS TEST |

| SCORE 2 |
|---|
| .......................... % |
| NO. CORRECT ÷ |
| NO. OF QUESTIONS ON THIS TEST |

| SCORE 3 |
|---|
| .......................... % |
| NO. CORRECT ÷ |
| NO. OF QUESTIONS ON THIS TEST |

## DENTAL ADMISSION TEST

# EXPLANATORY ANSWERS FOR ADVANCED BIOLOGY EXAMINATION

*Elucidation, clarification, explication and a little help with the fundamental facts covered in the Previous Test. These are the points and principles likely to crop up in the form of questions on future tests.*

1. **(B)** Pollination occurs only in plants that produce seeds. In order for seed formation to take place, pollen grains must come into effective contact with ovules. Pollination transfers the pollen from the anther to the stigma of a plant. Among the choices listed, only Angiosperms and Gymnosperms produce seeds, and as such exhibit the vital process of pollination.

2. **(D)** Normally, a "resting" nerve exhibits polarization with positive charges on the outside of the nerve fiber and negative charges on the inside. When an outside stimulus comes into contact with the nerve, sodium (positive) ions are permitted to infiltrate the fiber, leading to a wave of depolarization — becoming positively charged on the inside and negatively charged on the outside.

3. **(E)** Jacques Loeb compared the tropistic movements of plants to light with a behavioral pattern similar to that of the pill bug.

4. **(E)** Ferns, Gymnosperms and Angiosperms possess conducting tubes for transporting vital materials to all parts of the plant. This characteristic distinguishes a member of the Tracheophyta.

5. **(B)** Symbiotic bacteria inhabiting the alimentary canal secrete the enzyme cellulose, converting the polysaccharide cellulose into sugar, which is absorbed and utilized.

6. **(C)** Yeast will ferment molasses and other sugars under anaerobic conditions, producing alcohol and carbon dioxide. As this gas bubbles through colorless limewater, it turns the solution cloudy or milky white, as a precipitate of calcium carbonate is formed.

7. **(A)** It is stated in the passage that "with proper dilution for isotonicity it can be used even for cold-blooded forms." This statement implies that cells of cold-blooded forms must have their media adjusted with respect to isotonicity.

8. **(B)** The last sentence in the passage supports this statement.

9. **(D)** The final sentence states that, because of the exclusion principle, atoms tend to remain approximately the same in size.

10. **(C)** The large number of electrons orbiting the uranium nucleus are pulled closer to it. This causes all atoms to be approximately equal in size.

11. **(E)** No sentence in the passage suggests this statement.

12. **(A)** Photosynthetic bacteria possess an enzyme, different from chlorophyll, but still capable of enabling them to produce their own food.

13. **(B)** Phenylketonuria is caused by a lack of a single gene responsible for initiating the production of an enzyme that normally converts phenylalanine to tyrosine.

14. **(B)** Trace elements (copper, sulfur, iron, etc.) are present in protoplasm in very minute quantities — fractions of a per cent. However, even though present in trace quantity, their presence is vital to the normal functioning of the organism.

15. **(D)** The gram stain, routinely utilized in bacteriology, employs crystal violet, Lugol's iodine, 95% alcohol and safranin as part of its technique.

16. **(C)** The meaning of "homologous" is clearly stated in the second sentence of the second paragraph; in effect, the swim bladder and lungs arose from a modification of the primitive lung found in a common ancestor.

17. **(E)** The sturgeon is an elasmobranch possessing plates on its body, similar to those of armor-plated fish long extinct.

18. **(C)** See latter part of second paragraph: ". . . the lobe-finned fishes gave rise to the Amphibia and so to the land vertebrates," in which the mammals are included.

19. **(B)** The Devonian was one of six periods of the Paleozoic era in which fossils of the first amphibians are found.

20. **(E)** The definition of Osteichthyes is stated in the second sentence of the first paragraph: ". . . these bony fishes are separated . . ."

21. **(C)** This is stated in the next to last sentence of the passage: ". . . the gar pike . . . are ray-fins of primitive type . . ."

22. **(B)** *Hesperornis regalis* was found during the Cretaceous period and exhibited feathers and teeth. It is classified as a bird, but was wingless and inhabited coastal areas, diving for its food.

23. **(A)** Obelia and other colonial coelenterates include many specialized individuals who help the colony to function as a unit. These unusual members display polymorphism, or many body shapes.

24. **(B)** Bone tissue is composed of many Haversian systems, which comprise such parts as lamellae, lacunae and bone canals.

25. **(B)** The renal portal system gathers blood from the hind fin and posterior body wall, dividing into capillaries within the kidneys. The blood is then collected by renal veins and returned to the heart. Amphibians also possess a renal portal system, functioning in much the same manner.

26. **(E)** The planaria do not have complete digestive systems — that is, a separate mouth and anal opening. However, the digestive system does secrete enzymes which digest food sucked in through the proboscis. There are no specialized digestive organs like stomach, liver, esophagus, etc., but rather a diverse, branching intestine.

27. **(A)** This is stated in the third sentence: "As soon as the organic phosphates begin to break down in muscle contraction . . ."

28. **(B)** The third sentence from the end of the passage states that lactic acid undergoes change in an oxygen environment.

29. **(C)** Organic phosphates are composed chiefly of ATP and phospho-creatine which begin to break down in muscle contraction, only to be reformed after glycogen is changed to lactic acid. This sequence is described in the middle of the passage.

30. **(C)** The last sentence clearly states that "the energy is used to transform the remaining four-fifths of the lactic acid into glycogen again."

31. **(D)** The second sentence states that the organic phosphates are transformed anaerobically to organic compounds plus phosphates.

32. **(E)** Fibrinogen, a plasma protein, is vital for the clotting of blood. When acted upon by thrombin, fibrinogen causes threads of fibrin to be formed. It is this interlocking network of fibrin which traps red blood corpuscles, etc. and prevents the blood from flowing out of the wound.

33. **(C)** Protective mimicry is exhibited by several animals that inhabit the same environment. The monarch butterfly produces a chemical that does not appeal to most birds. Because the viceroy butterfly resembles it so perfectly, birds do not prey upon them. This evolutionary achievement has proved most beneficial to the survival and continuance of these insects.

34. **(E)** All animals evolved from a common ancestry. If we think of the trunk, or main part of a tree, as representing this original main line, the branches are all divisions or groupings from this origination point. Smaller branches and twigs are subgroups and constitute specific lines of evolutionary development from the aforesaid larger groupings.

35. **(A)** The male guppy is very brightly colored, while the female is dull and drab. This is known as a secondary sex characteristic directly controlled by the male sex hormone, androgen. If injected into the female, it will make these normally suppressed traits pronounced.

36. **(B)** If one link in a food chain is obliterated, the entire balance of nature is upset, causing all links to suffer. Coyotes, the natural enemy of sheep and rabbits, keep their numbers in check. If coyotes are destroyed, the birth rates of sheep and rabbits increase tremendously, causing a severe competition for the vital necessities of life, particularly food. Unfortunately, vegetation is the food source for both sheep and rabbits.

37. **(C)** The shrew is the smallest mammal in the world. Each day it must consume several times its own body weight in order to survive, insects supplying most of these demands. The great frequency of hunting, killing and feeding would make it almost impossible for any smaller mammal to exist.

38. **(C)** The achene dry fruit contains an individual seed attached at one point to the wall of the fruit, which does not split open. The dandelion is an example.

39. **(B)** In the Permian period, a group of reptiles possessing a few mammalian characteristics (therapsids) appeared. One representative member, *Cynognathus,* possessed teeth differentiated into incisors, canines and molars. In addition, the skull size was intermediate between that of a reptile and a mammal.

# ACHIEVEMENT TEST IN CHEMISTRY

*Directions for answering questions.* For each question, decide which is the best answer of the choices given. Note the capital letter preceding the best answer. On machine scored examinations you will be given an answer sheet and told to blacken the proper space on that answer sheet. At the end of this test we have provided a facsimile of such answer sheets. Tear it out, and mark your answers on it, just as you would do on an actual exam. It is most important that you learn to mark the answer sheet clearly.

1. Oxygen gas *cannot* be obtained in appreciable quantities by heating which one of the following?
   (A) $H_2O$  (B) $H_2O_2$
   (C) HgO  (D) $PbO_2$.

2. All of the reactions between the following pairs will produce hydrogen *except*
   (A) copper and hydrochloric acid
   (B) iron and sulfuric acid
   (C) magnesium and steam
   (D) sodium and alcohol.

3. When hydrochloric acid is added to sodium sulfite and the gas which is formed is bubbled through barium hydroxide, the salt which is formed is
   (A) $BaCl_2$  (B) $BaSO_3$
   (C) NaCl  (D) NaOH.

4. When chlorine and carbon tetrachloride are added to a solution of an iodide and shaken, the color produced is
   (A) brown  (B) orange
   (C) violet  (D) yellow.

5. An important use of silicon carbide is
   (A) as an abrasive
   (B) as a catalyst
   (C) as an explosive
   (D) in water purification.

6. If an eudiometer tube was filled with 26 ml of hydrogen and 24 ml of oxygen and the mixture exploded, there would remain uncombined
   (A) 2 ml hydrogen  (B) 14 ml hydrogen
   (C) 23 ml hydrogen  (D) 11 ml oxygen.

7. The gas evolved when hydrochloric acid is added to a mixture of iron filings and sulfur is
   (A) $H_2s$  (B) $SO_2$
   (C) $SO_3$  (D) $H_2$.

8. When a colorless gas is dissolved in water and the resulting solution turns red litmus blue, the gas may have been which one of the following?
   (A) HCl  (B) $NH_3$
   (C) $H_2S$  (D) $SO_2$.

9. Fluorine is the most active member of the halogen family because it
   (A) is a gas
   (B) has the smallest atomic radius
   (C) has no isotopes
   (D) combines with lithium.

10. In sulfuric acid the valence number of sulfur is
    (A) plus 2  (B) minus 2
    (C) minus 4  (D) plus 6.

11. In the fractional distillation of liquid air, the gas among the following which boils off last is
    (A) argon  (B) helium
    (C) nitrogen  (D) oxygen.

12. The element selenium is most closely related to which one of the following elements?
    (A) beryllium  (B) oxygen
    (C) silicon  (D) sulfur.

13. Baking soda is also called
    (A) washing soda  (B) caustic soda
    (C) soda ash  (D) bicarbonate of soda.

14. Solder is an alloy of
    (A) aluminum and copper
    (B) copper and tin
    (C) mercury and silver
    (D) tin and lead.

15. A lake is prepared by making a mixture of a colored dye with
    (A) $Al(OH)_3$  (B) $CaOCl_2$
    (C) $Na_2CO_3$  (D) $NH_4OH$.

16. A substance which will cause permanent hardness in water is
    (A) $Na_2SO_4$  (B) $H_2SO_4$
    (C) $MgSO_4$  (D) $Ca(HCO_3)_2$.

17. An apparatus which is used in the commercial preparation of sodium metal is named
    (A) Davy  (B) Downs
    (C) Glauber  (D) Hoffman.

18. Bleaching powder has the formula
    (A) $CaCl_2$  (B) CaOCl
    (C) $CaOCl_2$  (D) $Ca(ClO_3)_2$.

19. Pig iron is essentially the same as
    (A) low carbon steel  (B) wrought iron
    (C) cast iron    (D) Bessemer steel.

20. Of the following, an example of a transition element is
    (A) aluminum    (B) astatine
    (C) nickel    (D) rubidium.

21. A gas which is lighter than air is
    (A) $CH_4$    (B) $C_6H_6$
    (C) HCl    (D) $N_2O$.

22. Of the following gases, the one which is odorless and heavier than air is
    (A) CO    (B) $CO_2$
    (C) $H_2S$    (D) $N_2$.

23. The chief impurity in producer gas is
    (A) $CH_4$    (B) CO
    (C) $CO_2$    (D) $N_2$.

24. The weight in grams of 22.4 liters of nitrogen (atomic weight $= 14$) is
    (A) 3    (B) 7
    (C) 14    (D) 28.

25. One liter of a certain gas, under standard conditions, weighs 1.16 grams. A possible formula for the gas is
    (A) $C_2H_2$    (B) CO
    (C) $NH_3$    (D) $O_2$.

26. Of the following acids, the one which is most commonly found in the home is
    (A) $HC_2H_3O_2$    (B) $HNO_3$
    (C) $H_3PO_4$    (D) $H_2SO_4$.

27. Of the following, the one which is an aromatic compound is
    (A) benzene    (B) ethyl alcohol
    (C) iodoform    (D) methane.

28. The complete combustion of carbon disulfide would yield carbon dioxide and
    (A) sulfur    (B) sulfur dioxide
    (C) sulfuric acid    (D) water.

29. Alcoholic beverages contain
    (A) wood alcohol    (B) isopropyl alcohol
    (C) glyceryl alcohol  (D) ethyl alcohol.

30. Of the following compounds, the one which is more difficult to decompose than lithium fluoride is
    (A) lithium bromide  (B) lithium chloride
    (C) lithium iodide  (D) none of the above.

31. All of the following terms are associated with the manufacture of gasoline *except*
    (A) alkylation    (B) catalytic cracking
    (C) pickling    (D) polymerization.

32. Which one of the following will best show a substance in solution to be calcium nitrate?
    (A) The solution gives a green color in the cobalt nitrate test, and forms a white precipitate with $BaCl_2$
    (B) The solution gives a brown ring with $FeSO_4$ and $H_2SO_4$, and produces an orange-red flame
    (C) The borax bead test gives a green color, and the flame test is yellow
    (D) The solution turns tumeric paper red, and gives a blue flame.

33. The general formula for the acetylene series of hydrocarbons is
    (A) $C_nH_{2n+2}$    (B) $C_nH_{2n}$
    (C) $C_nH_{2n-2}$    (D) none of the above.

34. Of the following, the one which is a monosaccharide is
    (A) dextrose    (B) glycogen
    (C) lactose    (D) sucrose.

35. Fats belong to the class of organic compounds called
    (A) ethers    (B) soaps
    (C) esters    (D) lipases.

36. Of the following compounds, the one with the highest heat of formation is
    (A) NaCl    (B) NaI
    (C) NaF    (D) NaBr.

37. Of the following, the one which is a component of LP gas is
    (A) aviation gasoline
    (B) butane
    (C) liquid oxygen and kerosene
    (D) radioactive argon.

38. When a solution has a pH value of 9.2,
    (A) a drop of phenolphthalein indicator will redden it
    (B) magnesium will replace its hydrogen
    (C) litmus paper will turn red in it
    (D) the addition of calcium hydroxide will lower the pH value.

39. When a pale green coloration of the Bunsen flame is obtained during the performance of a flame test, it indicates the presence of a compound of which one of the following?
    (A) barium    (B) calcium
    (C) lithium    (D) potassium.

40. An oxide whose water solution will turn litmus red is
    (A) BaO
    (B) $Na_2O$
    (C) $P_2O_5$
    (D) CaO.

41. A compound which has a high heat of formation is normally
    (A) easy to form from its elements and easy to decompose
    (B) easy to form from its elements and difficult to decompose
    (C) difficult to form from its elements and easy to decompose
    (D) difficult to form from its elements and difficult to decompose.

42. A solution of zinc chloride should *not* be stored in a tank made of
    (A) aluminum
    (B) silver
    (C) copper
    (D) lead.

43. The valence number of sulfur in the ion $SO_5^{-2}$ is
    (A) —2
    (B) +2
    (C) +8
    (D) +10.

44. Of the following, the substance whose water solution will change color of litmus from red to blue is
    (A) $CuSO_4$
    (B) $K_2CO_3$
    (C) $NaNO_3$
    (D) $Zn(NO_3)_2$

45. The chemical name for sulfuric acid is
    (A) hydrogen sulfate
    (B) hydrogen sulfite
    (C) sulfur trioxide
    (D) hydrogen sulfide.

46. The number of grams of hydrogen formed by the action of 6 grams of magnesium (atomic weight = 24) on an appropriate quantity of acid is
    (A) 0.5
    (B) 8
    (C) 22.4
    (D) 72.

47. The symbol for two molecules of hydrogen is
    (A) $H_2$
    (B) 2H
    (C) $2H^+$
    (D) $2H_2$.

48. The formula for sodium bisulfate is
    (A) $NaBiSO_4$
    (B) $NaHSO_4$
    (C) $NaH_2SO_4$
    (D) $Na_2SO_4$.

49. The Law of Multiple Proportions was first enunciated by
    (A) Dalton
    (B) Davy
    (C) Priestley
    (D) Williams.

50. The per cent of oxygen in $Al_2(SO_4)_3$ (atomic weights: Al = 27, S = 32; O = 16) is approximately
    (A) 19
    (B) 21
    (C) 56
    (D) 92.

51. During the burning of one liter of carbon monoxide, the amount of oxygen consumed is
    (A) 0.5 liter
    (B) 1 liter
    (C) 2 liters
    (D) 4 liters.

52. Since the atomic weight of sulfur is *twice* that of oxygen, the percentage by weight of sulfur in sulfur dioxide is
    (A) 25%
    (B) 33%
    (C) 50%
    (D) 67%.

53. If a container is filled with hydrogen and another container of the same size is filled with carbon dioxide, both containers will, under normal air pressure, contain the same
    (A) number of atoms
    (B) number of molecules
    (C) weight of gas
    (D) number of neutrons.

54. 20 liters of hydrogen gas weigh about
    (A) 20 grams
    (B) 1.8 grams
    (C) 448 grams
    (D) 11.2 grams.

55. The density of krypton gas (atomic weight = 83.8) in grams per liter is
    (A) 1.28
    (B) 1.88
    (C) 3.7
    (D) 7.5.

56. If twenty-five ml of an acid are needed to neutralize exactly 50 ml of a 0.2N solution of a base, the normality of the acid is
    (A) 0.1
    (B) 0.2
    (C) 0.4
    (D) 2.0.

57. If an alloy consists of a mixture of 26 grams of chromium (atomic weight = 52) and 28 grams of iron (atomic weight = 56), the mole fraction of chromium equals
    (A) 0.48
    (B) 0.50
    (C) 0.52
    (D) 0.93.

58. An atom of chlorine, atomic number 17, and atomic weight 35, contains in its nucleus
    (A) 35 protons
    (B) 17 neutrons
    (C) 17 protons
    (D) 18 protons.

59. If the following, a particle which *cannot* be accelerated in a particle accelerator is
    (A) an alpha particle
    (B) an electron
    (C) an ion of carbon
    (D) a neutron.

60. After 40 days, the weight in grams of the pure radioisotope which remains of eight grams of a pure radioisotope with a half-life of 10 days is
    (A) 0.5          (B) 1.0
    (C) 2.0          (D) 6.0.

61. The electronic configuration of the element xenon is
    (A) 2-8-8          (B) 2-8-18-18-1
    (C) 2-8-18-18-8          (D) 2-8-18-28-8-2.

62. In the following incomplete nuclear equation, $_{29}Cu^{64} \rightarrow ? + _{28}Ni^{64}$, the missing term is
    (A) an electron          (B) a neutron
    (C) a positron          (D) a proton.

63. The element, californium, is a member of the
    (A) actinide series
    (B) alkali metal family
    (C) alkaline earth family
    (D) lanthanide series.

64. When a beam consisting of a mixture of alpha, beta, and gamma rays is passed at right angles through the magnetic field of a strong horseshoe magnet, the rays which are deflected to the N pole of the magnet are
    (A) alpha rays          (B) beta rays
    (C) gamma rays          (D) none of the above.

65. Plutonium for the Nagasaki bomb was produced from
    (A) graphite          (B) uranium-238
    (C) uranium-235          (D) strontium-90.

66. In the nuclear reaction
    $_3Li^7 + _1H^1 \rightarrow _2He^4 + X$,
    the term X represents
    (A) $_2He^4$          (B) $_1H^3$
    (C) $_3Li^6$          (D) $_1H^2$.

67. When strong acids are dissolved in water, a particle always formed is
    (A) $NH_4^+$          (B) $SO_4^=$
    (C) $NO_3^-$          (D) $H_3O^+$.

68. Of the following indicators, the one which will turn pink when NaOH solution is added to it is
    (A) litmus          (B) methyl orange
    (C) phenolphthalein          (D) methyl red.

69. The pH of pure water is
    (A) 3          (B) 5
    (C) 7          (D) 9.

70. An example of a proton donor is
    (A) $K_2SO_4$          (B) NaOH
    (C) CaO          (D) $HNO_3$.

71. The hydronium ion is usually written as
    (A) $HO^-$          (B) $H_3O^+$
    (C) $H_4N^+$          (D) $OH^-$

72. Of the following, an example of an anodic reaction is
    (A) $Cl^- - e \rightarrow Cl^\circ$
    (B) $Fe^{+3} + e \rightarrow Fe^{+2}$
    (C) $H_2O \rightarrow H^+ + OH^-$
    (D) $Na^+ + Cl^- \rightarrow NaCl$.

73. If a precipitate was formed when a crystal of hypo was placed in a clear solution of hypo, the solution must have been
    (A) contaminated          (B) saturated
    (C) supersaturated          (D) unsaturated.

74. Chemically pure water may be made from tap water by the process of
    (A) distillation          (B) boiling
    (C) electrolysis          (D) softening.

75. Tinctures always contain the solvent,
    (A) water          (B) iodine
    (C) alcohol          (D) glycerine.

76. The molecular weight of $Ba(NO_3)_2$ is 261.38. The approximate weight in grams needed to make 100 ml of a 0.1 N solution of $Ba(NO_3)_2$ is
    (A) 1.3          (B) 2.6
    (C) 13.1          (D) 26.1.

77. At about 4°C., water has its maximum
    (A) density          (B) vapor pressure
    (C) specific heat          (D) volume.

78. When sea water is boiled and passed through a filter, the material removed to the *least* extent is
    (A) air          (B) salt
    (C) bacteria          (D) suspended solids.

79. Real gases will approach the behavior of an ideal gas at
    (A) low temperatures and high pressures
    (B) high temperatures and low pressures
    (C) low temperatures and low pressures
    (D) high temperatures and high pressures.

80. When the temperature of 23 ml of dry $CO_2$ gas is changed from 10°C to 30°C, at a constant pressure of 760 m.m., the volume of gas becomes closest to which one of the following?
    (A) 7.7 ml          (B) 21.5 ml
    (C) 24.6 ml          (D) 69 ml.

81. Assume that a mole of gas "X" weighs 79 grams at S.T.P. The weight of 300 ml of this gas at 27°C and 760 m.m. pressure is
    (A) 0.853 grams
    (B) 0.938 grams
    (C) 1.030 grams
    (D) 2.330 grams.

82. If the analysis of a hydrocarbon is 83.6% carbon and 16.4% hydrogen, the most probable empirical formula is (Atomic Weights: $C = 12$; $H = 1$).
    (A) $C_3H_6$
    (B) $C_3H_8$
    (C) $C_6H_{14}$
    (D) $C_7H_{16}$.

83. If a compound contains 21.6% Na, 33.3% Cl and 45.1% O (Atomic Weights: $Na = 23$; $Cl = 35.5$; $O = 16$), the empirical formula of the compound is
    (A) $NaClO$
    (B) $NaClO_2$
    (C) $NaClO_3$
    (D) $NaClO_4$.

84. In the reaction given in unbalanced form below, the number of moles of $KClO_3$, needed to react with one mole of $C_{12}H_{22}O_{11}$ is
    $$KClO_3 + C_{12}H_{22}O_{11} \rightarrow KCl + CO_2 + H_2O$$
    (A) 2
    (B) 4
    (C) 6
    (D) 8.

85. If a 0.1 M solution of HCN is 0.01% ionized, the ionization constant for hydrocyanic acid is
    (A) $10^{-2}$
    (B) $10^{-3}$
    (C) $10^{-7}$
    (D) $10^{-9}$.

86. A colloidal solution of arsenious sulfide is most rapidly coagulated by the addition of a normal solution of which one of the following?
    (A) $NaCl$
    (B) $CaCl_2$
    (C) $Na_3PO_4$
    (D) $Al_2(SO_4)_3$.

87. Which one of the following carbon-carbon bonds has the highest energy?
    (A) single bond
    (B) covalent bond
    (C) triple bond
    (D) double bond.

88. Which one of the following best describes the double bond in ethylene, $C_2H_4$ ?
    (A) sigma bond
    (B) bond around which the carbon atoms are free to rotate
    (C) $sp^3$ hybrid orbital
    (D) pi bond.

89. The fact that carbon dioxide has no dipole moment indicates that the molecule is
    (A) covalently bonded
    (B) ionically bonded
    (C) angular
    (D) linear and symmetrical.

90. If seven millimoles of a base exactly neutralize 40 ml. of an acid, the normality of the acid is
    (A) 0.175
    (B) 0.280
    (C) 1.750
    (D) 7.000.

91. To which one of the following can the relatively great stability of the HCl molecule be attributed?
    (A) ability of chlorine to support combustion
    (B) ability of hydrogen gas to burn
    (C) non-ionic type of bonding
    (D) unequal sharing of the electron pair.

92. In the crystalline system if one axis of the simple cubic structure is extended in one direction, the unit cell produced is
    (A) body-centered cube
    (B) tetragonal
    (C) monoclinic
    (D) hexagonal.

93. Of the following groups, the one composed only of artificially produced elements is
    (A) polonium, francium, actinium
    (B) proactinium, neptunium, radon
    (C) berkelium, rhenium, hafnium
    (D) curium, californium, americium.

94. A major industrial use of the element bromine is to produce
    (A) dry cleaning fluids
    (B) a motor fuel additive
    (C) hydrobromic acid
    (D) sodium bromide.

95. Hydrazine has been used in rocket motors as a (an)
    (A) oxidizing agent
    (B) inert diluent
    (C) preheating agent
    (D) fuel.

96. Of the following elements to which one does the plastic "Teflon" owe many of its unique properties?
    (A) chlorine
    (B) nitrogen
    (C) sulfur
    (D) fluorine.

97. Which one of the following weights of nickel metal would be closest to the weight deposited by the passage of 24,125 coulombs through an aqueous solution of $NiI_2$ ? (Atomic wt. of $Ni = 58.7$)
    (A) 7.3g
    (B) 14.6g
    (C) 29.2g
    (D) 3.7g.

98. If a direct current deposits 11.5 grams of sodium (Atom weight = 23) in 1000 seconds, the number of grams of aluminum (Atomic weight = 27) deposited by the same current in the same period of time would be
(A) 4.5
(B) 9.0
(C) 11.5
(D) 13.5.

99. In the electrolysis of brine solution, an electron is lost by which one of the following?
(A) chloride ion
(B) hydroxyl ion
(C) hydrogen atom
(D) sodium hydroxide.

100. The mol fraction of nitrogen in a mixture containing 70g. of nitrogen, 128g. of oxygen, and 44g. of carbon dioxide (Atomic Weights: N = 14; O = 16, C = 12) is
(A) 0.29
(B) 0.33
(C) 0.36
(D) 0.50.

101. The percentage of hydrogen in the compound $NaHSO_4 \bullet H_2O$ (Na = 23, H = 1, S = 32, O = 16) is closest to which one of the following?
(A) 0.7%
(B) 1.4%
(C) 2.1%
(D) 4.2%.

102. Assume that air is 21.0% oxygen and 79.0% nitrogen by volume. If the barometric pressure is 740 m.m., the partial pressure of oxygen is closests to which one of the following?
(A) 155 m.m.
(B) 310 m.m.
(C) 580 m.m.
(D) 740 m.m.

103. The total number of types of water that can be made from $_1H^1$, $_1H^2$, $_1H^3$ and $_8O^{16}$, $_8O^{17}$ and $_8O^{18}$ is
(A) 3
(B) 9
(C) 18
(D) 27.

104. Of the following compounds, the one that hydrolizes to the greatest extent is
(A) Zns
(B) $Al_2O_3$
(C) $ZnSO_4$
(D) $Al_2S_3$.

105. Of the following formulas, the correct formula for periodic acid is
(A) HIO
(B) $HIO_2$
(C) $HIO_3$
(D) $H_5IO_6$.

106. Which one of the following men proposed the law that "The total pressure exerted by a mixture of gases is equal to the sum of the partial pressures of the various gases?
(A) Henry
(B) Avogadro
(C) Dalton
(D) Rayleigh.

107. Of the following valence numbers, the correct valence number of the element uranium in the formula $UO_2(NO_3)_2$ is
(A) +6
(B) +4
(C) +2
(D) —2.

108. The hydrogen halide whose water solution shows the highest acid strength is
(A) HF
(B) HBr
(C) HCl
(D) HI.

109. Of the following, one of the products of the reaction of magnesium nitride with water is
(A) magnesium oxide
(B) hydrogen
(C) ammonia
(D) nitrogen.

110. Which one of these following elements belongs to the family of elements that also includes the element gallium?
(A) carbon
(B) aluminum
(C) arsenic
(D) iron.

111. Which one of the following formulas is an example of a coordination compound?
(A) $[CO(NH_3)_6] Cl_3$
(B) NaCl
(C) $Na_2SO_4$
(D) $H_2O$.

112. Hydrogen bonding is shown most strongly in which one of the following?
(A) $H_2O$
(B) $H_2S$
(C) $H_2Se$
(D) $H_2Te$.

113. The mineral ore taconite, which is becoming important in our economy, is known chemically as a(an)
(A) sulfide
(B) silicate
(C) carbonate
(D) hydrated oxide.

114. In all of the following, water is employed as a reference substance *except* in
(A) molecular weights
(B) specific heats
(C) specific gravities
(D) thermometric scales.

115. Of the following metals, the two whose oxides are often reduced with hydrogen are
(A) iron and nickel
(B) titanium and zirconium
(C) tungsten and molybdenum
(D) vanadium and chromium.

116. Which one of the following pairs of metals has come to the fore in *recent* years because of the special properties of the two metals involved?
(A) titanium and zirconium
(B) chromium and vanadium
(C) aluminum and manganese
(D) technetium and rhenium.

117. Which one of the following formulas is the one for the ore molybdenite?
    (A) $MoO_3$  (B) $MoO_2Cl_2$
    (C) $MoS_2$  (D) $(NH_4)_2MoO_4$.

118. An isotone is a nucleous identical with a reference nucleus in
    (A) number of electrons
    (B) weight
    (C) number of protons
    (D) number of neutrons.

119. Assuming equal weights of radioactive elements, the most dangerous to approach immediately would be one having a half life of
    (A) 4.5 billion years  (B) 65 years
    (C) 12 days  (D) 0.001 minute.

120. The nuclear reaction $_3Li^7$ ( $2$ , n) $_5B^{10}$ can be used as a source of which one of the following?
    (A) alpha particles  (B) electrons
    (C) protons  (D) neutrons.

121. When a radioactive atom emits a beta particle from the nucleus, the new substance produced
    (A) has the same atomic number
    (B) gains one unit in atomic mass
    (C) gains one atomic number unit
    (D) gains one neutron.

122. In which one of the following fields would a machine using "magnetic mirrors" most likely be used for research?
    (A) optics  (B) magnetism
    (C) physical optics  (D) fusion reactors

123. Element 102, with a mass number of 253 was synthesized by bombarding $_{96}Cm^{240}$ with a single nuclear particle which it captured. The particle used was which one of the following?
    (A) $_{12}X^{13}$  (B) $_6X^{13}$
    (C) $_{13}X^6$  (D) $_{13}X^{12}$.

124. The radioactive disintegration of an atom of $_{14}Si^{27}$ yields $_{13}Al^{27}$ and a(an)
    (A) proton  (B) neutron
    (C) positron  (D) electron.

125. Which one of the following is an equivalent term to "mass-defect"?
    (A) average atomic weight
    (B) binding energy
    (C) crystal dislocation
    (D) Brillouin zone.

126. Which one of the following is a chemical name for the compound $(C_6H_5)_2AsCl$?
    (A) phenyldichlorarsine
    (B) diethyl chlorarsine
    (C) ethyl dichlorarsine
    (D) diphenyl chlorarsine.

127. An isomer of ethanol is
    (A) methanol  (B) dimethyl ether
    (C) diethyl ether  (D) ethylene glycol.

128. In cis-trans isomerism, the compound generally
    (A) rotates the plane of polarized light
    (B) exhibits enantiomorphism
    (C) possesses an asymmetric carbon atom
    (D) contains a double bond.

129. The degree of unsaturation in an organic compound may be found by shaking a specified weight of the substance with a standard solution of which one of the following?
    (A) sulfuric acid  (B) potassium hydroxide
    (C) acetone  (D) iodine.

130. The structural formula for $\alpha$-amino propionic acid is

131. Of the following, the tertiary alcohol is
    (A) $CH_3 \bullet CH_2 \bullet CH_2OH$
    (B) $(CH_3)_3 \bullet COH$
    (C) $(CH_3)_3C \bullet CH_2OH$
    (D) $CH_3 \bullet CHOH \bullet CH_3$.

132. Which one of the following is the empirical formula for ethyl cyclo pentane?
    (A) $C_7H_{13}$
    (B) $C_7H_9$
    (C) $C_7H_{14}$
    (D) $C_7H_{11}$.

133. The formula for xylene is
    (A) $C_6H_5CH_3$
    (B) $C_6H_3(CH_3)_3$
    (C) $C_6H_4(CH_3)_2$
    (D) $C_6(CH_3)_6$.

134. A solution of the compound D(—) glucose in water will rotate the plane of polarized light to which one of the following?
    (A) to the right
    (B) the left
    (C) either side
    (D) neither side.

135. Of the following substances, the one which could *not* be represented by the empirical formula $C_3H_6O$ is
    (A) acetone
    (B) propanol
    (C) vinyl methyl ether
    (D) ethinyl alcohol.

136. An acidified solution of sucrose on standing is converted into a mixture of which one of the following pairs?
    (A) mannose and talose
    (B) glucose and fructose
    (C) idose and gulose
    (D) altose and sorbose.

137. Which of the following are the chief products in the Fischer-Tropsch synthesis?
    (A) acids
    (B) alcohols
    (C) aldehydes
    (D) ketones.

138. The name of the substance $(NH_2)_2CO$ is
    (A) acetamide
    (B) methylamide
    (C) carbamide
    (D) urea.

139. Which one of the following molecules contains the greatest number of benzene rings?
    (A) quinone
    (B) naphthalene
    (C) phthalic anhydride
    (D) anthracene.

140. The reagent phthalic anhydride is obtained chiefly from the oxidation of
    (A) phthalic acid
    (B) turpentine
    (C) anthracene
    (D) naphthalene.

141. Of the following forms of sulfur, which one is most readily soluble in carbon disulfide?
    (A) amorphous
    (B) prismatic
    (C) rhombic
    (D) plastic.

142. Assume that solution "X" has a pH of 6.0. If solution "Y" has a hydronium ion concentration twice that of solution "X", its pH will be approximately
    (A) 3.0
    (B) 5.7
    (C) 6.0
    (D) 12.8.

143. The triple point for $CO_2$ is —57°C and 5.2 atmospheres. In order to obtain liquid $CO_2$, the
    (A) pressure must be below 5.2 atmospheres
    (B) temperature must be below —57°C
    (C) pressure must be below 5.2 atmospheres and temperature must be greater than —57°C
    (D) pressure must be below 5.2 atmospheres and temperature must be greater than —57°C.

144. The one of the following which is *not* an oxidation-reduction reaction is
    (A) the replacement of iodine by chlorine in sodium iodide
    (B) the Haber process
    (C) the softening of hard water
    (D) the reaction of iron and copper sulfate.

145. The nickel ion is usually identified by
    (A) cupferron
    (B) dimethylglyoxime
    (C) p—nitrobenzene azo resorcinol
    (D) diphenyl benzidine.

146. A mixture of $Al(OH)_3$ and $Fe(OH)_3$ can be separated easily by treatment with which one of the following?
    (A) sodium hydroxide solution
    (B) hydrochloric acid
    (C) sulfuric acid
    (D) ammonium hydroxide solution.

147. A saturated solution of $H_2S$ gas in water at atmospheric pressure and normal room temperature is approximately
    (A) 0.001 M
    (B) 0.1 M
    (C) 0.5 M
    (D) 1.0 M

148. By the addition of which one of the following can the blood-red color be produced in a confirmatory test for the $Fe^{+++}$ ion? A
    (A) cyanate
    (B) thiosulfate
    (C) sulfide
    (D) thiocyanate.

149. Of the following, the element which in solution will form a white precipitate with chloride ion which will turn black on the addition of aqueous ammonia is
    (A) lead
    (B) silver
    (C) tin
    (D) mercury.

150. When 27 grams of Al are added to one liter of 3N $CuSO_4$, the number of grams of Cu that will be displaced is (atomic weights: Cu = 64; AI = 27).
    (A) 32
    (B) 64
    (C) 96
    (D) 128.

151. The Fahrenheit and Centigrade scales of temperature have the same numerical reading at a temperature of
    (A) —40°
    (B) 0°
    (C) 32°
    (D) 212°.

152. When a gas expands adiabatically,
    (A) the temperature remains constant
    (B) energy is liberated
    (C) the pressure increases
    (D) the environment remains unchanged.

153. Of the following situations, the one in which no single electronic formula conforms both to the observed properties and to the octet rule is described as
    (A) isomerism
    (B) allotropism
    (C) enantiomorphism
    (D) resonance.

154. Assuming that 100 ml of a 0.1 solution of $H_2SO_4$ is needed to neutralize 200 ml of a $Ba(OH)_2$ solution, the normality of the $Ba(OH)_2$ solution is
    (A) 0.05
    (B) 0.10
    (C) 0.20
    (D) 0.50.

155. If 22.5 ml of HCl are needed to neutralize 25 ml of 0.1 N $Na_2CO_3$ solution, the normality of the acid is
    (A) 0.037
    (B) 0.056
    (C) 0.111
    (D) 0.167.

156. When a 0.1N solution of an acid of 25°C has a degree of ionization of 1%, the concentration of hydroxyl ions present is
    (A) $10^{-3}$
    (B) $10^{-11}$
    (C) $10^{-12}$
    (D) $10^{-13}$.

157. If a compound has a negative heat of solution, at high temperatures it dissolves
    (A) more rapidly and is more soluble
    (B) more rapidly and is less soluble
    (C) less rapidly and is less soluble
    (D) less rapidly and is more soluble

158. In general, a 1 molar solution of any substance, when converted into molalities at a fixed temperature, will be
    (A) less than 1 molal
    (B) 1 molal
    (C) more than 1 molal
    (D) indeterminate.

159. Eight liters of 0.86 N HBr solution contain
    (A) 6800 millimoles of HBr
    (B) 0.688 moles of HBr
    (C) 6.88 moles of HBr
    (D) 8000 millimoles of HBr.

160. A solution of 4.5g of a pure nonelectrolyte in 100.0g of water was found to freeze at —0.465°C. The molecular weight of the solute is closest to which one of the following?
    (A) 180
    (B) 172.4
    (C) 90
    (D) 86.2.

161. A saturated solution of $Ag_2SO_4$ is 2.5 x $10^{-2}$ M. The value of its solubility product is
    (A) 6.25 x $10^{7-}$
    (B) 1.6 x $10^{-5}$
    (C) 6.25 x $10^{-5}$
    (D) 1.25 x $10^{-3}$.

162. The concentration of hydronium ions in pure water, expressed in moles per liter, is
    (A) $10^{-7}$
    (B) 7
    (C) $1/10^{-7}$
    (D) $10^{-14}$.

163. If solid sodium acetate is added to a dilute solution of acetic acid the pH will
    (A) increase
    (B) be unaffected
    (C) decrease
    (D) first decrease, then increase.

164. The molality of a glucose solution containing 22.5 grams of glucose (atomic weights: C = 12; O = 16; H = 1) in 500 grams of water is closest to which one of the following?
    (A) 0.13
    (B) 0.25
    (C) 0.38
    (D) 0.50.

165. Silver chloride was precipitated by adding HCl to a solution of a silver salt until the concentration of chloride ions is 0.20 mole/liter. Ideally, the concentration of silver ions in this case should be:
    $$(K_{SpAgCl} = 1.56 \text{ x } 10^{-10})$$
    (A) $\sqrt{1.56}$ x $10^{-5}$
    (B) $\sqrt{7.8}$ x $10^{-10}$
    (C) 7.8 x $10^{-10}$
    (D) 1.56 x $10^{-10}$.

166. Of the following, the solvent which is *least* effective in dissolving fats is
    (A) alcohol
    (B) chloroform
    (C) ether
    (D) carbon tetrachloride.

167. Of the following, the compound in which oxygen exhibits an oxidation state of $+2$ is
    (A) $Cl_2O_6$
    (B) $BrO_2$
    (C) $HClO_2$
    (D) $F_2O$.

168. If 1.25 grams of a solid acid neutralize 25 ml of a 0.25 M $Ba(OH)_2$ solution, the equivalent weight of the acid will be
    (A) 25 grams
    (B) 50 grams
    (C) 100 grams
    (D) 200 grams.

169. When an element forms an oxide wherein the oxygen is 20% of the oxide by weight, the equivalent weight of the given element will be
    (A) 32
    (B) 40
    (C) 64
    (D) 128.

170. In the reaction given below, the equivalent weight of $HNO_3$ (Atomic Weights: $H = 1$; $N = 14$; $O = 16$) is closest to which one of the following?
    $$8HNO_3 + 3PbS \rightarrow 8NO + 3PbSO_4 + 4H_2O$$
    (A) 11.6
    (B) 21.0
    (C) 31.5
    (D) 63.0.

171. The oxidation number of nickel in the compound $K_4 [Ni(CN)_4]$ is
    (A) 0
    (B) $+2$
    (C) $-2$
    (D) $+3$.

172. Of the following, the compound whose color is *incorrectly* given is
    (A) $CrSO_4$ — red
    (B) $Cr_2 (SO_4)_3$ — purple
    (C) $K_2CrO_4$ — yellow
    (D) $K_2Cr_2O_7$ — orange.

173. According to the Bronsted Theory, which one of the following substances is classified as a base?
    (A) $Cl^-$
    (B) $H_3O^+$
    (C) $CH_3COOH$
    (D) $NH_4^+$.

174. Of the following, the acid that is most closely related chemically to $P_4O_6$ is
    (A) $HPO_3$
    (B) $H_3PO_3$
    (C) $H_3PO_4$
    (D) $H_4P_2O_7$.

175. According to the Lewis Theory of acids and bases, stannic chloride is
    (A) a base
    (B) neutral
    (C) an acid
    (D) amphoteric.

176. Of the following, the pair of reagents which can be used to separate cupric and aluminum ions from manganous ions is
    (A) $NaOH$ and $Na_2O_2$
    (B) $NaOH$ and tartrate ions
    (C) $NaOH$ and sodium bismuthate
    (D) $NaOH$ and $NH_4OH$.

177. Compounds of manganese that do *not* exhibit para-magnetism are those in which the oxidation state is which one of the following?
    (A) $+2$
    (B) $+4$
    (C) $+6$
    (D) $+7$.

178. An investigation of the energy sublevels of the electron shells in an atom discloses that the energy of the 3d subshell is greater than that of which one of the following?
    (A) 4f subshell
    (B) 4d subshell
    (C) 4p subshell
    (D) 4s subshell.

179. All of the following statements about the group of elements called the transitional elements are true *except* that
    (A) all of the transitional elements are predominantly metallic
    (B) in aqueous solution many of their simple ions are colored
    (C) most of the transitional elements show pronounced catalytic activity
    (D) most of the transitional elements show only one valence state.

180. When the specific heat of a metallic element is 0.214 calories/gram, the atomic weight will be closest to which one of the following?
    (A) 6.6
    (B) 12
    (C) 30
    (D) 66.

181. The most probable valence number for the atom with the total electron configuration, $1s^2 2s^2 2p^6 3s^2 3p^6 3d^{10} 4s^2 4p^5$, is
    (A) $-1$
    (B) $-3$
    (C) $+1$
    (D) $+3$.

182. Which one of the following groups of elements is analogous to the lanthanides?
    (A) halides
    (B) carbides
    (C) actinides
    (D) borides.

183. Heating ammonia with air in the presence of a platinum catalyst will produce
    (A) oxygen and nitrogen
    (B) hydrogen and nitrogen dioxide
    (C) water and nitric oxide
    (D) ammonium hydroxide and nitrous oxide.

184. Lavoisier's experiment to demonstrate the true nature of burning was made possible by the availability of which one of the following?
(A) the metal tin
(B) a lens for focusing sun's rays
(C) a glass retort
(D) a sensitive balance.

185. Hydrogen that is used commercially is frequently obtained from which one of the following?
(A) marsh gas      (B) coal gas
(C) producer gas    (D) water gas.

186. In general, a plastic shows greater strength and rigidity as the polymer molecules show more
(A) crystallinity
(B) amorphous nature
(C) random arrangement
(D) atactic nature.

187. An experiment designed to show the presence of water vapor in the air would probably employ which one of the following?
(A) phosphorus
(B) ammonium hydroxide
(C) hydrated copper sulfate
(D) sodium hydroxide.

188. The type of electronic bonding found in potassium hydride is
(A) covalent      (B) coordinate covalent
(C) metallic        (D) ionic.

189. If ammonium nitrate is heated, the principal product is
(A) $N_2O_5$      (B) $NO$
(C) $N_2O$       (D) $N_2$.

190. An example of a basic anhydride is
(A) $NH_3$      (B) $Na_2CO_3$
(C) $CO_2$       (D) $CaO$

191. Which one of the following substances can be used effectively as a water softener?
(A) sodium tetraborate
(B) calcium bicarbonate
(C) ferric chloride
(D) calcium silicate.

192. $CH_3COOC_2H_5$ is an example of which one of the following?
(A) alcohol      (B) soap
(C) acid         (D) ester.

193. Of the following, the formula which represents an unsaturated organic compound is
(A) $C_6H_{14}$      (B) $C_4H_8$
(C) $C_3H_7OH$    (D) $C_2H_4Cl_2$.

194. A device used to measure the number of nuclear disintegrations per minute is called a
(A) Geiger counter    (B) cyclotron
(C) cloud chamber    (D) electrometer.

195. Because of dangers inherent in the process, special precautions should be taken in diluting concentrated
(A) $HNO_3$      (B) $HCl$
(C) $H_2SO_4$      (D) $H_2C_2O_4$.

196. As the atomic number of the halogens increases, the halogens
(A) lose their outermost electrons less easily
(B) become less dense
(C) become lighter in color
(D) gain electrons less easily.

197. A water solution of which one of the following will have a pH of less than 7?
(A) $CuSO_4$      (B) $Na_3PO_4$
(C) $KCl$       (D) $Na_2CO_3$.

198. The emission of an alpha particle from the nucleus of $_{88}Ra^{226}$ will produce
(A) $_{88}Ra^{222}$      (B) $_{87}Fr^{222}$
(C) $_{87}Fr^{223}$      (D) $_{86}Rn^{222}$.

199. If under standard conditions of temperature and pressure, the weight of one liter of a certain gas is 1.25 grams, the molecular weight of this gas is
(A) 11.2      (B) 22.4
(C) 28        (D) 44.

200. Which one of the following substances is produced when ethyl alcohol in dilute solution is oxidized by action of "mother of vinegar" bacteria?
(A) glucose      (B) carbon monoxide
(C) acetaldehyde   (D) acetic acid.

**CHEMISTRY TEST**

# Correct Answers For The Foregoing Questions

*(Please make every effort to answer the questions on your own before looking at these answers. You'll make faster progress by following this rule.)*

| | | | | | | | | | |
|---|---|---|---|---|---|---|---|---|---|
| 1. A | 21. A | 41. B | 61. C | 81. C | 101. C | 121. C | 141. B | 161. B | 181. A |
| 2. A | 22. B | 42. A | 62. C | 82. C | 102. A | 122. D | 142. B | 162. A | 182. C |
| 3. B | 23. D | 43. C | 63. A | 83. C | 103. C | 123. B | 143. D | 163. A | 183. C |
| 4. C | 24. D | 44. B | 64. D | 84. D | 104. D | 124. C | 144. C | 164. B | 184. D |
| 5. A | 25. A | 45. A | 65. B | 85. D | 105. D | 125. B | 145. B | 165. C | 185. D |
| 6. D | 26. A | 46. A | 66. A | 86. D | 106. C | 126. D | 146. A | 166. A | 186. A |
| 7. D | 27. A | 47. D | 67. D | 87. C | 107. A | 127. B | 147. B | 167. D | 187. D |
| 8. B | 28. B | 48. B | 68. C | 88. D | 108. D | 128. D | 148. D | 168. C | 188. D |
| 9. B | 29. D | 49. A | 69. C | 89. D | 109. C | 129. A | 149. D | 169. A | 189. C |
| 10. D | 30. D | 50. C | 70. D | 90. A | 110. B | 130. B | 150. C | 170. A | 190. D |
| 11. D | 31. C | 51. A | 71. B | 91. D | 111. A | 131. B | 151. A | 171. A | 191. A |
| 12. D | 32. B | 52. C | 72. A | 92. C | 112. A | 132. A | 152. D | 172. A | 192. D |
| 13. D | 33. C | 53. B | 73. C | 93. D | 113. B | 133. C | 153. D | 173. A | 193. B |
| 14. D | 34. A | 54. B | 74. A | 94. B | 114. A | 134. B | 154. B | 174. B | 194. A |
| 15. A | 35. C | 55. C | 75. C | 95. D | 115. C | 135. B | 155. C | 175. A | 195. C |
| 16. C | 36. C | 56. C | 76. A | 96. D | 116. D | 136. B | 156. B | 176. D | 196. D |
| 17. B | 37. B | 57. B | 77. A | 97. A | 117. C | 137. B | 157. A | 177. D | 197. A |
| 18. C | 38. A | 58. C | 78. B | 98. A | 118. D | 138. D | 158. C | 178. D | 198. D |
| 19. C | 39. A | 59. D | 79. B | 99. A | 119. D | 139. D | 159. C | 179. D | 199. C |
| 20. C | 40. C | 60. A | 80. C | 100. B | 120. D | 140. D | 160. A | 180. C | 200. D |

| SCORE 1 | SCORE 2 | SCORE 3 |
|---|---|---|
| ............................ % | ............................ % | ............................ % |
| NO. CORRECT | NO. CORRECT | NO. CORRECT |
| NO. OF QUESTIONS ON THIS TEST | NO. OF QUESTIONS ON THIS TEST | NO. OF QUESTIONS ON THIS TEST |

# INTERPRETATION OF READING MATERIALS IN NATURAL SCIENCE

*We have good reason to believe that this kind of question will appear on your test. We want you to practice now and profit later. Guide and schedule your practice with the rules and tips you got in "Top Scores on Reading Tests." Go back to that chapter as often as needful in doing the questions that follow. If you can commit it to memory, it will help with any kind of reading question that may come up.*

*HERE'S HOW YOU SHOULD ANSWER THESE READING QUESTIONS. Each one is made up of a paragraph, followed by four or five statements based on the paragraph. You may never have seen the paragraph before, but you must now read it carefully so that you understand it. Then read the statements following. Any one of them might be right. You have to choose the one that is most correct. Try to pick the one that's most complete, most accurate ... the one that is best supported by and necessarily flows from the paragraph. Be sure that it contains nothing false so far as the paragraph itself is concerned. After you've thought it out, write the capital letter preceding your best choice in the margin next to the question. When you've answered all the questions, score yourself faithfully by checking with our answers that follow the last question. But please don't look at those answers until you've written your own. You just won't be helping yourself if you do that. Besides, you'll have ample opportunity to do the questions again, and to check with our answers, in the event that your first try results in a low score. If you'd really like to get into the swing of the thing while practicing, you might want to answer on facsimiles of the kind of answer sheets provided on machine-scored examinations. For practice purposes we have provided such facsimiles.*

A portion of the standard answer sheet is provided after each test for marking your answers in the way you'll be required to do on the actual exam. At the right of this answer sheet, to make the scoring job simpler (after you have derived your own answers), you'll find our correct answers.

# NATURAL SCIENCE INTERPRETATION TEST ONE

*DIRECTIONS: Below each of the following passages of natural science reading material you will find one or more incomplete statements about the passage. Select the words or expressions that most satisfactorily complete each statement in accordance with the meaning of the paragraph.*

*Correct key answers to all these test questions will be found at the end of the test.*

*Reading Passage*

Self-contained diving suits have made it possible for a diver to explore the depths without the local authorities' knowing very much about it. Should he be lucky enough to discover a wreck, a diver can recover the less cumbersome fragments, bronzes, marble, or bits of statuary, without attracting official attention. Today one can indulge in a secret treasure hunt right down to the seabed with the added advantage that it is far harder to keep a watch on sunken treasure than it is to protect excavations on shore. So the modern despoiler is as great a pest to the serious archaeologist at sea as he is on land. In Egypt and Syria he has deprived us of invaluable data. He nearly always ransacks his objective to take away some portable trophy which he thinks valuable, he keeps his treasure house a secret, and we must blame him for the appearance of various objects impossible to date or catalog.

1. The title below that best expresses the ideas of this passage is
   (A) Recovering ships
   (B) Modern diving suits
   (C) The irresponsible explorer
   (D) Cataloging long-lost objects
   (E) Concealing the truth in the Near East.

2. The passage suggests that the author is
   (A) opposed to excavations on shore
   (B) sympathetic to the officials
   (C) sympathetic to the divers
   (D) opposed to investigations in Syria and Egypt
   (E) opposed to the despoilers' cataloging their finds.

3. It is to the amateur archaeologist's advantage that local authorities
   (A) protect his findings on land
   (B) allow him to keep portable treasures

(C) provide catalogs of underwater treasures
(D) are sometimes unaware of his diving activities
(E) are ignorant of the true value of sunken treasures.

*Reading Passage*

The white man lapsed easily into an Indian. The mountain man's eye had the Indian's alertness, forever watching for the movement of boughs or grasses, for the passage of wildlife downwind, something unexplained floating in a stream, dust stirring in a calm, or the configuration of mere scratches on a cottonwood. His ear would never again hear church bells or the noises of a farm, but, like the Indian's, was tuned to catch any sound in a country where every sound was provisionally a death warning. He dressed like an Indian, in blankets, robes, buckskins, and moccasins. He lived like an Indian in bark huts or skin lodges. He thought like an Indian, propitiating the demons of the wild, making medicine, and consulting the omens.

4. The title below that best expresses the ideas of this passage is
   (A) Signs of an enemy
   (B) In praise of the Indian
   (C) Characteristics of a traitor
   (D) The white man turned Indian
   (E) Disadvantages of Indian life.

5. The author states that the mountain man was
   (A) homesick        (D) alert
   (B) patriotic        (E) learned.
   (C) humble

6. This passage suggests that the Indian is
   (A) careless
   (B) antisocial
   (C) contemptuous of the whites
   (D) a lover of his family
   (E) superstitious.

*Reading Passage*

We were about a quarter mile away when quiet swept over the colony. A thousand or more heads periscoped. Two thousand eyes glared. Save for our wading, the world's business had stopped. A thousand avian personalities were concentrated on us, and the psychological force of this was terrific. Contingents of homecoming feeders, suddenly aware of four strange specks moving across the lake, would bank violently and speed away. Then the chain reaction began. Every throat in that rookery let go with a concatenation of wild, raspy, terrorized trumpet bursts. With all wings now fully spread and churning, and quadrupling the color mass, the birds began to move as one, and the sky was filled with the sound of judgment day.

7. The title below that best expresses the idea of this passage is
    (A) Our shore birds
    (B) A quiet colony
    (C) Judgment day
    (D) Waiting
    (E) An unwelcome intrusion.

8. The passage indicates that the writer
    (A) was a psychologist
    (B) observed the fear of the flying birds
    (C) was terrified at the sounds
    (D) crossed the lake by boat
    (E) went alone to the rookery.

9. According to the passage, when they first noticed the visitors, the birds of the colony
    (A) flew away
    (B) became very quiet
    (C) churned their wings
    (D) set up a series of cries
    (E) glared at the homecoming birds.

10. The reaction of the visitors to the experience described in this passage was probably one of
    (A) impatience      (D) awe
    (B) fear            (E) sadness.
    (C) anger

*Reading Passage*

Lumbering in the Northwest in the early days was often a two-fisted business, in which one would say that neither the lumber barons nor the lumberjacks had learned a thing from the wastage, the fires, the boom-and-bust days, and stump counties of eastern history. Nothing, that is, except greatly increased efficiency at whirlwind exploitation. But that was in a cruder age, in the days when labor troubles went to the shooting stage, when pirates on

Puget Sound stole whole rafts of timber, when fires burned over forests the size of many a European principality, and when the Forest Service was jeered at and obstructed. Those days are gone. Progressive companies now hire their own trained foresters and follow practical conservation. Well-located lumber towns have become permanent cities with fine schools and churches. Employees are usually married, eat the best food, and own their homes. Fire is fought like the Devil.

11. The title below that best expresses the ideas of this passage is
    (A) Forestry today
    (B) The good old days
    (C) Lessons of history
    (D) Lumber baron and lumberjack
    (E) Improvement in the lumber industry.

12. Early methods of lumbering were
    (A) unplanned       (D) extravagant
    (B) impractical     (E) magnificent.
    (C) pugnacious

*Reading Passage*

The six year old is about the best example that can be found of that type of inquisitiveness that causes irritated adults to exclaim, "Curiosity killed the cat." To him, the world is a fascinating place to be explored and investigated quite thoroughly, but such a world is bounded by the environment in which he or the people he knows live. It is constantly expanding through new experiences, which bring many eager questions from members of any group of first graders, as each one tries to figure out new relationships—to know and accept his place within the family, the school, and the community—to understand all around him. There are adults who find it quite annoying to be presented with such rank inquisitiveness. But this is no purposeless prying, no idle curiosity! It is that quality, characteristic of the successful adult, inherent in the good citizen—intellectual curiosity.

13. The title below that best expresses the ideas of this passage is
    (A) A new-found world
    (B) New relationships
    (C) Wonders of growth
    (D) Purposeless prying
    (E) Curiosity—six-year-old style.

14. The author states that a successful adult inherently exhibits
  (A) irritation
  (B) questioning
  (C) curiosity
  (D) comprehension of change
  (E) understanding of machines.

15. In this passage the author's attitude toward children is one of
  (A) despair
  (B) confidence
  (C) indifference
  (D) sharp criticism
  (E) exaggerated optimism.

# Correct Answers For The Foregoing Questions

*To assist you in scoring yourself we have provided Correct Answers alongside your Answer Sheet. May we therefore suggest that while you are doing the test you cover the Correct Answers with a sheet of white paper.....to avoid temptation and to arrive at an accurate estimate of your ability and progress.*

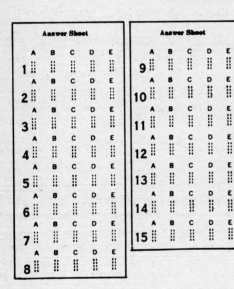

SCORE

_____ %

NO. CORRECT ÷

NO. OF QUESTIONS ON THIS TEST

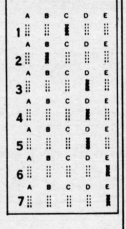

# NATURAL SCIENCE INTERPRETATION TEST TWO

*DIRECTIONS: Below each of the following passages of natural science reading material you will find one or more incomplete statements about the passage. Select the words or expressions that most satisfactorily complete each statement in accordance with the meaning of the paragraph.*

*Correct key answers to all these test questions will be found at the end of the test.*

*Reading Passage*

Observe the dilemma of the fungus: it is a plant, but it possesses no chlorophyl. While all other plants can put the sun's energy to work for them combining the nutrients of ground and air into body structure, the chlorophylless fungus must look elsewhere for an energy source. It finds it in those other plants which, having received their energy free from the sun, relinquish it at some point in their cycle either to other animals (like us humans) or to fungi.

In this search for energy the fungus has become the earth's major source of rot and decay. Wherever you see mold forming on a piece of bread, or a pile of leaves turning to compost, or a blowndown tree becoming pulp on the ground, you are watching a fungus eating. Without fungus action the earth would be piled high with the dead plant life of past centuries. In fact certain plants which contain resins that are toxic to fungi will last indefinitely; specimens of the redwood, for instance, can still be found resting on the forest floor centuries after having been blown down.

1. The title below that best expresses the ideas of this passage is
   (A) Life without cholorophyl
   (B) The source of rot and decay
   (C) The harmful qualities of fungi
   (D) The strange world of the fungus
   (E) Utilization of the sun's energy.

2. The statement ". . . you are watching a fungus eating" is best described as
   (A) figurative
   (B) ironical
   (C) parenthetical
   (D) joking
   (E) contradictory.

3. The author implies that fungi
   (A) are responsible for all the world's rot and decay
   (B) cannot live completely apart from other plants
   (C) attack plants in order to kill them
   (D) are poisonous to resin-producing plants
   (E) can survive indefinitely under favorable conditions.

4. The author uses the word "dilemma" to indicate that
   (A) the fungus is both helpful and harmful in its effects
   (B) no one really understands how a fungus lives
   (C) fungi are not really plants
   (D) the function of chlorophyl in producing energy is a puzzle to scientists
   (E) the fungus seems to have its own biological laws.

*Reading Passage*

It is here, perhaps, that poetry may best act nowadays as corrective and complementary to science. When science tells us that the galaxy to which our solar system belongs is so enormous that light, traveling at 186,000 miles per second, takes between 60,000 and 100,000 years to cross from one rim to the other of the galaxy, we laymen accept the statement but find it meaningless—beyond the comprehension of heart or mind. When science tells us that the human eye has about 137 million separate "seeing" elements, we are no less paralyzed, intellectually and emotionally. Man is appalled by the immensities and the minuteness which science has disclosed for him. They are indeed unimaginable. But may not poetry be a possible way of mediating them to our imagination?—of scaling them down to imaginative comprehension? Let us remember Perseus, who could not look directly at the nightmare Gorgon without being turned to stone, but could look at her image reflected in the shield the goddess of wisdom lent him.

5. The title below that best expresses the ideas of this passage is
   (A) Poetry and imagination
   (B) A modern Gorgon
   (C) Poetry as a mediator
   (D) The vastness of the universe
   (E) Imaginative man.

6. According to the passage, the average man
   (A) should have a better memory
   (B) is impatient with science
   (C) cannot trust the scientists
   (D) is overwhelmed by the discoveries of science
   (E) does not understand either science or poetry.

7. Perseus was most probably
   (A) a scientist
   (B) a legendary hero
   (C) an early poet
   (D) a horrible creature
   (E) a minor god.

8. This passage is chiefly developed by means of
   (A) examples          (D) definition
   (B) cause and effect   (E) anecdotes.
   (C) narration

*Reading Passage*

Hail is at once the cruelest weapon in Nature's armory, and the most incalculable. It can destroy one farmer's prospects of a harvest in a matter of seconds; it can leave his neighbor's unimpaired. It can slay a flock of sheep (it has killed children before now) in one field, while the sun continues to shine in the next. To the harassed meteorologist its behavior is even more Machiavellian than that of an ice storm. Difficult as it undoubtedly is for him to forecast the onset of an ice storm, he knows pretty well what its course and duration will be once it has started; just about all he can do with a hailstone is to measure the size of the stones—and they have a habit of melting as soon as he gets his hands on them. He is not even too sure any more about the way in which hail forms—and until he knows this, of course, he isn't likely to stumble upon any very satisfactory prognostic rules.

9. The title below that best expresses the ideas of this passage is
   (A) Forecasting ice storms
   (B) The way that hail forms
   (C) The harassed meteorologist
   (D) The unpredictability of hailstorms
   (E) Hail—the killer.

10. As used in the passage, the word "prognostic" (last line) most nearly means
   (A) restraining        (D) foretelling
   (B) breakable          (E) regular.
   (C) day-by-day

## Correct Answers For The Foregoing Questions

*To assist you in scoring yourself we have provided Correct Answers alongside your Answer Sheet. May we therefore suggest that while you are doing the test you cover the Correct Answers with a sheet of white paper.....to avoid temptation and to arrive at an accurate estimate of your ability and progress.*

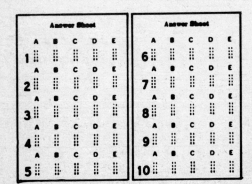

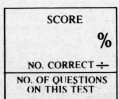

SCORE

%

NO. CORRECT ÷

NO. OF QUESTIONS ON THIS TEST

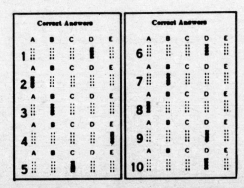

# NATURAL SCIENCE INTERPRETATION TEST THREE

*DIRECTIONS: Below each of the following passages of natural science reading material you will find one or more incomplete statements about the passage. Select the words or expressions that most satisfactorily complete each statement in accordance with the meaning of the paragraph.*

*Correct key answers to all these test questions will be found at the end of the test.*

*Reading Passage*

Lamarck's theory of evolution, although at one time pretty generally discredited, has now been revived by a number of prominent biologists. According to Lamarck, changes in an animal occur through use and disuse. Organs which are specially exercised become specially developed. The need for this special exercise arises from the conditions in which the animal lives; thus a changing environment, by making different demands on an animal, changes the animal. The giraffe, for instance, has developed is long neck in periods of relative scarcity by endeavoring to browse on higher and higher branches of trees. On the other hand, organs that are never exercised tend to disappear altogether. The eyes of animals that have taken to living in the dark grow smaller and smaller, generation after generation, until the late descendants are born eyeless.

The great assumption made by this theory is that the effects of personal, individual effort are transmitted to the offspring of that individual. This is a doctrine that is very much in dispute among modern biologists.

1. The title below that best expresses the ideas of this passage is
   (A) Why Lamarck's theory is valid
   (B) A changing environment
   (C) The modern biologist
   (D) The Lamarckian theory
   (E) An attack on Lamarck's theory.

2. According to the passage, most scientists today regard Lamarck's theory of evolution as
   (A) controversial      (D) important
   (B) disproved          (E) misunderstood.
   (C) accepted

3. The author's chief purpose in writing this passage was to

(A) discredit other theories of evolution
(B) indicate how heredity influences environment
(C) show why animals become extinct
(D) explain a concept of biology
(E) encourage the acceptance of Lamarck's theory.

4. Which pattern do the ideas of this passage follow?
   (A) general to particular, only
   (B) particular to general, only
   (C) general to particular to general
   (D) particular to particular to general
   (E) general to general to particular.

*Reading Passage*

The problems we face in conserving natural resources are laborious and complex. The preservation of even small bits of marshlands or woods representing the last stands of irreplaceable biotic communities is interwoven with the red tape of law, conflicting local interests, the overlapping jurisdiction of governmental and private conservation bodies, and an intricate tangle of economic and social considerations. During the time spent in resolving these factors, it often happens that the area to be preserved is swallowed up. Even more formidable is the broad-scale conservation problem raised by the spread of urban belts in such places as the northeastern part of the United States. The pressures of human growth are so acute in such instances that they raise issues which would tax the wisdom of Solomon.

5. The title below that best expresses the ideas of this passage is
   (A) Conservation's last stand
   (B) The encroaching suburbs
   (C) Hindrances to conservation

(D) How to preserve our resources
(E) An insoluble problem.

6. The most perplexing problem of conservationists is the one involving
   (A) population growth
   (B) public indifference
   (C) favorable legislation
   (D) division of authority
   (E) increased taxes.

7. The author's attitude toward the situation he describes is
   (A) optimistic
   (B) realistic
   (C) bitter
   (D) illogical
   (E) combative.

*Reading Passage*

It is perfectly clear that nature had no intention that any of her children would be monkeying around with radioactive elements, else she would have provided us with some sixth sense to protect us from running headlong into dangerous amounts of radiation. No, she evidently expected us to take our daily dose of cosmic and earth's radiation as we take the cuts and bruises of ordinary living. The idea of getting them out in the form of concentrated extracts was man's, and since the day when the Curies isolated radium from pitchblende, men have had to extend their perceptive capacities by means of various devices.

The earliest device, which indeed first aroused the Curies to pioneer the wilderness of radioactivity, was the fogging of photographic emulsion. Today it is still a very practical method of detecting radiation and is used universally by people working with radioactivity. Film, of course, is no good as a warning device. It can merely tell you later, when developed and compared to a standard, how much radiation you have been exposed to.

8. The title that best expresses the ideas of this passage is
   (A) Our sixth sense
   (B) The Curies' discovery
   (C) Detecting radiation
   (D) The wilderness of radioactivity
   (E) Radioactive elements.

9. The author implies that ever since the Curies isolated radium it has been necessary for scientists to
   (A) avoid radioactive elements
   (B) protect themselves from cosmic radiation
   (C) learn more about the art of photography
   (D) extend their use of concentrated extracts
   (E) be careful about overdoses of radiation.

10. The paragraph which follows this selection most probably deals with
    (A) further dangers in radioactive materials
    (B) a second device for measuring radioactivity
    (C) an explanation of the use of films as warning devices
    (D) the sources of pitchblende
    (E) the standard used to measure radioactivity.

## Correct Answers For The Foregoing Questions

*To assist you in scoring yourself we have provided, Correct Answers alongside your Answer Sheet. May we therefore suggest that while you are doing the test you cover the Correct Answers with a sheet of white paper.....to avoid temptation and to arrive at an accurate estimate of your ability and progress.*

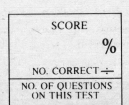

# NATURAL SCIENCE GLOSSARY

*This is some of the language you're likely to see on your examination. You may not need to know all the words in this carefully prepared glossary, but if even a few appear, you'll be that much ahead of your competitors. Perhaps the greater benefit from this list is the frame of mind it can create for you. Without reading a lot of technical text you'll steep yourself in just the right atmosphere for high test marks.*

This glossary was created to help you master some of the key words you will meet in the Natural Science section of the test. Generally, the test deals with four natural sciences: astronomy, biology, chemistry, and physics. You should know that astronomy is the study of celestial bodies, biology the study of living things, chemistry the study of the composition of different kinds of matter and the changes that happen to them, and physics the study of the actions of objects and the reasons behind their actions.

In the glossary, you will usually find a science in parenthesis after the word. This means that the word is by and large identified with that science. That does not mean that the word might not be used in other sciences, though. The word *element* refers to a chemical element and is used, of course, in connection with chemistry. But uranium is an element which is most important in nuclear fission, which is usually considered part of the field of physics.

You will notice that certain words or phrases have been italicized. These italicized words are defined in the glossary.

# [A]

**absolute zero**   (physics) The lowest temperature to which a gas can get. This is 460 degrees below zero on the *Fahrenheit* scale and 273 degrees below zero on the *centigrade* scale.

**acceleration**   (physics) A change in the speed of an object. If the object goes faster, this is called positive acceleration. If the object goes slower, it is called negative acceleration.

**acid**   (chemistry) A *compound* that dissolves in water, has a sour taste, and changes blue *litmus paper* to red.

**alchemy** (chemistry) The *theory* that less valuable metals can be transformed into gold or silver. This idea, popular during the Middle Ages, was false, but the *experiments* of alchemists laid the foundation of modern *chemistry*.

**alkali** (chemistry) A *base* that dissolves in water, has a bitter taste, and changes red *litmus paper* to blue.

**alkaline** (chemistry) The adjective form of *alkali*.

**ampere** (physics) A measurement of the *velocity* of electric current. It was named after a French scientist, Andre Marie Ampère.

**Ampère, Andre Marie** (physics) A French scientist (1775–1836) whose work and *theory* laid the foundation for the science of electrodynamics. His name lives on in the electrical measurement *ampere*, and its abbreviation, amp.

**amphipods** (biology) A *crustacean* group that includes sand fleas.

**anatomy** (biology) The study of the structure of living things. Usually anatomy refers to the structure of the human body.

**anemone** (biology) A sea animal that resembles the flower of the same name.

**aphid** (biology) A small insect which is destructive to crops. A fluid produced by aphids is eaten by ants.

**aquatic** (biology) An adjective referring to water, such as "aquatic sports" (diving, swimming, etc.)

**Aristotle** (biology) An ancient Greek philosopher whose active mind pondered all aspects of life and its processes. He is often called the "Father of Biology."

**asteroids** (astronomy) Small *planet*-like bodies that orbit around the sun.

**astrology** (astronomy) A false *theory* that the position of the stars, sun, moon and planets influence people's lives. Although this is false, the study of astrology was most helpful to the development of *astronomy*.

**astronomer** (astronomy) A person who studies the movements of *celestial* bodies.

**astronomy** The study of the movements of *celestial* bodies. This is a major science.

**atmosphere** (general) The air mass surrounding the earth.

**atom** (physics and chemistry) A small particle of matter. See *atomic energy*. Once it was thought that the atom was the smallest particle of matter that existed, but now it is known that atoms are made up of *protons*, *neutrons* and *electrons*.

**atomic energy** (physics) Power released when *atoms* are split or united. This is also called *nuclear* energy. Also see *nuclear fission* and *nuclear fusion*.

# [B]

**bacteria** (biology) Tiny *organisms* with one *cell*.

**bacteriology** (biology) The study of *bacteria*. Bacteriology is a branch of *biology*.

**base** (chemistry) A compound that can combine with an *acid* to make a *salt*.

**biochemistry** (biology and chemistry) The study of the chemical makeup of *organisms*. This science is a branch of both *chemistry* and *biology*.

**biology** The study of living things. This is a major science.

**botany** (biology) The study of plant life. Botany is a branch of *biology*.

**Brahe, Tycho** (astronomy) A Danish *astronomer* (1546–1601) who made the first systematic study of the movement of *celestial* bodies. He is often referred to only as Tycho.

# [C]

**carbohydrate** (biology) A food substance made up of *carbon*, *hydrogen* and *oxygen*.

**carbon** (chemistry) An important chemical *element*.

**carbon dioxide** (chemistry) A gas made up of *carbon* and *oxygen*.

**celestial** (astronomy) An adjective referring to the sky.

**cell** (biology) The basic and smallest part of living things.

**centigrade** (physics) A system of measurement of temperature. On the centigrade scale, the freezing point of water is zero degrees. The boiling point of water is 100 degrees. Another generally used temperature measurement is the *Fahrenheit* scale.

**chemistry** The study of the composition of different kinds of matter and the changes that happen to them. This is a major science.

**chlorophyll** (biology) The green coloring matter in the cells of living plants, caused by sunlight. Chlorophyll is the means by which all regular absorption and digestion of plant food is made.

**chromosome** (biology) The part of *cells* that determines heredity. Chromosomes contain *genes*.

**colloid** (chemistry) A substance that does not pass through *membranes* very quickly and may not pass through them at all.

**compound** (chemistry) The combining of two or more *elements* into a single unit.

**conduction** (physics) The process by which heat is carried from *molecule* to molecule.

**conservation of energy** (chemistry) The idea that *energy* changes its form but cannot be created or destroyed.

**conservation of matter** (chemistry) The idea that matter can change its form but cannot be created or destroyed.

**constellation** (astronomy) A particular grouping of stars.

**copepod** (biology) A small *crustacean* which is in the *plankton* family.

**Copernicus, Nicholas** (astronomy) A Polish astronomer (1473–1543) who put forth the idea that the earth moved through space. It was generally believed in this time that the earth was the center of the *universe* and did not move through space at all.

**cosmic year** (astronomy) The time it takes the sun to go around its *galaxy*.

**crop rotation** (biology) A method by which crops in an area are changed each year. This helps maintain the *fertility* of the soil.

**crustacean** (biology) A group of *aquatic* animals with a hard covering. They are often called "shellfish."

**crystal** (chemistry) The form many inanimate objects take.

# [D]

**Dalton, John** (physics) An English scientist (1766–1844) who set forth the idea that matter was made up of *atoms*.

**Darwin, Charles** (biology) The English scientist (1809–1883) who developed a *theory* of *evolution*.

**deforestation** (biology) The process by which land is cleared of forests.

**dorso-ventral** (biology) An adjective referring to the dorsal vertebrae. These are a set of bones which are found in the spinal column of the human body near the chest.

# [E]

**eclipse** (astronomy) The blotting out of light when one *celestial* object moves in front of another celestial object. When the moon comes between the earth and the sun it casts a shadow or an eclipse on part of the earth. During this time, the sun cannot be seen on that part of the earth. This is known as a *solar eclipse*. When the earth comes between the sun and the moon, it casts a shadow on the moon. The moon cannot be seen during this time. This is a *lunar eclipse*.

**Einstein, Albert** (physics) A German scientist (1879–1955) who lived the last years of his life in the United States. His *theories* changed the field of *physics*. He, more than any other scientist, was responsible for *nuclear fission*.

**electron** (physics) The smallest electrical charge known. It is part of every *atom*. See *proton* and *neutron*.

**electronics** (physics) The study of the motion of *electrons*.

**element** (chemistry) One of 102 known basic substances. These substances, or combinations of them, make up all matter as far as is known.

**embryology** (biology) The study of the early development of *organisms*, usually plant and animal.

**energy** (physics) The capacity to do *work*.

**enzyme** (biology) An *organic* substance that acts as an agent of change within cells.

**eugenics** (biology) A system it is thought will improve the human race by mating so-called superior men and women.

**evolution, theory of** (biology) Usually refers to *Darwin's theory* that living things change from generation to generation. Furthermore, the living things that survive, according to Darwin, manage to do so because they have acquired certain characteristics that make them more powerful or adaptable than others of their kind.

**evaporation** (biology and chemistry) The process by which liquids and solids change to gases.

**experiment** (general) A test to see if an idea is true or false.

# [F]

**Fahrenheit** (physics) The system of measurement of temperature which is generally used in the United States. It was developed by Gabriel Fahrenheit (1686–1736), a German scientist. On the Fahrenheit scale, 32 degrees is the freezing point of water and 98.6 degrees is the average temperature of the human body. Another widely used temperature measurement is the *centigrade* scale.

**Faraday, Michael** (physics) An English scientist (1791–1867) who discovered electricity could move through metal by the use of a magnet.

**fertility** (biology) The ability to reproduce. See *reproduction*.

**force** (physics) That which stops or creates motion, or changes the *velocity* of motion.

**friction** (physics) The resistance objects have when they are moved across other objects.

**fungi** (biology) A group of simple plants. Fungi do not have any leaves, flowers or color. Because they have no *chlorophyll*, they must feed on plants, animals or decaying matter.

**fungicides** (biology) Chemicals which kill *fungi*.

# [G]

**galaxy** (astronomy) A grouping of stars. Our sun is a star in the galaxy called the Milky Way.

**Galileo** (astronomy and physics) An Italian scientist (1564–1642) who made many contributions to science. He discovered that objects of different weights and shapes fall to the ground at the same rate of speed, attracted by *gravity*. He was a strong believer in *Copernicus'* theory that the earth moved in space and was persecuted for this belief.

**gene** (biology) A part of the *cell* found in the chromosome. Genes determine the traits of *heredity*.

**genetics** (biology) The study of the differences and similarities between living things and those living things that have reproduced them. See *reproduction*.

**geology**   (general) The study of how the earth has changed since its beginning.

**gravitation**   (physics and astronomy) The tendency of objects in space to move towards each other.

**gravity**   (physics and astronomy) Usually the tendency of smaller objects to move towards the earth.

# [H]

**Harvey, William**   (biology) An English scientist (1578–1657) who discovered the way blood moves through the body.

**heat**   (physics) The measurement of *kinetic energy*.

**hemoglobin**   (biology) A substance that gives blood its red color.

**heredity**   (biology) The way traits are carried from generation to generation.

**hormone**   (biology) An *organic* substance produced by the body. Hormones are responsible for many bodily functions.

**hydrogen**   (chemistry) One of the most important chemical *elements*.

**hypothesis**   (general) An unproved explanation of something that has happened or might happen.

# [I]

**inorganic**   (biology) An adjective meaning "not organic." See *organic*.

**insecticides**   (biology) Chemical combinations used to destroy harmful insects.

**interstellar**   (astronomy) An adjective meaning "between the stars."

**isotopes**   (physics) Atoms that belong to the same chemical element, but are different in weight or mass.

# [K]

**Kepler, Johannes**   (astronomy) A German *astronomer* (1571–1630) who made important discoveries about the *orbits* of *planets*.

**kinetic energy**   (physics) *Energy* that is in motion. The motion of the baseball between the pitcher's hand and the catcher's glove is an example of kinetic energy. See *potential energy*.

**Koch, Robert**   (biology) A German doctor (1843–1910) who studied bacteria. He and *Louis Pasteur* are considered the founders of the science of *bacteriology*.

# [L]

**Lamarck, Chevalier de** (biology) A French scientist (1744–1829) who developed a *theory* of *evolution*. See *Darwin*.

**Lavoisier, Antoine** (chemistry) A French scientist (1743–1794) who made important discoveries concerning fire and *conservation of matter*.

**light year** (astronomy) The distance it takes light to travel through *interstellar* space in one year.

**Linnaeus, Carolus** (biology) A Swedish scientist (1707–1778) best-known for developing a system to name animals and plants.

**litmus paper** (chemistry) A special paper used by chemists to test for *acid* and *alkalies*.

**lunar** (astronomy) An adjective referring to the moon. A lunar *eclipse* is an eclipse of the moon. See *solar*.

# [M]

**marine** (biology) An adjective meaning ''of the sea.'' Example: ''Fish are a form of marine life.''

**molecule** (physics and chemistry) A basic unit of matter made up of *atoms*.

**mechanics** (physics) The study of the effect force has on moving or motionless bodies. This is a branch of *physics*.

**membrane** (biology) Soft, thin sheet of tissue in an *organism*. A membrane acts as a wall between two different parts of the organism, or it covers a particular part of the organism.

**Mendel, Gregor Johann** (biology) An Austrian monk and scientist (1822–1844) who made important discoveries concerning *heredity*.

**metabolism** (biology) The process used by all living *organisms* to change food into tissue and *energy*.

**mercury** (chemistry) An important chemical *element*.

**meteorology** (general) A science that studies the weather and the *atmosphere*.

**mollusks** (biology) A family of animals usually found in water. Mollusks have no bones. Examples of mollusks are snails, oysters, and octopuses.

**mutation** (biology) A change from the parents in an offspring. If a rat was born with no tail although its parents had tails, this change would be a mutation.

# [N]

**nebula** (astronomy) A cloudy and gaseous mass found in *interstellar* space.

**neutron** (physics and chemistry) A small particle that is part of the *atom* and has no electrical charge. See *electron* and *proton*.

**Newton, Isaac** (physics and astronomy) An English scientist (1642–1727) who made major discoveries in *astronomy* and *physics*. His most important work was in his study of *gravitation* and *optics*.

**nuclear** (physics) An adjective referring to the *nucleus* of the *atom*.

**nuclear fission** (physics) The splitting of an *atom* in order to produce *energy*.

**nuclear fusion** (physics) The joining together of light-weight *atoms* resulting in the releasing of *energy*.

**nucleus** (physics and chemistry) The center or core of an object, necessary to maintain human life.

# [O]

**observatory** (astronomy) A specially constructed building containing one or more telescopes for observation of the heavens.

**optics** (physics) The study of light and its effect. Optics is a branch of *physics*.

**orbit** (astronomy) The route that an object in space (such as the moon) takes around another body (such as the earth).

**organic** (biology) An adjective referring to living things. See *inorganic*.

**organism** (biology) Living things, such as people, plants or animals.

**oxide** (chemistry) A compound made up of *oxygen* and another *element*. Water, for example, is a compound made up of 2 *atoms* of *hydrogen* for each atom of oxygen.

**oxygen** (chemistry) A very important chemical element. Oxygen, a gaseous element, makes up about 20% of air and is the supporter of ordinary combustion.

# [P]

**Pasteur, Louis** (biology) A French scientist (1822–1895) who made major discoveries in *chemistry* and *biology*, especially in the control of many diseases. He and Robert Koch were the founders of the science of *bacteriology*.

**physics** The study of the action of objects and the reasons behind these actions.

**phytogeographic map** (biology) A map showing plant life.

**Planck, Max** (physics) A German scientist (1858–1947) who did notable work in *thermodynamics*.

**planet** (astronomy) A large body that moves around the sun. The earth is a planet.

**plankton** (biology) A group of sea life—both plant and animal—which drifts with tides and currents. Jellyfish are an example of plankton.

**potential energy** (physics) *Energy* that is available for use. The baseball in the pitcher's hand is an example of potential energy. It becomes *kinetic energy* when it is thrown.

**Priestley, Joseph** (chemistry) The English chemist (1738–1804) who discovered *oxygen.*

**primeval** (general) An adjective meaning "the first" or "early."

**protein** (biology) A class of food necessary for life. Proteins build tissues and provide *energy.*

**proton** (physics) An electrically charged particle found in all *atoms.* See *electron* and *neutrons.*

**protoplasm** (biology) A substance necessary for life found in the *cells* of all *organisms.*

# [R]

**radio astronomy** (astronomy) The study of radio waves received from outer space.

**regeneration** (biology) The capacity of an *organism* to create new parts of itself.

**reproduction** (biology) The process by which *organisms* create offspring of their own species.

# [S]

**salinity** (chemistry) The degree of salt present. Usually refers to the amount of salt in a fluid.

**salt** (biology) A substance that is formed when an *acid* is mixed with a *base.*

**satellite** (astronomy) An object that *orbits* around a *planet,* such as a moon. In recent years, the earth has had man-made satellites.

**soluble** (chemistry) Able to be dissolved in a fluid. See *solute, solvent* and *solution.*

**solar** (astronomy) An adjective referring to the sun. A solar *eclipse* is an eclipse of the sun. See *lunar.*

**solar system** (astronomy) The sun, the *planets, satellites,* and the *asteroids.*

**solute** (chemistry) What is dissolved in a fluid to form a *solution.* See *solution, soluble,* and *solvent.*

**solution** (chemistry) A solution occurs when a liquid, solvent or gas mixes completely in a fluid. For example, when sugar is completely dissolved in hot water, the result is a solution. See *solute, solvent,* and *soluble.*

**solvent** (chemistry) The fluid in which a *solute* is dissolved to form a *solution.* Also see *soluble.*

**sonic** (physics) An adjective referring to sound.

**spawn** (biology) A noun referring to the eggs of certain *aquatic* animals, such as fish. Also a verb meaning to lay eggs, usually used in connection with fish.

**stimulus** (general) That which brings a response. If a person is hungry, the sight of food might make his mouth water. The stimulus is food, and the response, the watering of the mouth.

**substratum** (geology) A layer lying beneath the top layer.

**supersonic** (physics) An adjective meaning "faster than sound."

# [T, U]

**theory**  (general) An unproved explanation of something that has happened or might happen.

**thermodynamics**  (physics) The study of the actions of *heat*.

**ultrasonic**  (physics) An adjective referring to sound no person can hear because of its high frequency.

**unicellular**  (biology) An adjective meaning "one-celled." See *cell*.

**universe**  (astronomy) All things that exist in space taken as a whole.

# [V]

**velocity**  (physics) The rate of motion.

**Vesalius, Andreas**  (biology) An Italian scientist (1514–1564) who studied the body. His discoveries were so important that he is often referred to as "The Father of Anatomy." See *anatomy*.

**virus**  (biology) A tiny germ that attacks body *cells* and causes disease.

**vitamins**  (biology) Name for many special substances found in food which are necessary for the operation of particular functions of the body and to maintain health.

# [W, X, Y, Z]

**water table**  (general) The level nearest to the surface of the ground where water is found.

**work**  (physics) In science, work is what occurs when a *force* moves an object.

**zoology**  (biology) The study of animals. This science is a branch of *biology*.

# PART THREE

*Pinpoint Practice*
*For Verbal and Quantitative Ability*

3

# Practice Using Answer Sheets

Alter numbers to match the practice and drill questions in each part of the book.
Make only ONE mark for each answer. Additional and stray marks may be counted as mistakes.
In making corrections, erase errors COMPLETELY. Make glossy black marks.

# TOP SCORES ON VOCABULARY TESTS

*Although questions on vocabulary may not actually appear on your test, it is advisable to practice with the kind of material you have in this chapter. Words and their meanings are quite important in pushing up your score on tests of reading, comprehension, effective writing and correct usage. By broadening your vocabulary, you will definitely improve your marks in these and similar subjects.*

## INCREASE YOUR VOCABULARY

How is your vocabulary? Do you know the meanings of just about every word you come upon in your reading—or do you find several words that stump you? You must increase your vocabulary if you want to read with understanding. Following are six steps that you can take in order to build up your word power:

(a) Read as much as you have the time for. Don't confine yourself to one type of reading either. Read all kinds of things—newspaper, magazines, books. Seek variety in what you read—different newspapers, several types of magazines, all types of books (novels, poetry, essays, plays, etc.). If you get into the habit of reading widely, your vocabulary will grow by leaps and bounds. You'll learn the meanings of words *by context.* That means that, very often, even though you may not know the meaning of a certain word in a sentence, the other words that you are familiar with will help you get the meaning of the hard word.

(b) Take vocabulary tests. There are many practice books which have word tests. We suggest one of these: *2300 Steps to Word Power*—$1.45 (Arco Publishing Co.). These tests are fun to take—and they will build up your vocabulary fast.

(c) Listen to lectures, discussions, and talks by people who speak well. There are some worthwhile TV programs that have excellent speakers. Listen to such people—you'll learn a great many words from them simply by listening to them.

(d) Use a dictionary. Whenever you don't know the meaning of a word, make a note of it. Then, when you get to a dictionary, look up the meaning of the word. Keep your own little notebook—call it "New Words." In a month or two, you will have added a great many words to your vocabulary. If you do not have a dictionary at home, you should buy one. It is just as important in your life as pots and pans, furniture, or a television set. A good dictionary is not expensive. Any one of the following is highly recommended—and costs about five or six dollars:

*Standard College Dictionary* (Funk and Wagnalls)

*Seventh New Collegiate Dictionary* (Merriam-Webster)

*American College Dictionary* (Random House)

You'll never regret buying a good dictionary for your home.

(c) Play word games. Have you ever played Anagrams or Scrabble? They're really interesting. Buy one of these at a stationery store. They are quite inexpensive but effective in building up your vocabulary. Crossword puzzles will teach you new words also. Practically every daily newspaper has a crossword puzzle.

(f) Learn stems, prefixes, and suffixes. It is very important that you know these.

# BASIC LETTER COMBINATIONS

One of the most efficient ways in which you can build up your vocabulary is by a systematic study of the basic word and letter combinations which make up the greater part of the English language.

*Etymology* is the science of the formation of words, and this somewhat frightening-sounding science can be of great help to you in learning new words and identifying words which may be unfamiliar to you. You will also find that the progress you make in studying the following pages will help to improve your spelling.

A great many of the words which we use every day have come into our language from the Latin and Greek. In the process of being absorbed into English, they appear as parts of words, many of which are related in meaning to each other.

For your convenience, this material is presented in easy-to-study form. Latin and Greek syllables and letter-combinations have been categorized into three groups:

1. *Prefixes:* letter combinations which appear at the beginning of a word.

2. *Suffixes:* letter combinations which appear at the end of a word.

3. *Roots or stems:* which carry the basic meaning and are combined with each other and with prefixes and suffixes to create other words with related meanings.

With the prefixes and suffixes, which you should study first, we have given examples of word formation with meanings, and additional examples. If you find any unfamiliar words among the samples, consult your dictionary to look up their meanings.

The list of roots or stems is accompanied by words in which the letter combinations appear. Here again, use the dictionary to look up any words which are not clear in your mind.

Remember that this section is not meant for easy reading. It is a guide to a program of study that will prove invaluable if you do your part. Do not try to swallow too much at one time. If you can put in a half-hour every day, your study will yield better results.

After you have done your preliminary work and have gotten a better idea of how words are formed in English, schedule the various vocabulary tests and quizzes we have provided in this chapter. They cover a wide variety of the vocabulary questions commonly encountered on examinations. They are short quizzes, not meant to be taken all at one time. Space them out. Adhere closely to the directions which differ for the different test types. Keep an honest record of your scores. Study your mistakes. Look them up in your dictionary. Concentrate closely on each quiz . . . and watch your scores improve.

# ETYMOLOGY -
# A KEY TO WORD RECOGNITION

## PREFIXES

| PREFIX | MEANING | EXAMPLE |
|---|---|---|
| ab, a | away from | absent, amoral |
| ad, ac, ag, at | to | advent, accrue, aggressive, attract |
| an | without | anarchy |
| ante | before | antedate |
| anti | against | antipathy |
| bene | well | beneficent |
| bi | two | bicameral |
| circum | around | circumspect |
| com, con, col | together | commit confound, collate |
| contra | against | contraband |
| de | from, down | descend |
| dis, di | apart | distract, divert |
| ex, e | out | exit, emit |
| extra | beyond | extracurricular |
| in, im, il, ir, un | not | inept, impossible, illicit |
| inter | between | interpose |
| intra, intro, in | within | intramural, introspective |

| PREFIX | MEANING | EXAMPLE |
|---|---|---|
| mal | bad | malcontent |
| mis | wrong | misnomer |
| non | not | nonentity |
| ob | against | obstacle |
| per | through | permeate |
| peri | around | periscope |
| poly | many | polytheism |
| post | after | post-mortem |
| pre | before | premonition |
| pro | forward | propose |
| re | again | review |
| se | apart | seduce |
| semi | half | semicircle |
| sub | under | subvert |
| super | above | superimpose |
| sui | self | suicide |
| trans | across | transpose |
| vice | instead of | vice-president |

## SUFFIXES

| SUFFIX | MEANING | EXAMPLE |
|---|---|---|
| able, ible | capable of being | capable, reversible |
| age | state of | storage |
| ance | relating to | reliance |
| ary | relating to | dictionary |
| ate | act | confiscate |
| ation | action | radiation |
| cy | quality | democracy |

| SUFFIX | MEANING | EXAMPLE |
|---|---|---|
| ence | relating to | confidence |
| er | one who | adviser |
| ic | pertaining to | democratic |
| ious | full of | rebellious |
| ize | to make like | harmonize |
| ment | result | filament |
| ty | condition | sanity |

## LATIN AND GREEK STEMS

| STEM | MEANING | EXAMPLE | STEM | MEANING | EXAMPLE |
|------|---------|---------|------|---------|---------|
| ag, ac | do | agenda, action | arch | chief, rule | archbishop |
| agr | farm | agriculture | astron | star | astronomy |
| aqua | water | aqueous | auto | self | automatic |
| cad, cas | fall | cadence, casual | biblio | book | bibliophile |
| cant | sing | chant | bio | life | biology |
| cap, cep | take | captive, accept | chrome | color | chromosome |
| capit | head | capital | chron | time | chronology |
| cede | go | precede | cosmo | world | cosmic |
| celer | speed | celerity | crat | rule | autocrat |
| cide, cis | kill, cut | suicide, incision | dent, dont | tooth | dental, indent |
| clud, clus | close | include, inclusion | eu | well, happy | eugenics |
| cur, curs | run | incur, incursion | gamos | marriage | monogamous |
| dict | say | diction | ge | earth | geology |
| duct | lead | induce | gen | origin, people | progenitor |
| fact, fect | make | factory, perfect | graph | write | graphic |
| fer, lat | carry | refer, dilate | gyn | women | gynecologist |
| fring, fract | break | infringe, fracture | homo | same | homogeneous |
| frater | brother | fraternal | hydr | water | dehydrate |
| fund, fus | pour | refund, confuse | logy | study of | psychology |
| greg | group | gregarious | meter | measure | thermometer |
| gress, grad | move forward | progress, degrade | micro | small | microscope |
| homo | man | homicide | mono | one | monotony |
| ject | throw | reject | onomy | science | astronomy |
| jud | right | judicial | onym | name | synonym |
| junct | join | conjunction | pathos | feeling | pathology |
| lect, leg | read, choose | collect, legend | philo | love | philosophy |
| loq, loc | speak | loquacious, interlocutory | phobia | fear | hydrophobia |
| manu | hand | manuscript | phone | sound | telephone |
| mand | order | remand | pseudo | false | pseudonym |
| mar | sea | maritime | psych | mind | psychic |
| mater | mother | maternal | scope | see | telescope |
| med | middle | intermediary | soph | wisdom | sophomore |
| min | lessen | diminution | tele | far off | telepathic |
| | | | theo | god | theology |
| mis, mit | send | remit, dismiss | thermo | heat | thermostat |
| mort | death | mortician | sec | cut | dissect |
| mote, mov | move | remote, remove | sed | remain | sedentary |
| naut | sailor | astronaut | sequ | follow | sequential |
| nom | name | nomenclature | spect | look | inspect |
| pater | father | paternity | spir | breathe | conspire |
| ped, pod | foot | pedal, podiatrist | stat | stand | status |
| pend | hang | depend | tact, tang | touch | tactile, tangible |
| plic | fold | implicate | ten | hold | retentive |
| port | carry | portable | term | end | terminal |
| pos, pon | put | depose, component | vent | come | prevent |
| reg, rect | rule | regicide, direct | vict | conquer | evict |
| rupt | break | eruption | vid, vis | see | video, revise |
| scrib, scrip | write | inscribe, conscription | voc | call | convocation |
| anthrop | man | anthropology | volv | roll | devolve |

# TOP SCORES ON OPPOSITES TESTS

*It has been said, "Everything is known and better understood by its contrary." That may help explain why opposites are such a favorite with test-makers. Not only do they probe your knowledge of words, but also your flexibility in handling them and evaluating their meanings . . . your mental agility, so to speak. Skill in answering opposites questions boils down to knowing the meaning of a word; and then shifting "mental gears" to arrive at the correct opposite meaning. In studying vocabulary, opposites serve as an excellent counterpoint to straight-forward synonyms practice. Consequently, you'll be better prepared even if your test merely poses the simpler, synonyms questions. On the other hand, this chapter could be mighty helpful in case you do run into opposition. You can be thrown badly off balance when you encounter it for the first time. Proficiency comes with practice. And you're going to get plenty of it in this chapter.*

## FIVE TEST-TYPE QUIZZES FOR PRACTICE

*In vocabulary we have one of the most important of all test subjects. It appears in many forms on almost every examination. It will most certainly appear on yours. It's worth all the time you can give it. Not only will this chapter help you answer vocabulary questions as such . . . it will also help you with all the other question types which depend on a knowledge of vocabulary.*

Now, push forward! Test yourself and practice for your test with the carefully constructed quizzes that follow. Each one presents the kind of question you may expect on your test. And each question is at just the level of difficulty that may be expected. Don't try to take all the tests at one time. Rather, schedule yourself so that you take a few at each session, and spend approximately the same time on them at each session. Score yourself honestly, and date each test. You should be able to detect improvement in your performance on successive sessions.

A portion of the standard answer sheet is provided after each test for marking your answers in the way you'll be required to do on the actual exam. At the right of this answer sheet, to make the scoring job simpler (after you have derived your own answers), you'll find our correct answers.

S1219

# OPPOSITES TEST ONE

*DIRECTIONS: In each of the following questions, one word
. . . a numbered word . . . is followed by four or five lettered
words or expressions. Choose the lettered word or expression
that has most nearly the opposite meaning of the numbered word.
Mark the letter preceding that word as the answer to the question.*

1. incredulous
   (A) argumentative   (B) imaginative
   (C) indifferent   (D) irreligious
   (E) believing.

2. placate
   (A) amuse   (B) antagonize
   (C) embroil   (D) pity
   (E) reject.

3. cognizant
   (A) afraid   (B) ignorant
   (C) capable   (D) aware
   (E) optimistic.

4. dissonance
   (A) disapproval   (B) disaster
   (C) harmony   (D) disparty
   (E) dissimilarity.

5. torsion
   (A) bending   (B) compressing
   (C) sliding   (D) stretching
   (E) straightening.

6. accrued
   (A) subtracted   (B) incidental
   (C) miscellaneous   (D) special
   (E) unearned.

7. effrontery
   (A) bad taste   (B) conceit
   (C) dishonesty   (D) shyness
   (E) snobbishness.

8. acquiescence
   (A) advice   (B) advocacy
   (C) opposition   (D) friendliness
   (E) compliance.

9. reticent
   (A) fidgety   (B) repetitious
   (C) talkative   (D) restful
   (E) truthful.

10. pseudo
    (A) deep   (B) obvious
    (C) honest   (D) provoking
    (E) spiritual.

11. awry
    (A) straight   (B) deplorable
    (C) odd   (D) simple
    (E) striking.

12. nefarious
    (A) clever   (B) necessary
    (C) negligent   (D) short-sighted
    (E) kindly.

13. glib
    (A) cheerful   (B) delightful
    (C) dull   (D) quiet
    (E) gloomy.

14. paucity
    (A) lack   (B) ease
    (C) hardship   (D) abundance
    (E) stoppage.

15. lucrative
    (A) debasing   (B) fortunate
    (C) influential   (D) monetary
    (E) unprofitable.

16. indubitable
    (A) doubtful   (B) fraudulent
    (C) honorable   (D) safe
    (E) deniable.

17. savant
    (A) diplomat    (B) inventor
    (C) moron    (D) thrifty person
    (E) wiseacre.

18. incipient
    (A) concluding    (B) dangerous
    (C) hasty    (D) secret
    (E) widespread.

19. virile
    (A) honest    (B) loyal
    (C) effeminate    (D) pugnacious
    (E) virtuous.

20. assiduous
    (A) courteous    (B) careless
    (C) discouraged    (D) frank
    (E) slow.

21. eclectic
    (A) brilliant
    (B) not choosing
    (C) short pastoral poem
    (D) conclusive
    (E) reproaching.

22. truculent
    (A) brilliant    (B) fawning
    (C) automotive    (D) unruly.
    (E) grammatical

23. bibulous
    (A) biblical    (B) artistic
    (C) bookish    (D) non-absorbent.
    (E) devilish

24. discrete
    (A) prudent    (B) judicious
    (C) crooked    (D) stunted.
    (E) joined

25. poltroon
    (A) brave man    (B) colonial landowner
    (C) fool    (D) gambling resort
    (E) recipient.

26. lambent
    (A) cool and moist
    (B) warped
    (C) riding roughshod
    (D) shining brightly
    (E) chewing.

27. extrinsic
    (A) germ-proof    (B) eccentric
    (C) uncultivated    (D) internal.
    (E) terrifying

28. consensus
    (A) poll    (B) disharmony
    (C) conference    (D) attitude.
    (E) agreement

29. indigenous
    (A) elevating    (B) destitute
    (C) insulting    (D) livid.
    (E) foreign

30. desuetude
    (A) spasmodic action
    (B) languor induced by hot weather
    (C) state of use
    (D) harmlessness
    (E) platitude.

31. matutinal
    (A) growing and developing steadily
    (B) pertaining to the evening
    (C) pertaining to the afternoon
    (D) regularly established as an annual event.
    (E) offering a reward.

32. absolve
    (A) bless    (B) blame
    (C) melt    (D) repent.
    (E) recount

33. sacrosanct
    (A) sacerdotal    (B) sanctimonious
    (C) sacramental    (D) surreptitious.
    (E) unholy

34. polemic
    (A) arctic    (B) electro-chemical
    (C) agreeable    (D) statistical.
    (E) refundable

35. intransigent
    (A) impassable    (B) reconcilable
    (C) harsh    (D) fly-by-night.
    (E) corroborative

36. ingenuous
    (A) quick    (B) mischievous
    (C) talented    (D) plotting.
    (E) refulgent

37. canard
    (A) rebus
    (B) true story
    (C) scurrilous publication
    (D) flattery
    (E) blasphemy.

38. disinterested
    (A) opposed
    (C) superficial
    (E) partial
    (B) contemptuous
    (D) winsome.

SCORE

%

NO. CORRECT

NO. OF QUESTIONS
ON THIS TEST

## Correct Answers

*(You'll learn more by writing your own answers before comparing them with these.)*

# OPPOSITES TEST TWO

*DIRECTIONS: In each of the following questions, one word
. . . a numbered word . . . is followed by four or five lettered
words or expressions. Choose the lettered word or expression
that has most nearly the opposite meaning of the numbered word.
Mark the letter preceding that word as the answer to the question.*

1. cataclysm
   (A) blunder      (B) superstition
   (C) treachery    (D) triumph
   (E) status quo.

2. auspicious
   (A) condemnatory   (B) conspicuous
   (C) unfavorable    (D) questionable
   (E) spicy.

3. banter
   (A) conversation   (B) criticism
   (C) gossip         (D) irony
   (E) serious talk.

4. vernacular
   (A) literary speech   (B) correct usage
   (C) long words        (D) oratory
   (E) poetic style.

5. emolument
   (A) capital      (B) penalty
   (C) liabilities  (D) loss
   (E) output.

6. turgid
   (A) dusty    (B) muddy
   (C) rolling  (D) deflated
   (E) tense

7. expunge
   (A) clarify      (B) cleanse
   (C) perpetuate   (D) investigate
   (E) underline.

8. panoramic
   (A) brilliant  (B) pinpoint
   (C) pretty     (D) fluorescent
   (E) unique.

9. ignominy
   (A) fame       (B) isolation
   (C) misfortune (D) sorrow
   (E) stupidity.

10. relevant
    (A) ingenious  (B) inspiring
    (C) obvious    (D) inappropiate
    (E) tentative.

11. apposite
    (A) irrelevant  (B) contrary
    (C) different   (D) spontaneous
    (E) tricky.

12. ambulatory
    (A) confined to bed  (B) able to walk
    (C) injured          (D) quarantined
    (E) suffering from disease.

13. disparage
    (A) applaud  (B) degrade
    (C) erase    (D) reform
    (E) scatter.

14. limpid
    (A) calm     (B) turbid
    (C) crippled (D) delightful
    (E) sad.

15. derisive
    (A) dividing    (B) furnishing
    (C) reflecting  (D) laudatory
    (E) suggesting.

16. debilitate
    (A) encourage  (B) insinuate
    (C) prepare    (D) turn away
    (E) strengthen.

17. opulent
    (A) fearful   (B) free
    (C) oversized (D) trustful
    (E) impoverished.

18. blandishment
    (A) brunette     (B) criticism
    (C) ostentation  (D) praise
    (E) return.

19. cryptic
    (A) appealing      (B) arched
    (C) deathly        (D) revealing
    (E) intricate.

20. raucous
    (A) euphonious     (B) loud
    (C) querulous      (D) rational
    (E) violent

21. propitiate
    (A) anger          (B) approach
    (C) predict        (D) applaud.
    (E) promote

22. murrain
    (A) marsh land     (B) blessing
    (C) glacial ridge  (D) land held
    (E) subterranean       inalienably
        passage.

23. feral
    (A) iron-bearing   (B) panel
    (C) calm           (D) violent
    (E) ferrous.

24. somatic
    (A) sleepy         (B) spiritual
    (C) seminal        (D) psychogenic
    (E) traumatic.

25. ineluctable
    (A) avoidable      (B) inscrutable
    (C) approachable   (D) esoteric
    (E) applicable.

26. froward
    (A) complaisant    (B) cozy
    (C) candid         (D) precocious
    (E) cooperative.

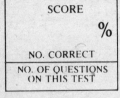

| SCORE |
| :---: |
| **%** |
| NO. CORRECT |
| NO. OF QUESTIONS ON THIS TEST |

## Correct Answers

*(You'll learn more by writing your own answers before comparing them with these.)*

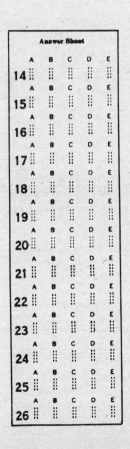

# OPPOSITES TEST THREE

*DIRECTIONS: In each of the following questions, one word . . . a numbered word . . . is followed by four or five lettered words or expressions. Choose the lettered word or expression that has most nearly the opposite meaning of the numbered word. Mark the letter preceding that word as the answer to the question.*

1. avidity
   - (A) friendliness
   - (B) generosity
   - (C) resentment
   - (D) speed
   - (E) thirst.

2. hiatus
   - (A) branch
   - (B) disease
   - (C) gaiety
   - (D) insect
   - (E) closing.

3. plenary
   - (A) easy
   - (B) stolid
   - (C) empty
   - (D) rewarding
   - (E) untrustworthy.

4. capricious
   - (A) active
   - (B) stable
   - (C) opposed
   - (D) sheeplike
   - (E) slippery.

5. specious
   - (A) scanty
   - (B) particular
   - (C) genuine
   - (D) suspicious
   - (E) vigorous.

6. extirpate
   - (A) besmirch
   - (B) clean
   - (C) renew
   - (D) favor
   - (E) subdivide.

7. equivocal
   - (A) positive
   - (B) medium
   - (C) monotonous
   - (D) musical
   - (E) well-balanced.

8. benison
   - (A) approval
   - (B) curse
   - (C) gift
   - (D) prayer
   - (E) reward.

9. sanguine
   - (A) limp
   - (B) mechanical
   - (C) muddy
   - (D) livid
   - (E) stealthy.

10. surcease
    - (A) inception
    - (B) hope
    - (C) resignation
    - (D) sleep
    - (E) sweetness.

11. sentient
    - (A) emotional
    - (B) callous
    - (C) hostile
    - (D) sympathetic
    - (E) wise.

12. obviate
    - (A) grasp
    - (B) reform
    - (C) simplify
    - (D) smooth
    - (E) make necessary.

13. rancor
    - (A) dignity
    - (B) affection
    - (C) odor
    - (D) spite
    - (E) suspicion.

14. dilatory
    - (A) hairy
    - (B) happy-go-lucky
    - (C) ruined
    - (D) punctual
    - (E) well-to-do.

15. ebullition
    - (A) bathing
    - (B) cooling
    - (C) refilling
    - (D) retiring
    - (E) returning

16. relegate
    - (A) welcome
    - (B) deprive
    - (C) designate
    - (D) report
    - (E) request.

17. recondite
    - (A) brittle
    - (B) exposed
    - (C) explored
    - (D) concealed
    - (E) uninformed.

18. sublime
    - (A) below par
    - (B) highly praised
    - (C) extreme
    - (D) ignoble
    - (E) settled.

19. termagant
   (A) fever    (B) quiet woman
   (C) sea bird    (D) sedative
   (E) squirrel.

20. sedulous
   (A) deceptive    (B) careless
   (C) grassy    (D) hateful
   (E) sweet.

21. simper
   (A) sniff    (B) frown
   (C) sob    (D) smile
   (E) blink.

22. redoubt
   (A) homestead    (B) weakness
   (C) supply dump    (D) sanctuary
   (E) reduction.

23. salad days
   (A) days of one's babyhood
   (B) days of yore
   (C) days of wide experience
   (D) halcyon days
   (E) eventide.

24. calumnious
   (A) disastrous    (B) conspiratorial
   (C) querulous    (D) complimenting
   (E) quarrelsome.

25. palled
   (A) exuberant    (B) shocked
   (C) pierced    (D) weighted
   (E) piled.

26. gaud
   (A) epithet    (B) simplicity
   (C) spur    (D) taunt.
   (E) fraud.

| SCORE | |
|---|---|
| | **%** |
| NO. CORRECT | |
| NO. OF QUESTIONS ON THIS TEST | |

## Correct Answers

*(You'll learn more by writing your own answers before comparing them with these.)*

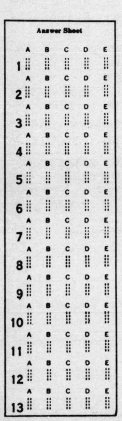

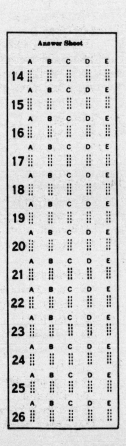

# OPPOSITES TEST FOUR

*DIRECTIONS: In each of the following questions, one word . . . a numbered word . . . is followed by four or five lettered words or expressions. Choose the lettered word or expression that has most nearly the opposite meaning of the numbered word. Mark the letter preceding that word as the answer to the question.*

1. alfresco
   (A) indoors    (B) art exhibit
   (C) sidewalk cafe    (D) charcoal sketch.

2. aliment
   (A) illness
   (B) non-support
   (C) sidewise motion
   (D) wing-formation.

3. animadversion
   (A) favorable remark
   (B) soul sickness
   (C) whole-heartedness
   (D) opposing clique.

4. antinomy
   (A) name-calling
   (B) agreement of two laws
   (C) contrary viewpoint
   (D) metallic alloy.

5. asyndeton
   (A) periodic in structure
   (B) lacking parallelism
   (C) faulty in conclusion
   (D) inclusion of conjunctions.

6. auscultation
   (A) religious veneration
   (B) refusal to listen
   (C) political intrigue
   (D) indoor horticulture.

7. basilic
   (A) fundamental    (B) deadly
   (C) slaggy    (D) lowly.

8. bowdlerized
   (A) uncensored
   (B) chopped fine
   (C) swallowed whole
   (D) criticized severely.

9. cabala
   (A) medieval tribunal
   (B) voodoo symbols
   (C) published doctrine
   (D) conspiratorial gathering.

10. canorous
    (A) extremely hungry
    (B) euphoniously sonorous
    (C) cacophonous
    (D) hound-like.

11. caveat
    (A) deception    (B) roe
    (C) invitation    (D) seizure.

12. cerement
    (A) death mask
    (B) garment for the living
    (C) inscription on tomb
    (D) refrain in threnody.

13. cicatrice
    (A) smooth surface  (B) house pest
    (C) fabulous serpent  (D) summer insects

14. congeneric
    (A) artificially reproduced
    (B) remotely related
    (C) carefree in nature
    (D) of a different kind.

15. contumelious
    (A) compromising
    (B) mildly reproachful
    (C) laudatory
    (D) genuinely contrite.

16. cupidity
    (A) passing fancy
    (B) restraint
    (C) foolish attraction
    (D) make-believe-tenderness.

17. demotic
    (A) tyrannical  (B) mobile
    (C) selective   (D) fiendish.

18. dissidence
    (A) propinquity  (B) efflorescence
    (C) dubiety      (D) concurrence.

19. divagation
    (A) operatic solo
    (B) adherence to topic
    (C) underwater study
    (D) summer travel.

20. epideictic
    (A) modest
    (B) concise
    (C) intended to edify
    (D) concentrated upon.

21. careen
    (A) hurtle
    (B) whirl around
    (C) blaspheme
    (D) move at break-neck speed
    (E) stand upright.

22. dolt
    (A) prankster   (B) clever fellow
    (C) manikin     (D) hobbledehoy.
    (E) dubiety.

23. ebullient
    (A) capricious  (B) bizarre
    (C) vapid       (D) destructive
    (E) cartographic.

24. apogee
    (A) introductory remarks  (B) zenith
    (C) figure of speech      (D) perigee.
    (E) sabot.

SCORE

%

NO. CORRECT

NO. OF QUESTIONS ON THIS TEST

## Correct Answers

*(You'll learn more by writing your own answers before comparing them with these.)*

# OPPOSITES TEST FIVE

*DIRECTIONS: In each of the following questions, one word
. . . a numbered word . . . is followed by four or five lettered
words or expressions. Choose the lettered word or expression
that has most nearly the opposite meaning of the numbered word.
Mark the letter preceding that word as the answer to the question.*

1. inamorata
   (A) nameless person
   (B) enemy
   (C) assumed name
   (D) lovelorn person.

2. inspissated
   (A) animated      (B) thickened
   (C) attenuated    (D) mixed thoroughly.

3. interpellate
   (A) alter by inserting
   (B) clarify
   (C) admonish
   (D) answer informally.

4. jardiniere
   (A) professional soldier
   (B) small flowerpot
   (C) female gardener
   (D) beekeeper.

5. lenitive
   (A) shortening    (B) emolient
   (C) painful       (D) elongating.

6. litigious
   (A) ornate in literary style
   (B) illegally threatening
   (C) agreeable
   (D) close to the shoreline.

7. lubricous
   (A) mercenary     (B) rough
   (C) tubular       (D) thrifty.

8. lucubrate
   (A) write stupidly
   (B) whine incessantly
   (C) sail nearer the wind
   (D) remove friction.

9. megacephaly
   (A) smallness of head
   (B) magnification of vision
   (C) malformation of feet
   (D) inordinate loss of hair.

10. mendicity
    (A) lying        (B) giving
    (C) venerating   (D) repairing.

11. nirvana
    (A) loss of auditory acuity
    (B) nervous tension
    (C) loss of courage
    (D) muscular atrophy.

12. objurgate
    (A) appeal       (B) forswear
    (C) praise       (D) importune.

13. oneiromancy
    (A) interpretation of actual occurrences
    (B) astrology
    (C) fortune-telling by cards
    (D) phrenology.

14. outré
    (A) barren       (B) out-of-bounds
    (C) usual        (D) stylish.

15. palinode
    (A) song of confirmation    (B) fence post
    (C) wedding hymm            (D) festival.

16. pelagic
    (A) landlocked   (B) horny
    (C) terrestrial  (D) furry.

17. pettifog
    (A) practice law in an honest way
    (B) spread smoke and haze
    (C) obstruct vision
    (D) shrink cloth

18. plashy
    (A) tawdry      (B) rainy
    (C) pretentious (D) dry.

19. repine
    (A) approve  (B) retract
    (C) relax    (D) confess.

20. raffish
    (A) dour   (B) carefree
    (C) sporty (D) reputable.

21. doughty
    (A) cowardly    (B) pasty
    (C) invincible  (D) vacillating.
    (E) uncanny.

22. contemn
    (A) recognize  (B) confine
    (C) sentence   (D) compete
    (E) relegate.

23. peculator
    (A) gambler    (B) herdsman
    (C) benefactor (D) finder
    (E) arraigner.

24. enclave
    (A) territory which is part of common group
    (B) settlement surrounded by palisades
    (C) papal summons to a consistory
    (D) prison yard
    (E) hustings.

SCORE

%

NO. CORRECT

NO. OF QUESTIONS ON THIS TEST

## Correct Answers

*(You'll learn more by writing your own answers before comparing them with these.)*

Answer Sheet

Answer Sheet

Correct Answers

Correct Answers

# SYNONYMS PRACTICE

**SYNONYMS TEST 1**

TIME : 20 minutes

*DIRECTIONS: For each question in this test select the appropriate letter preceding the word which is most nearly the same in meaning as the capitalized word.*

1. Pyrrhic victory
   - (A) victory gained at too great a cost
   - (B) victory as a result of encirclement
   - (C) total destruction of the enemy
   - (D) victory as a result of a complete surprise.

2. quirt
   - (A) riding-whip
   - (B) idiosyncrasy
   - (C) witty remark
   - (D) bludgeon.

3. rara avis
   - (A) cynosure
   - (B) nonentity
   - (C) gourmet
   - (D) unusual person.

4. sacerdotal
   - (A) pertaining to the priesthood
   - (B) pertaining to religious sacrifice
   - (C) pertaining to contributions for religious purposes
   - (D) pertaining to the lower back.

5. saraband
   - (A) stately dance
   - (B) tiara-like ornament
   - (C) small lute
   - (D) insignia worn on left arm.

6. saurian
   - (A) ape-like
   - (B) wicked
   - (C) winged
   - (D) lizard-like.

7. sloe-eyed
   - (A) of gentle look
   - (B) almond-eyed
   - (C) heavy-eyed
   - (D) black-eyed.

8. splayed
   - (A) hunched
   - (B) spread out
   - (C) splashed
   - (D) knobby.

9. Star Chamber
   - (A) secret tribunal
   - (B) royal manifesto
   - (C) illegal seizure
   - (D) special jury.

10. surrogate
    - (A) will
    - (B) substitute
    - (C) court clerk
    - (D) criminal court.

11. tertian
    - (A) recurring
    - (B) subordinate
    - (C) intermediate
    - (D) remote in time.

12. tessellate
    - (A) quiver uncontrollably
    - (B) arrange in a checkered pattern
    - (C) adorn with random scraps of material
    - (D) dry up rapidly.

13. trammel
    - (A) bore holes in
    - (B) stamp on
    - (C) impede
    - (D) blend into one mass.

14. truncated
    - (A) abused
    - (B) lopped off
    - (C) sharpened to a fine point
    - (D) columnar.

15. turbid
    - (A) insubordinate
    - (B) distended
    - (C) hooded
    - (D) muddy.

16. vitiate
    - (A) enliven
    - (B) create
    - (C) impair
    - (D) defame.

17. watershed
    - (A) artificial passage for water

(B) sudden copious rainfall
(C) drainage area
(D) line marking ebb or flow of tide.

19. welter
(A) ridge  (B) turmoil
(C) vault of heaven  (D) conglomeration.

18. welkin
(A) sky  (B) countryside
(C) fire gong  (D) church bells.

20. wherefore
(A) whilom  (B) why
(C) whence  (D) whither.

## CONSOLIDATE YOUR KEY ANSWERS HERE

## Correct Answers For The Foregoing Questions

*To assist you in scoring yourself we have provided Correct Answers alongside your Answer Sheet. May we therefore suggest that while you are doing the test you cover the Correct Answers with a sheet of white paper.....to avoid temptation and to arrive at an accurate estimate of your ability and progress.*

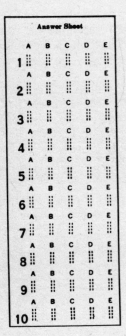

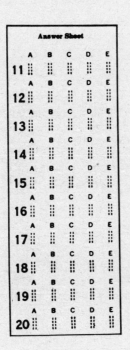

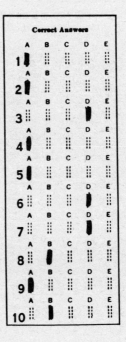

| SCORE 1 | .......................... % |
| --- | --- |
| NO. CORRECT ÷ | |
| NO. OF QUESTIONS ON THIS TEST | |

| SCORE 2 | .......................... % |
| --- | --- |
| NO. CORRECT ÷ | |
| NO. OF QUESTIONS ON THIS TEST | |

**SYNONYMS TEST 2**

TIME : 20 minutes

*DIRECTIONS: For each question in this test select the appropriate letter preceding the word which is most nearly the same in meaning as the capitalized word.*

*Correct key answers to all these test questions will be found at the end of the test.*

# A FAIR SAMPLING OF THE QUESTIONS YOU'LL BE ASKED

1. acanthus
   (A) leaf-like architectural ornamentation
   (B) gummy substance used in stiffening fabrics
   (C) ethereal spirit
   (D) ornamental vessel.

2. alfresco
   (A) fresh food        (B) spring flood
   (C) water color       (D) in the open air.

3. animadversion
   (A) vitality          (B) ire
   (C) taboo             (D) stricture.

4. aplomb
   (A) self-assurance    (B) stodginess
   (C) foppishness       (D) sturdiness.

5. apocryphal
   (A) awesome
   (B) disease-bearing
   (C) of doubtful authority
   (D) threatening.

6. artifact
   (A) product of human workmanship
   (B) stratagem
   (C) duplication
   (D) artful or skillful contrivance.

7. atavistic
   (A) overeager
   (B) narrow-minded
   (C) reverting to a primitive type
   (D) pertaining to an uncle.

8. baize
   (A) cereal plant      (B) medicinal plant
   (C) tree marking      (D) soft fabric.

9. bowdlerize
   (A) ratiocinate       (B) interpolate
   (C) asseverate        (D) expurgate.

10. carafe
    (A) glass water bottle
    (B) means of transportation
    (C) wineskin
    (D) bony case covering back of animal.

11. carte blanche
    (A) demerit
    (B) symbol of cowardice
    (C) unconditional authority
    (D) press card.

12. chapbook
    (A) style book used by publishers and printers
    (B) small book of popular literature
    (C) missal
    (D) compendium of usage.

13. cicerone
    (A) orator           (B) guide
    (C) buffoon          (D) cavalier.

14. colander
    (A) species of lizard
    (B) upright of a sluice
    (C) baking dish
    (D) vessel perforated for use as a sieve or strainer.

15. complaisant
    (A) discontented     (B) smug
    (C) obliging         (D) satisfied.

16. congeries
    (A) intricate plots    (B) aggregation
    (C) clique             (D) leave-takings.

17. contumacious
    (A) stubbornly disobedient
    (B) deservedly disgraced
    (C) unduly pompous
    (D) gravely libelous.

18. coryphee
    (A) shepherdess       (B) priestess
    (C) ballet dancer     (D) small fishing
                              boat.

19. covert
    (A) envious           (B) secret
    (C) timid             (D) protected.

20. crepitate
    (A) enfeeble          (B) worsen
    (C) depreciate        (D) crackle.

## CONSOLIDATE YOUR KEY ANSWERS HERE

# Correct Answers For The Foregoing Questions

*To assist you in scoring yourself we have provided Correct
Answers alongside your Answer Sheet. May we therefore suggest
that while you are doing the test you cover the Correct Answers
with a sheet of white paper.....to avoid temptation and to arrive at
an accurate estimate of your ability and progress.*

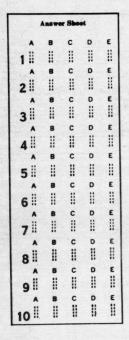

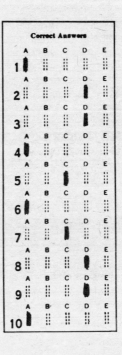

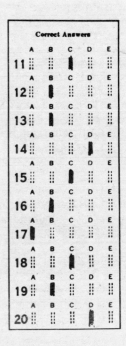

| SCORE 1 |
| :---: |
| **%** |
| ............................ |
| NO. CORRECT |
| NO. OF QUESTIONS ON THIS TEST |

| SCORE 2 |
| :---: |
| **%** |
| ............................ |
| NO. CORRECT |
| NO. OF QUESTIONS ON THIS TEST |

## SYNONYMS TEST 3

### TIME : 20 minutes

*DIRECTIONS: For each question in this test select the appropriate letter preceding the word which is most nearly the same in meaning as the capitalized word.*

*Correct key answers to all these test questions will be found at the end of the test.*

# A FAIR SAMPLING OF THE QUESTIONS YOU'LL BE ASKED

1. unassuaged
   (A) unseen          (B) unrelieved
   (C) unconvinced     (D) unwashed

2. coadjutor
   (A) assistant       (B) partner
   (C) arbitrator      (D) extra judge

3. doughty
   (A) flabby and pale
   (B) strong and valiant
   (C) weak and craven
   (D) crude and boorish.

4. durance
   (A) penance         (B) imprisonment
   (C) strength        (D) toughness.

5. entomology
   (A) study of plant fossils
   (B) study of relics of man
   (C) study of insects
   (D) study of derivatives.

6. euphemistic
   (A) having good digestion
   (B) less offensive in phrasing
   (C) exhibiting great enjoyment
   (D) excessively elegant in style.

7. euphoria
   (A) sense of well-being
   (B) assumption of friendliness
   (C) ability to speak well
   (D) eagerness to agree.

8. exceptionable
   (A) not better than average
   (B) objectionable
   (C) out of the ordinary
   (D) captious.

9. excoriate
   (A) rack           (B) expel
   (C) disembarrass   (D) flay.

10. farrier
    (A) ship's carpenter   (B) litter of pigs
    (C) blacksmith         (D) trainman.

11. fecund
    (A) fruitful       (B) decaying
    (C) offensive      (D) feverish.

12. fettle
    (A) gala occasion
    (B) shackle
    (C) thriving condition
    (D) part of a horse's leg.

13. fey
    (A) appearing to be under a spell
    (B) happy-go-lucky
    (C) not clairvoyant
    (D) lacking vision.

14. fiduciary
    (A) faithful         (B) speculative
    (C) yielding interest (D) holding in trust.

15. atelier
    (A) hat shop       (B) tea shop
    (C) jeweler        (D) workshop

16. fulminating
   (A) hurling denunciation
   (B) reaching the highest point
   (C) fulfilling acceptably
   (D) remonstrating gently.

17. halcyon days
   (A) period of sowing wild oats
   (B) period of storms and turbulence
   (C) period of ominous portents
   (D) period of tranquility and peace.

18. hyperbole
   (A) exaggeration      (B) plane curve
   (C) onomatopoeia      (D) assumption

19. immure
   (A) ossify      (B) enclose
   (C) fertilize   (D) inhere.

20. indefeasible
   (A) not probable      (B) not justifiable
   (C) not practicable   (D) not annullable.

## CONSOLIDATE YOUR KEY ANSWERS HERE

## Correct Answers For The Foregoing Questions

*To assist you in scoring yourself we have provided Correct Answers alongside your Answer Sheet. May we therefore suggest that while you are doing the test you cover the Correct Answers with a sheet of white paper.....to avoid temptation and to arrive at an accurate estimate of your ability and progress.*

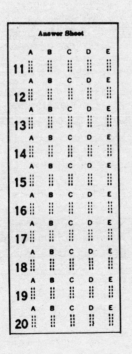

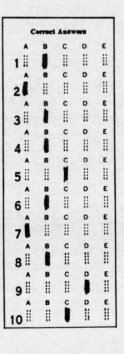

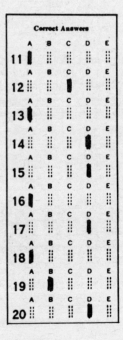

| SCORE 1 |
| --- |
| .......................... % |
| NO. CORRECT ÷ |
| NO. OF QUESTIONS ON THIS TEST |

| SCORE 2 |
| --- |
| .......................... % |
| NO. CORRECT ÷ |
| NO. OF QUESTIONS ON THIS TEST |

## SYNONYMS TEST 4

TIME : 20 minutes

*DIRECTIONS: For each question in this test select the appropriate letter preceding the word which is most nearly the same in meaning as the capitalized word.*

*Correct key answers to all these test questions will be found at the end of the test.*

# A FAIR SAMPLING OF THE QUESTIONS YOU'LL BE ASKED

1. indurate
   (A) harden          (B) prolong
   (C) endow           (D) suffer.

2. internecine
   (A) pertaining to fraternal strife
   (B) mutually destructive
   (C) pertaining to sibling competition
   (D) excessively diffident.

3. jeremiad
   (A) dolorous tirade
   (B) optimistic prophecy
   (C) prolonged journey
   (D) religious pilgrimage.

4. kelp
   (A) military cap       (B) sharp cry
   (C) disembodied spirit (D) seaweed ash.

5. hegemony
   (A) body of officials disposed according to rank
   (B) preponderant influence
   (C) tendency to evade
   (D) protection against fluctuation in stock prices.

6. lissom
   (A) supple         (B) beautiful
   (C) strong         (D) rippling.

7. lodestar
   (A) guiding star
   (B) vein of ore
   (C) central star of constellation
   (D) celestial body exercising magnetic force.

8. lucubrate
   (A) illuminate brilliantly
   (B) lament unduly
   (C) work or study laboriously
   (D) deprecate unceasingly.

9. maunder
   (A) weep sentimentally
   (B) talk incoherently
   (C) flow swiftly
   (D) act insincerely.

10. mead
    (A) upland        (B) fermented drink
    (C) reward        (D) fallow soil.

11. nexus
    (A) gist
    (B) central portion of atom
    (C) opposing argument
    (D) connection.

12. nubile
    (A) obscure       (B) voluptuous
    (C) marriageable  (D) oriental

13. obloquy
    (A) sacrifice     (B) forgetfulness
    (C) calumny       (D) indirectness.

14. orthography
    (A) beautiful handwriting
    (B) correct spelling
    (C) autobiography
    (D) illegibility.

15. otiose
    (A) long-winded   (B) thick-skinned
    (C) inactive      (D) hateful.

16. panoply
    (A) comprehensive survey
    (B) full suit of armor
    (C) overhanging projection
    (D) elaborate display.

17. patois
    (A) inner court
    (B) perfume
    (C) sympathetic sorrow
    (D) provincial speech.

18. pertinacious
    (A) persistent     (B) relevant
    (C) saucy          (D) cohesive.

19. potsherd
    (A) primitive agricultural implement
    (B) herdsman
    (C) fragment of earthen pot
    (D) caretaker.

20. pragmatic
    (A) smoothly        (B) practical
        rehearsed       (D) bookish.
    (C) absolute

## CONSOLIDATE YOUR KEY ANSWERS HERE

## Correct Answers For The Foregoing Questions

*To assist you in scoring yourself we have provided Correct Answers alongside your Answer Sheet. May we therefore suggest that while you are doing the test you cover the Correct Answers with a sheet of white paper.....to avoid temptation and to arrive at an accurate estimate of your ability and progress.*

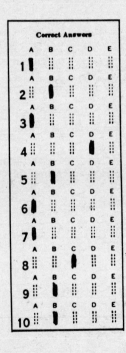

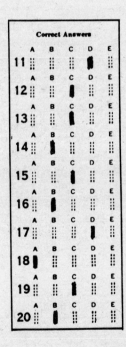

| SCORE 1 | ........................... % |
|---|---|
| NO. CORRECT ÷ NO. OF QUESTIONS | |

| SCORE 2 | ........................... % |
|---|---|
| NO. CORRECT ÷ NO. OF QUESTIONS | |

## SYNONYMS TEST 5

### TIME : 20 minutes

*DIRECTIONS: For each question in this test select the appropriate letter preceding the word which is most nearly the same in meaning as the capitalized word.*

*Correct key answers to all these test questions will be found at the end of the test.*

# A FAIR SAMPLING OF THE QUESTIONS YOU'LL BE ASKED

1. proclivity
   (A) propensity
   (B) rapid descent
   (C) devoted adherence
   (D) buoyancy.

2. prosthesis
   (A) attempt to convert
   (B) addition of an artificial part to the human body
   (C) complete exhaustion
   (D) figure of speech.

3. pundit
   (A) prosy speaker  (B) witty saying
   (C) learned man  (D) harsh judge.

4. quondam
   (A) which was to be done
   (B) having been formerly
   (C) to this extent
   (D) cited as an authority.

5. recidivist
   (A) one who receives
   (B) one who relapses into criminality
   (C) one who remains behind
   (D) one who reciprocates.

6. rubric
   (A) footnote
   (B) enigmatic representation of a word
   (C) manuscript title or heading
   (D) medicinal application.

7. satrap
   (A) subordinate ruler
   (B) male woodland deity

   (C) form of basalt rock
   (D) device for entangling small game.

8. sawbuck
   (A) antler  (B) bucksaw
   (C) male deer  (D) rack.

9. sobriquet
   (A) musical comedy actress
   (B) nickname
   (C) puppet
   (D) habitual temperance.

10. spoliate
    (A) decay  (B) besmirch
    (C) wind on a bobbin  (D) plunder.

11. spoor
    (A) mutation
    (B) trail of wild animal
    (C) unicellular reproductive body
    (D) fetid odor.

12. tamp
    (A) pound down  (B) tread clumsily
    (C) curl  (D) bind firmly.

13. "cross the Rubicon"
    (A) pass into oblivion
    (B) overcome almost insurmountable difficulties
    (C) take an irrevocable step
    (D) change one's identity.

14. "send to Coventry"
    (A) doom to destruction
    (B) reduce in rank
    (C) send on a fool's errand
    (D) ostracize.

15. touchstone
    (A) instrument for sharpening tools
    (B) material for cleaning decks of chips
    (C) test for worth
    (D) fundamental cause.

16. truckle
    (A) transport
    (B) submit obsequiously
    (C) tighten securely
    (D) barter.

17. turgid
    (A) distended      (B) muddy
    (C) agitated       (D) sluggish.

18. viable
    (A) not excusable
    (B) open to corrupt influence
    (C) easily pulverized
    (D) capable of living.

19. vouchsafe
    (A) scort          (B) acknowledge openly
    (C) grant          (D) attest the truth of.

20. wraith
    (A) anger          (B) perversity
    (C) calamity       (D) apparition.

## CONSOLIDATE YOUR KEY ANSWERS HERE

# Correct Answers For The Foregoing Questions

*To assist you in scoring yourself we have provided Correct Answers alongside your Answer Sheet. May we therefore suggest that while you are doing the test you cover the Correct Answers with a sheet of white paper.....to avoid temptation and to arrive at an accurate estimate of your ability and progress.*

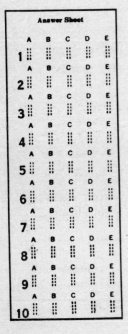
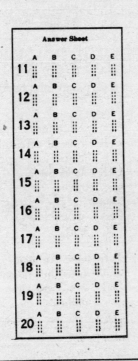
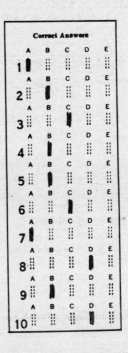
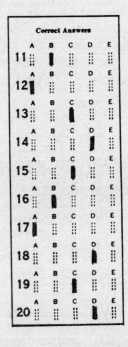

SCORE 1 .............................. %

NO. CORRECT ÷ NO. OF QUESTIONS

SCORE 2 .............................. %

NO. CORRECT ÷ NO. OF QUESTIONS

# SENTENCE COMPLETIONS

*Here is a most effective measure of your mental agility and verbal imagination. Although this type of question is sometimes used to test vocabulary, grammar, or even your knowledge of factual material in general, in its truest form it is a test of your ability to think of words and to grasp ideas quickly and easily.*

### Many Tests. . .

. . . pose questions requiring you to complete a sentence in which one or two words are represented by blank spaces. Here it is necessary to look for the implication of a sentence, the underlying meaning. Usually this understanding does not require any special knowledge, but it does require a solid vocabulary background.

*Directions:* Select from the lettered word or sets of words which follow, the word or words which best fit the meaning of the quotation as a whole. For each question read all the choices carefully. Then select that answer which you consider correct or most nearly correct. Write the letter preceding your best choice next to the question.

You may want to answer on facsimiles of the kind of answer sheets provided on machine-scored examinations. For practice purposes we have provided several such facsimiles throughout the book. Tear one out if you wish, and mark your answer on it . . . just as you would do on an actual exam.

## Sentence Completion Tests by Levels

### Level One—Easy Completions

1. Through his _____, he deceived us all.
   (A) whit
   (B) selvage
   (C) canard
   (D) petard

2. The lover of democracy has an _____ toward totalitarianism.
   (A) antipathy
   (B) empathy
   (C) antipode
   (D) idiopathy

3. An _____ may connect the names of members of a partnership.
   (A) addendum
   (B) ampersand
   (C) epigram
   (D) encomium

4. A _____ person cannot be expected to resist _____.
   (A) profligate-money
   (B) raucous-temptation
   (C) recreant-aggression
   (D) squalid-quarreling

5. He hated his father so intensely that he committed _____.
   (A) parricide
   (B) fratricide
   (C) genocide
   (D) matricide

6. Being very _____, he knew what was going on about him.
   (A) circumlocutory
   (B) choleric
   (C) caustic
   (D) circumspect

7. The convicted man resorted to _____ in attacking his accusers.
   (A) nepotism
   (B) anathema
   (C) panoply
   (D) bravura

8. The _____ woman was the _____ of all eyes.
   (A) tilted-cupola
   (B) lonely-sinecure
   (C) ugly-doggerel
   (D) attractive-cynosure

5910

9. A _____ is likely to give you the wrong advice.
   (A) nuance    (C) charlatan
   (B) panacea   (D) virago

10. The _____ professor put his wife out and went to sleep with the cat.
    (A) diurnal    (B) distrait

(C) dubious    (D) dilatory

## Correct Answers For Level One

| | | | |
|---|---|---|---|
| 1. C | 4. C | 7. B | 9. C |
| 2. A | 5. A | 8. D | 10. B |
| 3. B | 6. D | | |

## Level Two—Easy Completions

1. Art is long and time is _____.
   (A) fervid     (C) nebulous
   (B) fallow     (D) evanescent

2. The _____ flower was also _____.
   (A) pretty-redolent
   (B) drooping-potable
   (C) pale-opulent
   (D) blooming-amenable

3. The _____ effects of the drug made her very weary.
   (A) succinct    (C) soporific
   (B) spurious    (D) supine

4. Being _____, the child was not permitted to have his supper.
   (A) refractory    (C) vernal
   (B) reticent      (D) unctuous

5. The chairman's _____ speech swayed the audience to favor his proposal.
   (A) cursory    (C) ancillary
   (B) blatant    (D) cogent

6. He is quite _____ and, therefore, easily _____.
   (A) callow-deceived    (B) lethal-perceived

(C) fetal-conceived    (D) limpid-received

7. That _____ seems so out of place with those lovely little girls.
   (A) shard    (C) tyro
   (B) hoyden   (D) vanguard

8. The sculptor will convert this _____ piece of clay into a beautiful bust.
   (A) virulent    (C) taciturn
   (B) amorphous   (D) salient

9. His _____ had no place in our serious conversation.
   (A) badinage    (C) concatenation
   (B) viscosity   (D) valence

10. Her _____ manner embarrassed the others at the party.
    (A) affable     (C) sapid
    (B) tractable   (D) gauche

## Correct Answers For Level Two

| | | | |
|---|---|---|---|
| 1. D | 4. A | 7. B | 9. A |
| 2. A | 5. D | 8. B | 10. D |
| 3. C | 6. A | | |

## Level Three—Difficult Completions

1. In a state of _____, we are likely to have _____.
   (A) ochlocracy-havoc
   (B) bureaucracy-respect
   (C) theocracy-sin
   (D) desuetude-activity

2. Knowledge cannot thrive where there is _____.
   (A) parturition    (C) protocol
   (B) nescience      (D) neoclassicism

3. _____ is a phase of the study of penology.
   (A) recidivism    (C) hematosis
   (B) eclecticism   (D) hydrometry

4. The _____ of war is death and cruelty.
   (A) sirocco    (C) beldam
   (B) rutabaga   (D) quiddity

5. The conceited soldier was forward and _____ in his attitude.
   (A) mundane      (C) gratuitous
   (B) thrasonical  (D) laconic

6. Being a man of maxims, he was _____ in what he said.
   (A) sententious     (C) sebaceous
   (B) transmogrified  (D) sentient

7. His _____ remarks are too stupid to be taken _____.
   (A) empyreal-lightly
   (B) puerperal-slowly
   (C) lacunal-violently
   (D) vapid-seriously

8. The _____ was very informative during the trip.
   (A) censer          (C) cicerone
   (B) centaur         (D) burgeon

9. A _____ and the principle of monogamy are poles apart.

   (A) seraglio        (C) shallop
   (B) purlieu         (D) benison

10. The mourning throng was preparing for a _____.
    (A) wimple         (C) riposter
    (B) cirque         (D) monody

## Correct Answers For Level Three

| | | | |
|---|---|---|---|
| 1. A | 4. D | 7. D | 9. A |
| 2. B | 5. B | 8. C | 10. D |
| 3. A | 6. A | | |

## Level Four—Difficult Completions

1. The will did not require _____ of witnesses since it was holographic.
   (A) subornation     (C) attestation
   (B) bribery         (D) consternation

2. Man's fate is _____.
   (A) ineluctable     (C) estivated
   (B) ceruleant       (D) spatulated

3. How can you depend upon a person who is so _____?
   (A) protean         (C) pensile
   (B) somatic         (D) empirical

4. A _____ would be interested in a _____ of that type.
   (A) botanist-vignette
   (B) soldier-maverick
   (C) musician-caterwaul
   (D) butcher-brioche

5. In India, a wealthy person may travel in a _____ borne by means of poles resting on men's shoulders.
   (A) palanquin       (C) gambrel
   (B) bibelot         (D) lampoon

6. Suffering from _____, he decided to stay indoors.
   (A) claustrophobia  (C) chicanery
   (B) agoraphobia     (D) patois

7. _____ that my uncle is, he can do just about everything.
   (A) Dipsomaniac     (C) Numismatist
   (B) Factotum        (D) Pachyderm

8. His _____ features reminded me of the missing link.
   (A) simian          (C) vicarious
   (B) euphemistic     (D) vertiginous

9. For insisting on "It is I" instead of "It is me," he was charged with _____.
   (A) calligraphy     (C) bellicosity
   (B) anomaly         (D) preciosity

10. In certain tropical areas, malaria is an _____ disease.
    (A) endocrine      (C) endemic
    (B) introversive   (D) interstitial

## Correct Answers For Level Four

| | | | |
|---|---|---|---|
| 1. C | 4. A | 7. B | 9. D |
| 2. A | 5. A | 8. A | 10. C |
| 3. A | 6. B | | |

# VERBAL ABILITY : SENTENCE COMPLETIONS

*DIRECTIONS: Each of the completion questions in this test consists of an incomplete sentence. Each sentence is followed by a series of lettered words, one of which best completes the sentence. Select the word that best completes the meaning of each sentence, and mark the letter of that word opposite that sentence.*

*Correct key answers to all these test questions will be found at the end of the test.*

1. Publication of the article was timed to _____ with professor's fiftieth birthday.
   (A) coincide      (B) harmonize
   (C) amalgamate      (D) terminate
   (E) elucidate.

2. Few institutions are more _____ than France's provincial museums, but lately an effort has been made to rouse them from their lethargy.
   (A) resistant      (B) conformist
   (C) conservative      (D) mellifluous
   (E) somnolent.

3. The early part of the performance may prove to be only the lively _____ to a more sumptuous drama.
   (A) fissure      (B) consummation
   (C) prelude      (D) diversion
   (E) incarceration.

4. He owes most of his success to his calm, measured, analytical attack on the problems of advertising making order out of _____.
   (A) procedure      (B) chaos
   (C) anathema      (D) propulsion
   (E) miscellany.

5. Genius, according to Schopenhauer, is _____ to the opinions of others—notably of authorities.
   (A) response      (B) condolence
   (C) pertinence      (D) malice
   (E) imperviousness.

6. His productions are not _____. The ideas usually are slow in building up.
   (A) comprehensible      (B) conducive
   (C) matriarchal      (D) spontaneous
   (E) mortified.

7. The fact is so _____ that no one has ever succeeded even in defining it.
   (A) fragmentary      (B) morbid
   (C) elusive      (D) mortification
   (E) mastoidal.

8. One of the few hard and fast "musts" around here is _____, which Webster defines as the ability to live, grow, and develop.
   (A) malleability      (B) viability
   (C) flexibility      (D) retention
   (E) latency.

9. Honors go to Insley's drawings which have an unusual _____ quality, as if they had been traced by a misunderstanding hand, by a mind utterly unaccustomed to Western pictorial representation and haltingly trying to understand through copying.
   (A) dilettante      (B) professional
   (C) primitive      (D) snide
   (E) gauche.

10. Discretion and a gift for compensating a basic monotony of composition by subtle _____ also characterize his paintings.
    (A) modulations      (B) aberrations
    (C) consolidations      (D) analogies
    (E) complications.

**Answer Sheet**

|   | 1 | 2 | 3 | 4 | 5 |
|---|---|---|---|---|---|
| 1 | ⋮ | ⋮ | ⋮ | ⋮ | ⋮ |
| 2 | ⋮ | ⋮ | ⋮ | ⋮ | ⋮ |
| 3 | ⋮ | ⋮ | ⋮ | ⋮ | ⋮ |
| 4 | ⋮ | ⋮ | ⋮ | ⋮ | ⋮ |
| 5 | ⋮ | ⋮ | ⋮ | ⋮ | ⋮ |

**Answer Sheet**

|    | 1 | 2 | 3 | 4 | 5 |
|----|---|---|---|---|---|
| 6  | ⋮ | ⋮ | ⋮ | ⋮ | ⋮ |
| 7  | ⋮ | ⋮ | ⋮ | ⋮ | ⋮ |
| 8  | ⋮ | ⋮ | ⋮ | ⋮ | ⋮ |
| 9  | ⋮ | ⋮ | ⋮ | ⋮ | ⋮ |
| 10 | ⋮ | ⋮ | ⋮ | ⋮ | ⋮ |

# Correct Answers For The Foregoing Questions

*(Please make every effort to answer the questions on your own before look-ing at these answers. You'll make faster progress by following this rule.)*

**Completions Test**

| 1. A | 4. B | 6. D | 8. B |
|------|------|------|------|
| 2. E | 5. E | 7. C | 9. E |
| 3. C |      |      | 10. A |

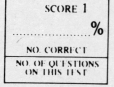

SCORE 1

.................... %

NO. CORRECT

NO. OF QUESTIONS ON THIS TEST

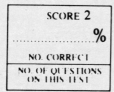

SCORE 2

.................... %

NO. CORRECT

NO. OF QUESTIONS ON THIS TEST

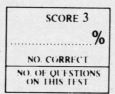

SCORE 3

.................... %

NO. CORRECT

NO. OF QUESTIONS ON THIS TEST

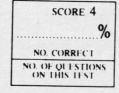

SCORE 4

.................... %

NO. CORRECT

NO. OF QUESTIONS ON THIS TEST

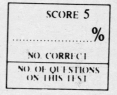

SCORE 5

.................... %

NO. CORRECT

NO. OF QUESTIONS ON THIS TEST

# Practice Using Answer Sheets

Alter numbers to match the practice and drill questions in each part of the book.
Make only ONE mark for each answer. Additional and stray marks may be counted as mistakes.
In making corrections, erase errors COMPLETELY. Make glossy black marks.

TEAR OUT ALONG THIS LINE AND MARK YOUR ANSWERS AS INSTRUCTED IN THE TEXT

# SKILL WITH VERBAL ANALOGIES

*This is an interesting variation of the vocabulary question, often encountered on intelligence tests. It tests your understanding of word meanings and your ability to grasp relationships between words and ideas. We expect this kind of question on your test, so you can be sure that this chapter is worthwhile. But even more important is the practice in mental agility which will carry over to better results with all the other questions on the test.*

IN addition to their simple meanings, words carry subtle shades of implication that depend in some degree upon the relationship they bear to other words. There are various classifications of relationship, such as similarity (synonyms) and opposition (antonyms). The careful student will examine each word in these analogy questions for the exact shade of meaning indicated.

The ability to detect the exact nature of the relationship between words is a function of your intelligence. In a sense, the verbal analogy test is a vocabulary test. But it is also a test of your ability to analyze meanings, think things out and to see the relationships between ideas and words, and avoid confusion of ideas. In mathematics, this type of situation is expressed as a ratio and proportion problem: $3:5 = 6:X$. Sometimes verbal analogies are written in this mathematical form:

CLOCK: TIME—THERMOMETER: (A) hour (B) degrees (C) temperature (D) climate (E) weather.

Or the question may be put:

CLOCK is to TIME as THERMOMETER is to (A) hour (B) degrees (C) temperature (D) climate (E) weather.

The problem is to determine which of the lettered words has the same relationship to thermometer as time has to clock.

The best way of determining the correct answer is to provide the word or phrase which shows the relationship between these words. In the example above, the word is measures. However, this may not be enough. The analogy must be correct in exact meaning. Climate or weather would not be exact enough. Temperature, of course, is the correct answer.

You will find that many of the choices you have to select from have some relationship to the third word. You must select the one with a relationship most closely approximating the relationship between the first two words.

## What the Analogy Question Measures

The analogy question tests your ability to see a relationship between words and to apply this relationship to other words. Although the verbal analogy test is, to some degree, an indicator of your vocabulary, it is essentially a test of your ability to think things out. In other words, analogy questions will spotlight your ability to think clearly—your ability to sidestep confusion of ideas. In mathematics, this type of situation is expressed as a proportion problem—for example, $3:5 :: 6:X$. Verbal analogy questions, are written in this mathematical form.

# Three Forms of the Analogy Question

*Type 1. Example:*

From the four (or five) pairs of words which follow, you are to select the pair which is related in the same way as the words of the first pair.

> SPELLING : PUNCTUATION :: (A) pajamas : fatigue (B) powder : shaving (C) bandage : cut (D) biology : physics

*SPELLING* and *PUNCTUATION* are elements of the mechanics of English; *BIOLOGY* and *PHYSICS* are two of the subjects that make up the field of science. The other choices do not possess this PART : PART relationship. Therefore, (D) is the correct choice.

*Type 2. Example:*

Another popular form is the type in which two words are followed by a third word. The latter is related to one word in a group of choices in the same way that the first two words are related.

WINTER is to SUMMER as COLD is to
> (A) wet (B) future (C) warm (D) freezing

*WINTER* and *SUMMER* bear an opposite relationship. *COLD* and *WARM* have the same type of opposite relationship. Therefore, (C) is the correct answer.

*Type 3. Example:*

Still another analogy form is that in which *one* of the four relationship elements is not specified. From choices offered—regardless of the position—you are to select the one choice which completes the relationship with the other three items.

SUBMARINE : FISH as (A) kite (B) limousine (C) feather (D) chirp : BIRD

Both a *SUBMARINE* and a *FISH* are found in the water; both a *KITE* and *BIRD* are customarily seen in the air. (A), consequently, is the correct answer.

This third type is used in the Miller Analogy Test, considered one of the most reliable and valid tests for selection of graduate students in universities, and high-level personnel in government, industry, and business.

# Kinds of Relationship

In analogy questions, the relationship between the first two words may be one of several kinds. Following are relationship possibilities.

1. *Purpose Relationship*
   GLOVE : BALL :: (A) hook : fish (B) winter : weather (C) game : pennant (D) stadium : seats

2. *Cause and Effect Relationship*
   RACE : FATIGUE :: (A) track : athlete (B) ant : bug (C) fast : hunger (D) walking : running

3. *Part : Whole Relationship*
   SNAKE : REPTILE :: (A) patch : thread (B) removal : snow (C) struggle : wrestle (D) hand : clock

4. *Part : Part Relationship*
   GILL : FIN : (A) tube : antenna (B) instrument : violin (C) sea : fish (D) salad : supper

5. *Action to Object Relationship*
   KICK : FOOTBALL :: (A) kill : bomb (B) break : pieces (C) question : team (D) smoke : pipe

6. *Object to Action Relationship*
   STEAK : BROIL :: (A) bread : bake (B) food : sell (C) wine : pour (D) sugar: spill

7. *Synonym Relationship*
   ENORMOUS : HUGE :: (A) rogue : rock (B) muddy : unclear (C) purse : kitchen (D) black : white

8. *Antonym Relationship*
   PURITY : EVIL :: (A) suavity : blunt-
   ness (B) north : climate (C) angel :
   horns (D) boldness : victory

9. *Place Relationship*
   MIAMI : FLORIDA :: (A) Chicago :
   United States (B) New York : Albany
   (C) United States : Chicago (D) Albany
   : New York

10. *Degree Relationship*
    WARM : HOT :: (A) glue : paste (B)
    climate : weather (C) fried egg : boiled
    egg (D) bright : genius

11. *Characteristic Relationship*
    IGNORANCE : POVERTY :: (A) blood
    : wound (B) money : dollar (C) schools
    : elevators (D) education : stupidity

12. *Sequence Relationship*
    SPRING : SUMMER :: (A) Thursday :
    Wednesday (B) Wednesday : Monday
    (C) Monday : Sunday (D) Wednesday
    : Thursday

13. *Grammatical Relationship*
    RESTORE : CLIMB :: (A) segregation
    : seem (B) into : nymph (C) tearoom :
    although (D) overpower : seethe

14. *Numerical Relationship*
    4 : 12 :: (A) 10 : 16 (B) 9 : 27 (C) 3
    : 4 (D) 12 : 6

15. *Association Relationship*
    DEVIL : WRONG :: (A) color : sidewalk
    (B) slipper : state (C) ink : writing
    (D) picture : bed

## Correct Answers

*(You'll learn more by writing your own an-
swers before comparing them with these.)*

| | | | |
|---|---|---|---|
| 1. A | 5. D | 9. D | 13. D |
| 2. C | 6. A | 10. D | 14. B |
| 3. D | 7. B | 11. A | 15. C |
| 4. A | 8. A | 12. D | |

SCORE ............................. %

NO. CORRECT ÷ NO. OF QUESTIONS

*Note 1:* In many analogy questions, the incorrect choices may relate in some way to the first two words. Don't let this association mislead you. For example, in Number 4 above (PART : PART RELATIONSHIP example), the correct answer is (A) tube : antenna. The choice (C) sea : fish is incorrect, although these two latter words are associated in a general sense with the first two words (gill : fin).

*Note 2:* Very often, the relationship of the first two words may apply to more than *one* of the choices given. In such a case, you must "narrow down" the initial relationship in order to get the correct choice. For example, in Number 6 above (OBJECT : ACTION RELATIONSHIP), a STEAK is something that you BROIL. Now let us consider the choices: BREAD is something that you BAKE; FOOD is something that you SELL; WINE is something that you POUR; and SUGAR is something that you (can) SPILL. Thus far, each choice seems correct. Let us now "narrow down" the relationship: a STEAK is something that you BROIL with *heat*. The only choice that fulfils this *complete* relationship is (A) BREAD — something that you BAKE with *heat*. It follows that (A) is the correct choice.

## Two Important Steps to Analogy Success

Step One—Determine the relationship between the first two words.
Step Two—Find the same relationship among the choices which follow the first two words.

NOW LET US APPLY THESE TWO STEPS

1. *Determining the relationship.*

*Directions:* Each question consists of two words which have some relationship to each other. From the five following pairs of words, select the one which is related in the same way as the words of the first pair:

ARC : CIRCLE :: (A) segment : cube
   (B) angle : triangle (C) tangent : circum-
   ference (D) circle : cube (E) cube : square
   An arc is part of a circle, just as an angle is part of a triangle. The other choices do not bear this PART : WHOLE relationship. Therefore, (B) is correct.

With the foregoing line of reasoning, you probably eliminated choice (A) immediately. Choice (B) seemed correct. Did you give it *final* acceptance without considering the remaining choices? In this analogy question, choice (B), as it turned out, was the correct choice. However, let us change the question slightly:

ARC : CIRCLE :: (A) segment : cube
(B) angle : triangle (C) tangent : circumference (D) circle : cube (E) line: square

Note that the (E) choice has been changed. (E)— not (B)— is now the correct answer. REASON: An arc is *any* part of the drawn circle. Likewise, a line is *any* part of the drawn square. However, an angle is *not* any part of the drawn triangle. The correct answer is, therefore, (E) line : square.

This illustration should caution you not to "jump to conclusions." Consider *all* choices carefully before you reach your conclusion.

## 2. *Use the word that shows the relationship.*

The best way of determining the correct answer to an analogy question is to *provide the word or phrase* which shows the relationship that exists between the first two words. Let us illustrate with the following analogy question:

CLOCK : TIME :: (A) hour : latitude
(B) thermometer : temperature (C) weather : climate (D) tide : moon

The problem here is to determine which choice has the same relationship that *clock* has to *time*. Let us, now, provide the word or phrase which shows the relationship between *clock* and *time*. The word is *measures*. Choice B, then, is the correct answer since a thermometer *measures* temperature.

You will find that many of the choices which you are given have some relationship to the opening pair. You must be sure to select *that* choice which bears a relationship most closely approximating the relationship between the opening two words.

## ANALYSIS OF ANALOGY PITFALLS

*DIRECTIONS: In each of the following questions the FIRST TWO words in capital letters go together in some way. Find how they are related. Then write the correct letter to show which one of the last five words goes with the THIRD word in capital letters in the same way that the second word in capital letters goes with the first.*

The important rule to remember in answering an analogy question is to determine the specific relationship of the first two words of the analogy, and then choose the word given in the alternatives bearing a similar relationship to the third member of the analogy.

It is also important to point out some of the more important pitfalls involved in answering this type of question. Let us take some sample questions:

I.   FOOD is to HUNGER as SLEEP is to
     (A) night          (B) dream
     (C) weariness      (D) health
     (E) rest

Obviously, all of the words are related to sleep in some way. None of them except weariness bears the same relationship to sleep as hunger does to food. Before answering one of these questions, then, we must fix in our minds the relationship that the first two words of the analogy bear to each other.

(A) although one sleeps at night, it is not the night that is relieved by sleep.

(B) sleep is certainly related to dream because people dream when they sleep. But again, it is not dreams that are relieved by sleep.

(C) food relieves hunger and sleep relieves weariness. Therefore weariness is correct.

(D) sleep is productive, in part, of health, but this is not the relationship that we are seeking.

(E) sleep results in rest but food does not result in hunger.

II.  CUP is to DRINK as PLATE is to
     (A) supper         (B) fork
     (C) dine           (D) earthenware
     (E) silver

What is the relationship between cup (noun) and drink (verb)?

It is obvious that one DRINKS from a cup.
What does one do from a plate in the same manner that one drinks from a cup?
It becomes apparent that of the five choices offered, (C) dine, is the only one which bears a similar relationship, since one dines from a plate.

A closer analogy would have been one EATS from a plate, but since this word is not offered, the best of the five choices is DINE.
Notice that all of the remaining choices bear some relationship to the word plate but not the same that cup bears to drink.

(A) supper is related to plate since one's supper may be eaten from a plate. Supper, however, is a noun, and the part of speech required is a verb.

(B) fork is related to plate since both are eating utensils, but this is not the relationship required, so it must be eliminated.

(C) earthenware is related to plate since many plates are made of earthenware, but this also is not the relationship called for.

(D) silver is related to plate since in one sense they are synonyms. There is also a relationship established in the word "silver-plated," but neither of these is the relationship required.

III. GUILLOTINE is to DECAPITATE as RAZOR is to

(A) beard      (B) hair
(C) shave     (D) cut
(E) steel

This is the type of analogy which deals with the use, purpose or function of an object or instrument.
The purpose of a guillotine is to decapitate.
What is a razor used for?
It is obvious that the most important use of the razor is to shave, so (C) is the correct answer.
Notice the relationships of the remaining choices:

(A) razor is related to beard, since it is used to cut beards, but it is not the relation-

ship required. Also, the sense of the analogy calls for a verb, not a noun.

(B) razor is related to hair, since it cuts hair, but hair is not the purpose of razor.

(C) cut is one of the uses of a razor, but it is not its primary function. Relatively it is not as important as shave.

(E) steel is related to razor in the sense that some razors are made of steel, but since steel is not the function of a razor, it must be eliminated as incorrect.

IV. ADDER is to SNAKE as CROCODILE is to

(A) ruminant     (B) marsh
(C) reptile      (D) carnivore
(E) rapacious

This is a type of analogy question frequently met on examinations. The candidate must learn to distinguish between a specific and a general. In many cases it is a question of comparing a specie of an animal, plant, tree, bird, etc. to its broader classification.
An adder is a kind or type of snake.
Snake is a general term including many different species, of which adder is only one.
In the same way, which of the five choices is the general classification under which the specie crocodile can be classified?

(A) a ruminant is an animal that chews the cud, as a goat or a sheep. A crocodile is not a ruminant.

(B) a marsh is a tract of low, miry land. It has no connection with types of crocodiles.

(C) reptile is a broad classification of animals including the crocodile. It has the same relation to crocodile as adder has to snake, and is therefore the correct choice.

(D) a carnivore is a mammalian animal which lives on flesh for food. The crocodile is not of this type.

(E) rapacious is an adjective meaning subsisting on prey or animals seized by violence." Since rapacious is not a type of crocodile, it could not possibly be the correct choice.

V. BREAKABLE is to FRANGIBLE as GULLIBLE is to

(A) credulous  (B) deceptive
(C) capable   (D) lurid
(E) marine

This is an analogy formed by comparing two adjectives.

They are synonymous since they have the same meanings.

Inasmuch as the first words of the analogy are adjectives the second pair must also be adjectives.

Gullible is an exact synonym of credulous and is therefore the most correct choice.

None of the other choices bears any resemblance in meaning to gullible.

Now, push forward! Test yourself and practice for your test with the carefully constructed quizzes that follow. Each one presents the kind of question you may expect on your test. And each question is at just the level of difficulty that may be expected. Don't try to take all the tests at one time. Rather, schedule yourself so that you take a few at each session, and spend approximately the same time on them at each session. Score yourself honestly, and date each test. You should be able to detect improvement in your performance on successive sessions.

A portion of the standard answer sheet is provided after each test for marking your answers in the way you'll be required to do on the actual exam. At the right of this answer sheet, to make the scoring job simpler (after you have derived your own answers), you'll find our correct answers.

# ANALOGY TEST

*DIRECTIONS: In these test questions each of the two CAPI-TALIZED words have a certain relationship to each other. Following the capitalized words are other pairs of words, each designated by a letter. Select the lettered pair wherein the words are related in the same way as the two CAPITALIZED words are related to each other*

## EXPLANATIONS OF KEY POINTS BEHIND THESE QUESTIONS ARE GIVEN WITH THE ANSWERS WHICH FOLLOW THE QUESTIONS.

1. JAIL : CRIME ::

   (A) judge : criminal
   (B) freedom : bird
   (C) prison : thief
   (D) cemetery : death
   (E) victim : intruder

2. DESCRIPTION : CHARACTERIZATION ::

   (A) novel : narration
   (B) biographer : author
   (C) artist : writer
   (D) composition : argumentation
   (E) picture : portrait

3. MUMBLE : TALK ::

   (A) orate : speak
   (B) scrawl : write
   (C) bumble : buzz
   (D) yell : shout
   (E) mumbo : jumbo

4. HYBRID : THOROUGHBRED ::

   (A) steel : iron
   (B) fruit : tree
   (C) stallion : mare
   (D) highbrow : lowbrow
   (E) superficiality : thoroughness

5. FRAGILE : CRACK ::

   (A) potent : enervate
   (B) irreducible : reduce
   (C) frangible : strengthen
   (D) odorous : spray
   (E) pliable : bend

6. FULLBACK : FIELD ::

   (A) halfback : infield
   (B) baseball : stadium
   (C) boxer : ring
   (D) medal : winner
   (E) helmet : pad

7. HYDRO : WATER ::

   (A) helio : sun
   (B) Reno : divorce
   (C) canto : score
   (D) hydrophobia : dog
   (E) Hires : root beer

8. 3 : 3's ::

   (A) three : six
   (B) trio : quartet
   (C) singular : possessive
   (D) salmon : salmon
   (E) number : letter

9. SONG : SWAN ::

   (A) tune : goose
   (B) speech : orator
   (C) bird : tweet
   (D) call : telephone
   (E) sandwich : ham

10. PEACH : BEET ::

    (A) grape : apple
    (B) potato : tomato
    (C) currant : raspberry
    (D) banana : plum
    (E) cherry : radish

11. SMILE : AMUSEMENT ::

    (A) yell : game
    (B) guffaw : laughter
    (C) yawn : ennui
    (D) wink : vulgarity
    (E) cry : havoc

12. MINK : LION ::

    (A) chicken : wolf
    (B) tiger : zebra
    (C) farm : zoo
    (D) lady : gentleman
    (E) timidity : daring

13. DREDGE : SILT ::

    (A) tug : gravel
    (B) train : plane
    (C) scoop : ice cream
    (D) distance : sequence
    (E) drudge : sludge

14. SHONE : DISHONEST ::

    (A) lest : candlestick
    (B) seen : revelation
    (C) concealed : honesty
    (D) caught : thief
    (E) neither : innocence

15. WOOD : CHARCOAL ::

    (A) bonfire : marshmallow
    (B) grill : oven
    (C) coal : coke
    (D) furniture : portrait
    (E) light : heavy

16. MICROMETER : BURETTE ::

    (A) microscope : germ
    (B) hydrometer : water
    (C) microbe : thorn
    (D) chemist : biologist
    (E) ruler : dropper

17. MOLD : DIE ::

    (A) cast : stamp
    (B) fungus : death
    (C) form : destroy
    (D) hold : defeat
    (E) imprison : execute

18. DOOR : PORTAL ::

    (A) opening : closing
    (B) doorway : living room
    (C) house : ship
    (D) knob : key
    (E) porch : portico

19. DUNE : SAND ::

    (A) hill : beach
    (B) wind : grain
    (C) salt : air
    (D) glazier : glass
    (E) glacier : snow

20. LAWYER : CLIENT ::

    (A) doctor : patient
    (B) teacher : pupil
    (C) mother : child
    (D) country : inhabitant
    (E) Hindu : Moslem

# Correct Answers For The Foregoing Questions

*(Check your answers with these that we provide. You should find considerable correspondence between them. If not, you'd better go back and find out why. On the next page we have provided concise clarifications of basic points behind the key answers. Please go over them carefully because they may be quite useful in helping you pick up extra points on the exam.)*

**Answer Sheet** / **Answer Sheet** / **SCORE** **%** / NO. CORRECT / NO. OF QUESTIONS ON THIS TEST / **Correct Answers** / **Correct Answers**

Correct Answers (left column):
1. C
2. E
3. B
4. A
5. E
6. B
7. A
8. E
9. C
10. E

Correct Answers (right column):
11. C
12. B
13. A
14. A
15. B
16. E
17. A
18. E
19. E
20. C

# EXPLANATORY ANSWERS

*Elucidation, clarification, explication and a little help with the fundamental facts covered in the Previous Test. These are the points and principles likely to crop up in the form of questions on future tests.*

1. **(D)** Crime usually lands a person in jail; death usually lands a person in a cemetery.

2. **(E)** A characterization is a kind of description—usually a description of a person; a portrait is a kind of picture—usually a picture of a person.

3. **(B)** To mumble is to talk carelessly, thus making it difficult to be understood; to scrawl is to write carelessly so that it is difficult to be understood.

4. **(A)** A hybrid is of mixed origin or of different elements—a thoroughbred is of pure stock; steel is an alloy of iron.

5. **(E)** One can crack something that is fragile; one can bend something that is pliable.

6. **(C)** A fullback plays on a football field; a boxer "operates" in a ring.

7. **(A)** Hydro is a combining form meaning water; helio is a combining form meaning sun.

8. **(D)** The plural form of 3 is 3's; the plural form of salmon is salmon.

9. **(D)** We listen to a swan song and a telephone call.

10. **(E)** A peach grows above the ground—a beet below; a cherry grows above the ground—a radish underground.

11. **(C)** A smile indicates amusement; a yawn indicates ennui.

12. **(B)** The mink and lion are brown; the tiger and zebra are striped.

13. **(C)** One dredges silt and scoops ice cream.

14. **(A)** Shone is an integral part of the word dishonest; lest is an integral part of the word candlestick.

15. **(C)** Charcoal is made by burning wood; coke is made by heating coal.

16. **(E)** A micrometer is used instead of a ruler for measuring small distances; a burette is used instead of a dropper for delivering small quantities of a liquid.

17. **(A)** One casts a mold and stamps a die.

18. **(E)** A portal is a fancy type of door; a portico is a fancy type of porch.

19. **(E)** A dune is a hill of loose sand heaped by the wind; a glacier is a field of ice formed from compacted snow.

20. **(C)** A lawyer protects his client; a mother protects her child.

# DAT WORD LIST

*There are over two thousand words in this list. And every one of them has been included because it has appeared in the past on a vocabulary test similar to the one you're going to take. Many thousands of people have used the list successfully. And they have sent us hundreds of letters testifying to its value in raising their scores. Please note that the words are in alphabetic order; that each one is defined briefly; and that the important synonyms and antonyms are given wherever they are helpful.*

## A

**abase**—to degrade
**abash**—to embarrass
**abate**—to decrease
**aberration**—variation
**abeyance**—temporary suspension
**abject**—miserable
**abjure**—to renounce
**ablution**—cleansing
**abnegate**—to reject
**abominate**—to abhor
**aborigine**—original inhabitant
**abortive**—futile
**abrade**—to rub off
**abrogate**—to abolish
**absolve**—to acquit
**absolution**—forgiveness
**abstemious**—sparing in diet
**abstruse**—difficult to understand
**abut**—to adjoin
**accolade**—praise
**accoutre**—to equip
**acerbity**—bitterness
**acolyte**—assistant
**acrimony**—bitterness

**actuary**—insurance computer
**actuate**—to incite
**acumen**—sharpness of mind
**adage**—proverb
**adamant**—inflexible
**adduce**—to bring forth proof
**adipose**—fatty
**adjunct**—attachment
**adjure**—to demand, request
**admonish**—to warn
**adroit**—skillful
**adulation**—praise
**adumbration**—omen, warning
**advent**—coming
**adventitious**—accidental
**adversity**—misfortune
**affable**—friendly
**affected**—assumed artificially
**affidavit**—sworn statement in writing
**affinity**—relationship
**affirmation**—positive statement
**affluent**—plentiful

**agenda**—things to be done
**agglomerate**—to gather into one mass
**aggrandize**—to increase
**aggregate**—total
**agnostic**—doubter
**agrarian**—rural
**akimbo**—with hands on hips
**alacrity**—speed
**albino**—white
**alchemy**—medieval chemistry
**alienist**—psychiatrist
**alimentary**—pert. to food
**allay**—to calm
**allocate**—to apportion
**allude**—to refer
**alluvial**—left by departing water
**altercate**—to quarrel
**altruism**—unselfishness
**amatory**—loving
**ambidextrous**—versatile, skillful
**ambrosia**—food for ancient gods
**ambulant**—able to walk

**ameliorate**—to improve
**amenable**—submissive
**amenity**—pleasing manner
**amnesty**—pardon
**amulet**—charm
**anachronism**—something out of time
**analgesic**—pain-reliever
**analogous**—corresponding (to)
**anathema**—curse
**anchorite**—hermit
**aneroid**—using no fluid
**aneurism**—swelling of artery
**animadversion**—criticism
**animalcule**—microscopic animal
**annals**—records by the year
**anneal**—to toughen
**anomaly**—irregularity
**antediluvian**—old
**anterior**—front; earlier
**anthropoid**—resembling man
**anthropology**—the science of man

antithesis—direct opposite
antipathy—dislike
apartheid—South African racial segregation
apathetic—indifferent
aperture—opening
apex—peak
aphorism—proverb
apiary—place where bees are kept
aplomb—poise
apocalypse—revelation
apocryphal—of doubtful authority
apogee—highest point
apostasy—forsaking one's religion
apothegm—aphorism
apotheosis—deification
appall—to horrify
appellation—name; title
append—to attach
apposite—appropriate
apprise—to give notice
aquiline—hooked
arabesque—ornament; ballet position
arable—plowable
arbiter—judge
arboreal—living among trees
archetype—example
archipelago—group of islands
archive—record
arduous—laborious
argot—slang
armada—fleet of armed ships
arraign—to bring before a court
arrogate—to claim without right
arroyo—dry river bed
artifacts—products of primitive art
artifice—deception
ascetic—practicing self-denial
aseptic—free from bacteria
asperity—harshness
aspersion—slanderous remark

assay—to evaluate
asseverate—to assert
assiduous—constant; devoted
assimilate—to absorb
assuage—to ease
astral—relating to stars
astute—shrewd
athwart—in opposition to
atoll—a ring-shaped island
atrophy—wasting away
attenuate—to make slender
attest—to bear witness to
attrition—rubbing against
atypical—not normal
augur—to foretell
aural—pert. to hearing
aureate—gilded
auspices—protection
auspicious—indicating success
austerity—severity
austral—southern
autocrat—absolute monarch
autonomy—self-government
autopsy—inspection of corpse
avarice—greed
averse—reluctant
avocation—hobby
avoirdupois—system of weights
avuncular—like an uncle
awry—in the wrong direction

## B

badger—to tease or annoy
badinage—playful teasing
baleful—destructive
banal—commonplace
bandy—to give and take
baneful—evil
banter—good-natured ridicule
baroque—highly ornate
barrister—counselor-at-law
bastion—fortification

bauble—trinket
beatify—to make happy
bedizen—to adorn gaudily
beguile—to cheat
belabor—to beat soundly
belle-lettres—literature
bellicose—warlike
benediction—blessing
beneficence—charity
benign—kindly
berate—to scold vehemently
besom—a broom
bestride—to straddle
bicameral—consisting of two branches
biennial—every two years
biped—two-footed animal
blanch—to bleach
blasphemy—contempt for God
blatant—noisy
blithe—joyous
bluster—to be noisy
bombastic—pompous
bourgeois—pert. to the middle class
bourne—boundary
bourse—a foreign exchange
bovine—cowlike
brigand—bandit
broach—introduce
bromidic—tiresome; dull
bruit—to rumor
brusque—blunt in manner
bucolic—rustic
buffoon—a clown
bull—a papal letter
bullion—gold or silver in bars
burgeon—to sprout
burnish—to polish by rubbing

## C

cabal—conspiracy
cabala—any occult science
cache—hiding place
cacophony—discord
cadaver—dead body

cadence—rhythm
cadre—framework
caduceus—symbol of the medical profession
cairn—heap of stones used as a tombstone
caitiff—scoundrel
cajole—coax
caliph—Moslem head
calk, caulk  to fill a seam
calligraphy—penmanship
callow—immature; innocent
calumniate—to slander
camaraderie—fellowship
canaille—rabble; mob
cant—slang; pretense
canter—easy gallop
cantilever—type of bridge
canvass—to solicit (note spelling)
capacious—spacious
capitulate—to surrender
capricious—whimsical; fickle
captious—faultfinding
carafe—coffee bottle
carcinoma—cancer
careen—to tip to one side
carnal—of the body
carnivorous—flesh-eating
carrion—decaying flesh
carte blanche—unrestricted authority
cassock—long church garment
castigate—to criticize; punish
casuistry—false reasoning
cataclysm—sudden, violent change
catalyst—substance causing change
catastrophe—calamity
catechism—elementary religious book
categorical—certain
cathartic—cleansing
catholic—universal
caudal—near the tail
causerie—a chat

**cauterize**—to cut with a hot iron
**caveat**—warning
**cavil**—to find fault
**celerity**—swiftness
**celibacy**—unmarried state
**cenotaph**—monument for the dead
**cephalic**—pert. to the head
**cerebral**—pert. to the brain
**cerebration**—process of thought
**cervical**—pert. to the neck
**chaff**—rubbish; to tease
**chagrin**—disappoint-ment, vexation
**challis**—soft cotton fabric
**chamberlain**—official
**chameleon**—lizard
**champ**—to bite
**chandler**—dealer in candles
**charlatan**—impostor
**charnel**—burial place
**chary**—careful, stingy
**chaste**—pure
**chastisement**—punish-ment
**chattel**—property
**chauvinism**—zealous patriotism
**chicanery**—fraud
**chide**—to rebuke
**chimerical**—imaginary
**chiropractic**—healing by manipulating
**chivalrous**—gallant
**chrysalis**—the pre-butterfly stage
**churlish**—rude
**chutney**—seasoning
**cicada**—locust
**circuitous**—roundabout
**circumlocution**—talking around a subject
**circumspect**—watchful
**circumvent**—to go around
**cirrus**—thin, fleecy cloud
**citadel**—fortress
**cite**—to quote

**clack**—to chatter
**clairvoyant**—foretelling the future
**clandestine**—secret
**claque**—hired applauders
**claustrophobia**—fear of enclosed places
**clavicle**—collarbone
**clavier**—musical keyboard
**cleave**—to adhere; to split
**cliché**—overworked expression
**climacteric**—critical
**coadjutor**—helper
**coalesce**—to grow together
**coddle**—to boil gently
**codicil**—addition
**coerce**—to compel
**coffer**—box
**cogent**—convincing
**cogitate**—to think
**cognate**—related
**cohesion**—sticking together
**cohort**—a company or band
**colander**—strainer
**collateral**—accompany-ing
**collate**—to collect in order
**collation**—a light meal
**colligate**—arrange in order
**collocation**—arrange-ment
**colloquialism**—informal conversation
**colloquy**—conference
**collusion**—secret agree-ment
**colophon**—inscription in a book
**comatose**—lethargic
**comity**—friendly feeling
**commensurate**—equal; corresponding
**comminuted**—reduced to fine particles
**commiseration**—sym-pathy
**commodious**—roomy
**commutation**—substitu-

tion
**compact**—agreement
**complacent**—self-satisfied
**complaisant**—calm
**complement**—full quantity
**component**—ingredient
**compunction**—remorse
**concatenate**—to connect
**concentric**—with the same center
**conclave**—a private meeting
**concomitant**—accom-panying
**concordat**—covenant
**concupiscent**—lustful
**concurrent**—running together
**condign**—well-deserved
**condiment**—spice
**condole**—to express sympathy
**condone**—to pardon
**conduce**—to lead to
**conduit**—pipe
**confidant**—one confided in
**configuration**—form resulting from arrangement of parts
**conflagration**—large fire
**confute**—to overwhelm by argument
**congeal**—to change from a fluid to a solid
**congenital**—dating from birth
**conglomerate**—mixture
**congruent**—in agreement
**congruous**—becoming
**conic**—cone-shaped
**conifer**—cone-bearing tree
**conjecture**—guess
**conjoin**—to unite
**conjugal**—pert. to marriage
**conjure**—to produce by magic
**connive**—to assist in wrong-doing
**connubial**—pert. to marriage
**consanguinity**—blood relationship

**consecrate**—to dedicate
**consign**—to transfer merchandise
**consonance**—agreement
**consort**—wife or husband
**constituency**—body of voters
**constrain**—to compel
**consummate**—to complete
**contemn**—to despise
**contentious**—quarrel-some
**contiguous**—next to
**contingent**—conditional
**contravene**—to oppose
**contrition**—repentance
**controvert**—to dispute
**contumacious**—stub-bornly disobedient
**contumely**—contempt
**contusion**—bruise
**conundrum**—puzzle
**conversant**—having knowledge of
**convivial**—gay,
**convoke**—to call together
**copious**—plentiful
**cordillera**—chain of mountains
**cordovan**—type of leather
**cornucopia**—horn of plenty
**coronary**—pert. to the arteries
**corporeal**—bodily
**corpulent**—very fat
**correlate**—to have a relationship
**corroborate**—to confirm
**corollary**—something that follows; result
**corona**—crown
**cortege**—procession
**cosmopolitan**—belonging to the world
**coterie**—small informal group
**cotillion**—a social dance
**cotter**—pin
**couchant**—lying down
**coulee**—gulch
**countermand**—to revoke an order

coup d'état—overthrow of government
couplet—two lines that rhyme
couturier—dressmaker
cozen—to cheat
covenant—agreement
covert—hidden
covetous—envious
cower—to shrink from fear
crag—rock
crass—stupid
craven—cowardly
credence—belief
credulous—inclined to believe
cremate—to burn a dead body
cretinism—dwarfism
crimp—to make wavy
criterion—standard of judging
crouton—piece of toasted bread
cruciate—cross-shaped
crux—vital point
cryptic—mysterious
cudgel—thick stick
culinary—relating to the kitchen
culmination—acme
culpable—guilty
cuneate—wedge-shaped
cumulus—rounded cloud
cupidity—greed
curmudgeon—churlish person
cursory—superficial
cygnet—young swan

## D

dactyl—a metrical foot
daguerreotype—type of early photograph
dale—valley
dalliance—dawdling
damask—a figured fabric
dank—damp
dappled—marked with small spots
dastard—coward
davit—crane for hoisting boats
dawdle—to waste time

dearth—scarcity
debase—to reduce in dignity
debauch—to corrupt
debilitate—to weaken
debonair—courteous
decadence—deterioration
decamp—to depart; flee
decant—to pour off gently
decanter—ornamental wine bottle
deciduous—leaf-shedding
declivity—downward slope
décolleté—low-necked
decorous—proper
decrepit—old
decry—to clamor against
deduce—to derive by reasoning
de facto—actual
defalcation—embezzlement
defamation—slander
defection—desertion
deference—act of respect
definitive— final
defunct—dead
deify—to make as a god
deign—to condescend
de jure—according to law
delectable—delightful
delete—to erase; remove
deleterious—harmful
delineate—to mark off
delta—flat plain at river mouth
demagogue—leader who incites
demean—to debase
demesne—possession of land
demur—to hesitate
demure—serious
denizen—inhabitant
dénouement—solution
deposition—testimony outside court
deprecate—to belittle

depreciate—decrease in value
depredation—plundering
derelict—something abandoned
derogatory—disparaging
descant—to talk or write lengthily
descry—to spy out
desecrate—to profane
despicable—contemptible
despoil—to plunder
desultory—aimless
deterrent—thing which discourages
detonate—to explode
deviate—to stray
devolve—to hand down
dexterity—skill
diabolic—devilish
diadem—a crown
diapason—full range of notes
diaphanous—translucent; filmy
dichotomy—division
dictum—authoritative statement
didactic—instructive
diffidence—timidity
diffuse—to spread out
digress—to wander
dilate—to expand
dilatory—dawdling
dilettante—a dabbler
diluvial—pert. to the flood
diminution—reduction in size
diocese—district of bishop
dipsomaniac—an alcoholic (person)
dirk—a kind of dagger
discernible—identifiable
disciple—student
disclaim—to renounce
discomfit—to defeat
disconcert—to throw into confusion
disconsolate—hopeless
discordant—not harmonious

discountenance— to disapprove
discursive—rambling
disdain—to reject
disingenuous—not innocent
disinterested—unprejudiced
disjoin—to separate
disparage—to belittle
disparity—inequality
disputation—controversy
disquisition—discussion of a subject
dissemble—to disguise
disseminate—to spread
dissertation—formal essay
dissimulation—disguise
dissipate—to squander
dissolute—immoral
dissonant—inharmonious
dissuade—to advise against
distend—to stretch
distortion—twisting out of shape
distraught—bewildered
dithyramb—choral song
diurnal—daily
diva—prima donna
diverge—to extend in different directions
diversity—variety
divest—to deprive
divination—foreseeing the future
divot—turf cut out by a stroke
docile—easily led
doctrinate—impractical theorist
doggerel—poorly written poetry
dogma—system of beliefs
dogmatic—arbitrary
doldrums—boredom
dole—free food or money
doleful—sorrowful
dolorous—grievous
dolphin—porpoise
dolt—blockhead

doomsday—day of judgment

dormant—sleeping

dorsal—referring to the back

dossier—file on a person

dotage—senility

dotard—senile person

doublet—man's coat

doughty—valiant

dour—sullen

dowry—money given at time of marriage

doxology—hymn praising God

dray—open cart

drivel—foolish talk

droll—amusing

dross—waste matter

dryad—wood nymph

dubiuos—doubtful

ductile—able to be molded

dudgeon—resentment

duenna—Spanish chaperone

dupe—to deceive

duplicity—hypocrisy

durance—imprisonment

## E

ebullience—boiling up

ecclesiastical—pert. to the church

eclat—brilliancy of achievement

ecology—science of environment

eclogue—pastoral poem

electic—selective

ecstasy—extreme happiness

ecumenical—general

edict—public notice

edifice—a building (especially large)

edify—to instruct

educe—to bring out

efface—to wipe out

effete—worn-out

effigy—image

effluence—a flowing out

effrontery—boldness

effulgent—illuminated

effusive—gushing

egocentric—self-centered

egotism—conceit

egress—exit

elated—elevated in spirit

electorate—voting body

eleemosynary—devoted to charity

elegy—mournful poem

elicit—to draw out

elucidate—to make clear

emanate—to issue forth

embellish—to adorn

embody—to render concrete

embolism—blood clot

embrocate—to rub with a lotion

emendation—a correction

emetic—inducing vomiting

emissary—messenger

emollient—soothing

empirical—pert. to experience

emporium—trade center

empyreal—celestial

empyrean—heavenly

emulate—to try to equal

enclave—area within foreign territory

encomium—praise

encroach—to infringe

encyclopedic—covering a wide range

endemic—pecular to an area

endive—lettuce-like plant

endogenous—originating from within

enervate—to weaken

enfranchise—to give the right to vote; set free

engender—to produce

engrossed—fully absorbed

engulf—to swallow up

enhance—to improve; add to

ennui—weariness

enormity—outrageous offense

ensnare—to trap

enteric—intestinal

enthrall—to charm; subjugate

entrepreneur—employer

enunciate—to pronounce clearly

envenom—to embitter

eolithic—stone age

epic—long poem of grandeur

epicure—lover of good food

epigram—witty thought

epilogue—concluding literary portion

epistle—a letter

epithet—descriptive adjective

epitome—condensation

equanimity—calm temper

equestrian—pert. to horses

equinox—equal day and night

equipoise—equilibrium

equivocate—to deceive

ergo—therefore

erode—to wear away

erotic—amatory

eruct—to belch

erudite—scholarly

escadrille—airplane squadron

escarpment—a steep slope

eschew—to avoid

escritoire—writing desk

esculent—edible

escutcheon—shield

esoteric—secret

esthetic—beautiful; artistic

estuary—river mouth

ethereal—spirit-like

ethnic—referring to a race

ethnology—study of origin of races

etiolate—to whiten

etiology—study of causes of disease

etude—musical composition

etymology—derivation of words

eugenics—improvement in offspring

eulogy—praise

euphemism—mild expression

euphonious—pleasant-sounding

euphoria—sense of well-being

euphuism—affected way of writing

euthanasia—painless death

evacuate—to empty

evanescent—transitory

evasion—a subterfuge

evince—to make evident

eviscerate—to disembowel

evoke—to call forth

evolve—to develop gradually

exacting—severe

exchequer—treasury

excise—indirect tax

excoriate—to skin; denounce

execrable—extremely bad

execrate—to abhor

exemplary—deserving imitation

exhort—to incite

exhortation—recommendation

exhume—to dig out

exigency—necessity

existentialism—philosophy of a purposeless world

exodus—a going forth

exogenous—derived externally

exonerate—to free from guilt

exorbitant—unreasonable

exorcise—to expel evil spirits

exordium—beginning part of an oration

expatiate—to elaborate (especially in speech)
expedient—advantageous
expedite—to speed up
expiate—to atone
expeditious—prompt
explicate—to explain
expostulate—to protest
expound—to state in detail
expulsion—driving out
expunge—to erase or delete
expurgate—to remove objectionable matter
exquisite—carefully selected
extant—still existing
extemporaneously—on the spur of the moment
extirpate—to destroy entirely
extol—to praise
extort—to obtain by threat of violence
extradite—to transfer a prisoner
extricate—to free
extrinsic—foreign; external
extrude—to expel

### F

fabricate—to build
facade—front of a building
facetious—humorous
facilitate—to make easy
facile—expert
factious—contrary; petulant
factotum—employee with many duties
faculty—a natural or acquired ability
fallible—capable of erring
fallow—lying idle
falter—to hesitate
farraginous—mixed; jumbled
farrier—blacksmith
fasces—emblem of power

fastidious—very critical
fathom—six feet
fatuous—foolish
feasible—suitable
feckless—ineffective
feculent—foul; impure
felicitate—to congratulate
ferret—to search
ferrous—containing iron
fetid—stinking
fetish—superstition
fettle—state of fitness
fetus—unborn babe
fiasco—ridiculous failure
fief—estate under feudal control
finesse—subtlety; craftiness
fiord—sea inlet
firth—narrow inlet
fissure—crack
flaccid—not firm
flagitious—wicked
flagrant—openly disgraceful
flail—to beat
flatulent—causing gas
flaunt—to show off
fledge—to furnish with feathers
flex—to bend
florescence—flowering
florid—flowery; having a ruddy color
flotsam—ship wreckage
flout—to scoff at; mock or jeer
fluctuate—to rise and fall
flume—valley
foible—weakness
foliaceous—leaflike
font—religious receptacle; type assortment
foray—plundering raid
forensic—pert. to debate
foresquare—direct
formidable—frightening; impressive
fortuitous—accidental

fractious—unruly
fray—fight
frenetic—frantic
frivolous—not serious
frizzle—to make crisp or curly
frond—divided leaf
frugal—thrifty
fugue—musical composition
fulminate—to denounce loudly
fulsome—objectionably excessive
furbelow—trimming
fustian—worthless

### G

gabble—to talk without meaning
galaxy—large system of stars
gall—to wear away
gallinaceous—pert. to fowl
gainsay—to deny
gambol—to frolic
gamut—the complete range
garble—to confuse such as facts
garish—flashy; showy
garrulous—talkative
gauntlet—type of glove
generic—pert. to a race or kind
genus—a kind or class
geriatrics—care for the aged
germane—pertinent
gerund—a verbal noun
gestation—pregnancy
ghoul—grave-robber
gibber—to talk foolishly
gird—to encircle
gist (jist)—essence
glaucous—sea-green
glib—speaking fluently without sincerity
glucose—sugar
gluttonous—greedy for food
gnostic—wise
goad—to urge on

golgotha—a place of sacrifice; cemetery
gonad—sex gland
gossamer—sheer
gourmet—a judge of food
gradient—degree of rising or falling
grail—a shallow vessel
grandee—person of high rank
grandeur—splendor
granular—grain-like
graphology—study of handwriting
gratuitous—free
gratuity—tip
gregarious—sociable
grimace—to distort the features
grimalkin—old cat
grimly—fiercely
grist—a thing used to one's advantage
grommet—a metal ring
grouse—to complain
grub—to toil unceasingly
gudgeon—simpleton
guile—deceit
gull—to swindle
gut—to destroy
guzzle—to drink much
gynecology—science of women's diseases
gyrate—to spin
gyroscope—rotating wheel
gyve—shackle

### H

habiliment—clothes
habitable—livable
haft—handle
haggard—gaunt; careworn
halberd—axlike weapon
halcyon—peaceful
hale—to compel to go
hallow—to make holy
hallucination—delusion
harass—to annoy
harbinger—forecast
harridan—vicious old woman

hassock—cushion used as stool
hauteur—pride
hawser—a large rope
hearth—floor of fireplace
hedonist—lover of pleasure
hegemony—leadership
heinous—hateful; atrocious
helix—coil of wire
heptagon—seven-sided polygon
herbivorous—feeding on herbs
heretical—not agreeing
hermitage—monastery
heterodox—having unorthodox opinions
heterogeneous—different
hexapod—having six feet
heyday—period of great vigor
hidalgo—Spanish nobleman
hieratic—prestly
hinder—to retard
hirsute—hairy
histology—science of organic tissue
histrionic—theatrical
hoary—white with age
holocaust—great destruction
holograph—personally handwritten document
homage—respect
homeopathy—method of treating disease
homiletics—art of preaching
homily—sermon
homogeneous—essentially alike
homogenous—derived from the same source
homologous—similar
homunculus—dwarf
hone—to sharpen
hormone—internal secretion
hortatory—encouraging

horticulture—the science of gardening
hoyden—tomboy
humanist—classical scholar
humerus—arm bone
hummock—small hill
humus—fertilizer
hurtle—to clash; rush headlong
husbandry—occupation of farming
hustings—electioneering platform
hydrophobia—rabies; fear of water
hydrous—containing water
hygroscope—instrument indicating humidity
hymeneal—pert. to marriage
hyperbole—exaggeration
hypertension—high blood pressure
hypochondria—fancies of bad health
hypothesis—assumption

I

ichthyology—science fish
iconoclast—image breaker
ideology—body of ideas
idiosyncrasy—peculiar tendency
idyllic—simple or poetic
igneous—of volcanic origin
ignoble—base, unworthy
ignominious—contemptible
illusory—unreal
imbibe—to drink in
imbrue—to stain or drench
imbue—to saturate
impale—to fix on a point
impalpable—not evident
impassioned—animated; excited
impeach—to accuse (not to find guilty)

impeccable—faultless
impecunious—poor
impede—to hinder
imperceptible—not easily seen
imperishable—indestructible
imperturbable—tranquil
impervious—not to be penetrated
impetuous—impulsive
implicit—absolute; implied
importune—to beg
impotent—incapable
imprecation—curse
impresario—manager
imprimatur—license to publish
impudence—shamelessness
impugn—to question
impunity—exemption from punishment
impute—to blame
inadvertence—carelessness
inalienable—not transferable
inarticulate—not distinct
incarcerate—to imprison
incarnadine—flesh-colored
incendiary—inflammatory
incognito—with identity concealed
incommensurate—not adequate
incongruous—not suitable
inconsiderable—trivial
incorrigible—beyond reform
incubus—burden
inculpate—to blame
indenture—contract
indigenous—native
indigent—poor
indiscriminate—not selective
indite—to write
indolent—lazy
indubitable—undeniably true
indurate—hardened

inebriated—drunk
ineffable—indescribable
inert—sluggish
inexorable—unyielding
inference—conclusion
inflammable—burnable
ingenuous—innocent
ingratiate—to establish in favor
iniquitous—sinful
innocuous—harmless
innuendo—insinuation
inscrutable—unfathomable
insensate—without sensation
insidious—treacherous
insinuate—to suggest subtly
insolvent—bankrupt
insouciant—carefree
insular—pert. to an island
intangible—not touchable
interdict—official order
interpolate—to insert new material
interregnum—interval between reigns
intractable—stubborn
intransigent—uncompromising
intravenous—through a vein
intrepid—brave
intrinsic—essential
introvert—to turn inward
inveigh—to attack
investiture—act of giving an office or right to
inveterate—firmly established
invidious—odious
invocation—calling on God
ionosphere—outer layers
isobar—weather map line
isotope—chemical element
isthmus—narrow land strip

iterate—to repeat
itinerant—traveling on a circuit

### J

jaded—worn out
jargon—confused talk
jaundiced—envious
jeremiad—lamentation
jettison—to cast overboard
jocose—humorous
jodhpurs—riding pants
juridical—legal
juxtaposed—close together

### K

kaleidoscope—optical instrument
karat—1/24 part gold
kinetics—science of pure motion
kiosk—stand which is open on one side
kith—friends

### L

lacerate—to tear
laconic—brief
lachrymose—tearful
laity—the people collectively as distinguished from clergymen
lampoon—satire or ridicule
landed—having an estate in land
languish—to become weak
lascivious—lewd
lassitude—weariness
latent—concealed
latex—milky fluid
latitude—allowance
legerdemain—trickery
lethargic—drowsy
lexicon—dictionary
libel—defamation
libretto—verbal text of an opera
licentiate—one who has a license
liege—feudal lord

limn—to portray
litany—prayer
lithe—supple
litigation—legal action
liturgy—religious ritual
livid—black and blue
loquacious—talkative
lucid—clear
lucre—money or riches
ludicrous—ridiculous
lugubrious—sad
lymph—transparent body fluid

### M

macabre—gruesome
macadamize—to cover with broken stones
macerate—to soften by dipping
madrigal—short musical poem
maelstrom—whirlpool
magisterial—authoritative
magnanimous—generous
mahatma—extraordinary person
mahout—elephant driver
maladroit—clumsy
malaise—discomfort
malapropism—word misused ridiculously
malfeasance—wrongful act
mandate—a specific order
mange—skin disease
mantilla—head scarf
marline—a nautical cord
marquee—canopy
marsupial—pert. to animals such as kangaroos
martinet—disciplinarian
matrix—a mold
masticate—to chew
maw—mouth of a voracious animal
mawkish—nauseating
maxim—proverb
medley—mixture

mega—million
megrim—low spirits
melange—mixture
mellifluent—sweetly flowing
menage—household
mendacious—lying
mendicant—beggar
meniscus—crescent-shaped
mercurial—lively
meretricious—showily attractive
mesa—high, wide tableland with rocky slopes
metamorphose—to transform
metaphor—a comparison
mete—to distribute
mettle—courage
microcosm—a little world
mien—manner or bearing
militate—to operate against
misanthropy—dislike mankind
miscegenation—interbreeding of races
misconstruction—wrong interpretation
miscreant—villain
missal—prayer book
mistral—cold dry northerly wind
mitigate—to lessen
mnemonics—memory device
modicum—small quantity
modulate—to soften
monolith—large piece of stone
montage—blending of pictures
mordant—biting; sarcastic
moribund—dying
mortar—container for crushing
mosque—Moslem temple
motley—miscellaneous

mufti—civilian dress
mulct—to defraud
mummery—pretentious ritual
murrain (mur-rin)—cattle disease
muzhik—Russian peasant
myopia—nearsightedness
myriad—a great many

### N

nacre—mother-of-pearl
nadir—lowest point
naiad—mythical water nymph
nape—back of neck
narcissism—love of oneself
natatorial—pert. to swimming
nebulous—hazy
nefarious—wicked
neophyte—new convert
neolithic—pert. to later Stone Age
neurasthenia—nervous exhaustion
niggardly—stingy
nihilism—disbelief in religion
nimbus—halo
nirvana—freedom from pain
noctambulist—sleepwalker
nocturne—a piece of dreamy music
node—knob
noisome—offensive
nomenclature—names of things
nonagenarian—person in his 90's
nonpareil—without equal
nonplus—to perplex
non sequitur—illogical argument
nosegay—bouquet
noxious—harmful
nuncio—representative of Pope

nurture—to provide food

## O

obdurate—callous; hardened
obeisance—bowing
obelisk—four-sided pillar
obesity—excessive fatness
obfuscate—to confuse
oblation—solemn offering
obloquy—disgrace
obsequious—servile
obsolescent—becoming out-of-date
obstreperous—noisy
obtrude—to thrust forth
obturate—to stop or close
obtuse—dull
obviate—to prevent
occidental—Western
occipital—pert. to back of head
occlude—to close
ocellated—having eyelike spots
octamerous—having eight parts
odoriferous—fragrant
officious—meddling
oleaginous—oily
olfactory—pert. to sense of smell
oligarchy—rule by a few
omega—last letter
ominous—threatening
omnipotent—all-powerful
omnivorous—eating everything
onerous—difficult
opprobrious—shameful
optimum—the best
opulence—riches
oracular—prophetic
orbicular—circular
ordnance—military weapons
ordinance—law
ordure—filth

oriel—a bay window
orifice—opening
orthography—science of spelling
oscillate—to vibrate
ossify—to become rigid or bonelike
ostensible—apparent
ostentatious—pretentious
overt—open to view

## P

pachyderm—elephant
pacific—calm
paisley—colorful fabric
paean—song of praise
palanquin—bed carried on poles
palatable—tasty
palaver (puh-**lav**-ur)—smooth or empty talk
pall—to become dull
palliate—to mitigate (see)
palpable—evident
panacea—remedy for all ills
panegyric—eulogy
panoply—set of armor
pantheism—belief of God-nature unity
paradigm—model
paradox—contradiction
parapet—barricade
paregoric—pain-reliever
pariah—outcast
parietal—pert. to side of skull
parity—equality
parochial—provincial
paroxysm—a fit
parsimonious—stingy
pastoral—pert. to rural life
patriarch—leader of a tribe
patrimony—an inheritance
pavilion—a large tent
peccadillo—a small fault
pectoral—pert. to chest
peculate—to embezzle

pecuniary—financial
pedantic—bookish
pediculous—infested with lice
peduncle—flower stalk
peignoir—dressing gown
pejorative—disparaging
pelagic—pert. to ocean
pelf—stolen property
penchant—strong inclination
pendant—anything hanging from something
pensile—hanging
pennate—winged
penurious—stingy
perambulate—to walk about
perception—awareness
percussion—impact
peregrination—traveling
peremptory—positive
perigee—point nearest earth
periphery—external surface
peristaltic—pert. to alternate waves
permeable—penetrable
permutation—changing
perquisite—incidental compensation
peroration—last part of a speech
perspective—the effect of distance
perspicuity—clearness of style or expression
pert—saucy
peruse—to read carefully
pervade—to spread to every part
perverse—contrary
pestle—that which pounds
petulance—peevishness
phalanx—any massed body
philistine—narrow-minded person
philology—study of words or literature
phylum—grouping in biology

picaresque—pert. to rogues
pilaster—part of a column
pileous—pert. to hair
pillory—structure for exposing to scorn
piquant—pungent
pique—to wound
piscatorial—pert. to fishing
pixilated—amusingly eccentric
plagiarism—stealing ideas from someone else
plait—to braid or pleat
platitude—trite remark
plectrum—small piece used to pluck
plenipotentiary—possessing full power
plethora—oversupply
plinth—lower part of column
plumb—to test the depth of
plutocracy—rule by the rich
poach—to trespass
pogrom—organized massacre
poignant—keenly affecting
polemics—art of disputing
polity—method of government
polonaise—slow Polish dance
polymer—chemical compound
pontificate—to speak pompously
porringer—soup plate
posterity—succeeding generations
portend—to warn
pottage—a stew
poultice—a soft moist mass
pragmatic—practical
prate—chatter
precarious—uncertain
precipitous—steep
preclude—to prevent

**precursor**—predecessor
**predatory**—plundering
**predilection**—preference
**preeminent**—superior
**premeditation**—forethought
**preposterous**—very absurd
**prerogative**—privilege
**presbyter**—ordained clergyman
**prescience**—foresight
**presentiment**—foreboding
**presentment**—report made by a grand jury
**preternatural**—supernatural
**prevaricate**—to lie
**primogeniture**—state of being first-born
**primordial**—first in order
**pristine**—primitive; unspoiled
**probity**—integrity
**proclivity**—tendency
**procrastinate**—to put off
**prodigious**—large
**proffer**—to offer
**profligate**—utterly immoral
**progeny**—offspring
**proletarian**—pert. to workers
**prolix**—long-winded
**promontory**—a high point of land
**propinquity**—nearness
**propitious**—favorable
**proscenium**—front stage
**proselyte**—a convert
**prosody**—science of verse forms
**protagonist**—leading character
**prototype**—example
**protuberance**—projection
**provender**—food for animals
**providential**—fortunate
**psychoneurosis**—emotional disorder

**puissant**—powerful
**punctilious**—exact
**purloin**—to embezzle
**purulent**—discharging pus
**pusillanimous**—afraid
**putative**—supposed
**putrefy**—to decay
**Pyrrhic victory**—victory at great cost
**pythonic**—prophetic

## Q

**quadrennial**—comprising four years
**qualm**—feeling of fear
**quandary**—doubt
**quasi**—resembling but not genuine
**query**—question
**quidnunc**—curious person
**quiescent**—inactive
**quietus**—a silencing
**quintessence**—concentrafed essence
**quirk**—a turn
**quixotic**—visionary
**quotidian**—daily

## R

**rabbet**—groove
**rabble**—vulgar, noisy people
**rabid**—furious
**raillery**—banter
**raiment**—clothing
**ramification**—a division
**rampant**—springing; climbing
**ramshackle**—out of repair
**rancor**—anger
**rankle**—to irritate
**rapacity**—greediness
**ratiocination**—reasoning
**recalcitrant**—stubborn
**recapitulate**—to summarize
**reciprocal**—in return
**recitative**—ordinary speech set to music
**recrimination**—countercharge

**rectitude**—uprightness
**refractory**—obstinate
**regale**—to entertain
**regicide**—killing of a king
**regimen**—manner of living
**relegate**—to assign
**reliquary**—receptacle
**remission**—pardon
**remonstrate**—to protest
**renascent**—being reborn
**renegade**—deserter
**repine**—to complain
**replete**—full
**reprehension**—rebuke
**reprisal**—injury in return
**reproof**—a scolding
**respite**—pause or rest
**repudiate**—to refuse
**requital**—repayment
**resilient**—rebounding
**resplendent**—shining
**restitution**—compensation
**résumé**—summary
**resurgent**—rising again
**resuscitate**—to revive
**reticulate**—net-like
**retroactive**—applying to the past
**retrogression**—going back
**retrousse**—turned up
**revile**—to scold
**rhesus**—type of monkey
**rhinitis**—inflammation of nose
**risibility**—disposition to laughter
**rote**—mechanical routine
**rubicund**—red
**rudiment**—first stage; non-functioning organ

## S

**sable**—black
**sabot**—wooden shoe
**saccharine**—pert. to sugar
**sagacious**—wise
**salacious**—obscene
**salient**—prominent
**saline**—salty

**salubrious**—healthful
**salutary**—wholesome
**salutatory**—pert. to a greeting
**sanctimonious**—affectedly holy
**sanctity**—holiness
**sanguine**—confident
**saponify**—to make fat into soap
**sardonic**—ironical
**satiate**—to supply to excess
**satrap**—governor of province
**saturate**—to fill
**saturnine**—gloomy
**scapular**—pert. to shoulder
**scarab**—ornament
**scarify**—to make scratches
**schism**—division
**schist**—a type of rock
**sciatic**—pert. to the hip
**scintilla**—bit
**scintillation**—a sparkling
**scrip**—paper money less than a dollar
**scruple**—reluctance
**scurrilous**—insulting
**secular**—not religious
**sedentary**—sluggish
**sedulous**—painstaking
**seismic**—caused by an earthquake
**semantic**—pert. to meanting
**senescent**—growing old
**sententious**—magisterial
**sentient**—feeling
**sequester**—to seclude
**seraglio**—harem
**serrated**—saw-toothed
**shamble**—something detroyed or in disorder
**shibboleth**—a pet phrase
**shunt**—to turn aside
**sidereal**—pert. to stars
**silicosis**—lung disease
**simian**—pert. to a monkey

**simile**—comparison using as or like

**simony**—profit from sacred things

**simper**—self-conscious smile

**sinecure**—job requiring little work

**sinuous**—with many curves

**slake**—to lessen

**slatternly**—sloppy

**slothful**—lazy

**slough**—soft, muddy ground

**sluice**—a water channel

**sojourn**—temporary residence

**solicitude**—concern

**soliloquy**—monologue

**somatic**—bodily

**sonorous**—resonant

**sophism**—fallacy

**spatula**—flat, broad instrument

**specious**—deceptive

**spectre**—ghost

**speculum**—mirror

**splenetic**—peevish

**spontaneous**—unconstrained

**sporadic**—occasional

**spume**—foam

**stalactite**—hanging calcium deposit

**stalagmite**—calcium deposit on cave floor

**steppe**—vast treeless plain

**sternum**—the breastbone

**stigma**—blemish

**stilted**—elevated

**stint**—to be frugal

**stoical**—impassive

**stratagem**—scheme

**stricture**—severe criticism

**strident**—grating

**suave**—smoothly polite

**subcutaneous**—beneath the skin

**subjoin**—to add

**sublimate**—to purify or refine

**subpoena**—summons for witness

**subsidy**—financial aid

**subterfuge**—a false excuse

**succinct**—brief

**succor**—comfort; aid

**succulence**—juiciness

**suffuse**—to overspread

**sully**—to soil

**supercilious**—proud and haughty

**supernal**—heavenly

**supersede**—to take the place of

**supervene**—to interrupt

**supplicate**—to beg

**surfeit**—excess

**surreptitious**—secret

**surrogate**—deputy

**surveillance**—watching

**swathe**—to bind or wrap

**sybarite**—person devoted to luxury

**sycophant**—flatterer

**syllogism**—deductive reasoning

**sylvan**—pert. to woods

**symposium**—meeting for discussion

**syncope**—contraction of a word

**synonymy**—the quality of being the same

**synthesis**—combination

## T

**tableau**—a striking scene

**taboret**—small stool

**tachometer**—instrument for measuring speed

**taciturn**—silent

**talus**—slope

**tankard**—large drinking vessel

**tantamount**—equal to

**tautology**—needless repetition

**temerity**—rashness

**terminus**—limit

**thesaurus**—treasury

**thoracic**—between neck and abdomen

**thrall**—slave

**threnody**—song of lamentation

**thrombosis**—blood clot

**tiara**—headdress

**tirade**—vehement speech

**tithe**—tax of one-tenth

**tocsin**—bell

**tome**—volume

**toque**—hat without a brim

**torpor**—dullness

**tortilla**—large round thin cake

**trachea**—windpipe

**tractable**—easily led

**traduce**—to slander

**tranquillity**—calmness

**transcendent**—surpassing others

**transfuse**—to pour from one to another

**transmute**—to change

**transpire**—to become known

**transubstantiation**—to change to another substance

**transverse**—lying across

**trauma**—wound

**travail**—labor

**treacle**—molasses

**treble**—triple

**tremulous**—shaking

**trenchant**—sharp

**trepidation**—trembling from fear

**tribulation**—trouble

**truncheon**—club

**trundle**—small wheel

**tumbrel**—farmer's cart

**tumid**—swollen

**turbulent**—violent

**turgid**—swollen

**turpitude**—shameful depravity

**tutelage**—instruction

**twit**—to tease

**tyke**—mischievous child

**tyro**—novice

## U

**ubiquity**—omnipresence

**ukase**—Russian government order

**ululation**—a wailing

**umbilicus**—navel

**umbrage**—offense

**unctuous**—oily or smooth

**undulating**—waving

**ungainly**—clumsy

**upbraid**—to reproach

**uproarious**—noisy

**urbane**—refined

**ursine**—pert. to bears

**usurpation**—wrongful seizure

**uxorious**—fond of a wife

## V

**vacuous**—empty

**vapid**—dull

**varicosity**—swollen veins

**vacillation**—unsteadiness

**vacuity**—stupidity

**vagary**—whim

**vanguard**—leaders

**vaquero**—cowboy

**variegate**—to diversify

**vaunt**—to boast

**vendetta**—feud

**venerate**—to revere

**venous**—pert. to veins

**ventricle**—cavity

**verdant**—green; fresh

**verisimilitude**—appearance of truth

**verity**—honesty

**vernacular**—native language

**vernal**—pert. to spring

**vertex**—top

**vertigo**—dizziness

**vestige**—trace

**viable**—capable of living

**vicissitude**—change

**vilify**—to defame

**vindicate**—to uphold

**viridity**—greenness

**vituperate**—to defame

**vociferate**—to shout

**volatility**—frivolity

**volition**—will

**voracious**—ravenous
**votary**—devoted person

# W

**waft**—current of wind
**waggery**—mischievous merriment
**wainscot**—wood paneling

**wassail**—a toast
**wastrel**—spendthrift
**wean**—to detach
**welter**—to roll about
**wheedle**—to coax
**whimsical**—fantastic; quaint
**whey**—milk water
**wizened**—withered
**wont**—custom

**woof**—fabric
**wraith**—ghost

# X

**xylem**—woody tissue of plants

# Y

**yak**—species of ox

**yen**—monetary unit of Japan
**yogi**—an ascetic

# Z

**zany**—clown
**zeal**—enthusiasm
**zenith**—highest point

# QUANTITATIVE ABILITY

*Based on all the information available before going to press we have constructed this examination to give you a comprehensive and authoritative view of what's in store for you. To avoid any misunderstanding, we must emphasize that this test has never been given before.*

## MATHEMATICS TEST

### (75 minutes)

DIRECTIONS: *For each of the following questions, select the choice which best answers the question or completes the statement.*

## EXPLANATIONS ARE GIVEN WITH THE ANSWERS WHICH FOLLOW THE QUESTIONS

1. In two hours, the minute hand of a clock rotates through an angle of

   (A) 60°
   (B) 90°
   (C) 180°
   (D) 360°
   (E) 720°

2. Which of the following fractions is less than one-third?

   (A) $22/63$
   (B) $4/11$
   (C) $15/46$
   (D) $33/98$
   (E) $102/303$

3.

   The length of each side of the square above is $\frac{2x}{3} + 1$. The perimeter of the square is

   (A) $\dfrac{8x + 4}{3}$
   (B) $\dfrac{8x + 12}{3}$
   (C) $\dfrac{2x}{3} + 4$
   (D) $\dfrac{2x}{3} + 16$
   (E) $\dfrac{4x}{3} + 2$

4. An individual intelligence test is administered to John A when he is 10 years 8 months old. His recorded M.A. (mental age) is 160 months. What I.Q. should be recorded?

   (A) 80
   (B) 125
   (C) 128
   (D) 148
   (E) 160.

5. When it is noon at prime meridian on the equator, what time is it at 75° north latitude on this meridian?

   (A) 12 noon
   (B) 3 P.M.
   (C) 5 P.M.
   (D) 7 A.M.
   (E) Midnight.

*Questions 6-9 are to be answered with reference to the following diagram:*

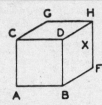

The diagram shows a cube. Each corner has been identified by a letter. Corner E is not shown, but its location is the one corner not shown in the diagram. The cube has a 1″ side.

6. The distance from A to D is

(A) 1 inch
(B) 2 inches
(C) $\sqrt{2}$ inches
(D) $\sqrt{3}$ inches
(E) $\dfrac{1}{\sqrt{2}}$ inches

7. There is a dot X on the BDHF face of the cube. If we let the cube rotate 180° in a clockwise direction on an axis running through A and H, the

(A) cube will be standing on corner C
(B) dot X will appear in the plane where face ABCD is now shown
(C) dot X will be in the plane where face CDGH is now shown
(D) cube will return to its position as shown in the diagram
(E) corner C will appear in the place where corner F is now shown.

8. The distance from A to X is

(A) more than 2 inches
(B) less than 1 inch
(C) between 1 and $\sqrt{3}$ inches
(D) between $\sqrt{3}$ and 2 inches
(E) exactly $\sqrt{3}$ inches.

9. If the cube is successively rotated 180° on axes going through the center of faces ABCD and EFGH, faces AECG and BFDH, and faces CDGH and ABEF, where will the face containing point X be?

(A) where face BDHF was at the start of the operation
(B) Where face AECG was at the start of the operation
(C) Where face EFGH was at the start of the operation

(D) Where face ABEF was at the start of the operation
(E) Where face ABCD was at the start of the operation.

10. A carpenter needs four boards, each 2 feet, 9 inches long. If wood is sold only by the foot, how many feet must he buy?

(A) 9
(B) 10
(C) 11
(D) 12
(E) 13

11. CMXLIX in Roman numerals is the equivalent of

(A) 449
(B) 949
(C) 969
(D) 1149
(E) 1169.

*Questions 12-16 are to be answered with reference to the graph below:*

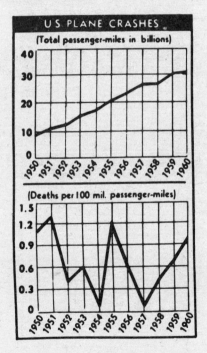

12. The period with the smallest increase in total passenger-miles was

(A) 1951-52
(B) 1954-55
(C) 1955-56
(D) 1957-58
(E) 1958-59.

13. It is *not* true that

(A) excluding 1960, there were more deaths in the aggregate, per 100 million passenger-miles, during the odd years than during the even years

(B) there was an increase in passenger-miles flown from 1950 to 1957

(C) there has been an increase in passenger-deaths every year since 1950

(D) there were more passenger-deaths in 1960 than in 1950

(E) 30 billion passenger-miles were flown in 1959

14. The greatest and the least number of passenger-deaths occurred during

(A) 1950 and 1957
(B) 1954 and 1960
(C) 1952 and 1955
(D) 1953 and 1956
(E) 1954 and 1957

15. In 1955, passenger-deaths numbered approximately

(A) 24
(B) 240
(C) 2400
(D) 24,000
(E) 240,000

16. The sharpest drop in passenger-deaths was during the period of

(A) 1951-1952
(B) 1953-1954
(C) 1954-1955
(D) 1955-1956
(E) 1957-1958

*Questions 17-21 are to be answered with reference to the following paragraph:*

Five geometric figures have been drawn: An isosceles triangle with base equal to its altitude = a, a square with side = a, a circle with a radius = a, a regular hexagon with each side = a, and a semicircle with a diameter = a. (The figures are not drawn to scale. All the questions assume the stated dimensions.)

17. Which figure has the greatest area?

(A) △      (B) □
(C) ○      (D) ○
       (E) ◠

18. Which figure has the shortest perimeter?

(A) □      (B) △
(C) ○      (D) ○
       (E) ◠

19. Which of the following statements is true?

(A) ○ can be inscribed inside □
(B) □ can be inscribed inside △
(C) ○ can be inscribed inside □
(D) ○ can be inscribed inside ○
(E) △ can be inscribed inside ◠

20. Which of these statements is true? The area of

(A) △ is just ⅙ the area of ○
(B) △ is just ½ the area of □
(C) □ is just ½ the area of ○
(D) ○ is just ¾ the area of ○
(E) ◠ is just ½ the area of O ○

21. The ratio of the areas of ◠ and ○ is

(A) 1:8      (B) 1:6
(C) 1:4      (D) 1:2
       (E) 1:1

22. A motorist travels 120 miles to his destination at the average speed of 60 miles per hour and returns to the starting point at the average speed of 40 miles per hour. His average speed for the entire trip is

(A) 53 miles per hour
(B) 50 miles per hour
(C) 48 miles per hour
(D) 45 miles per hour
(E) 52 miles per hour

23. A snapshot measures 2½ inches by 1⅞ inches. It is to be enlarged so that the longer dimension will be 4 inches. The length of the enlarged shorter dimension will be

(A) 2½ inches      (B) 3 inches
(C) 3⅜ inches      (D) 2⅝ inches
       (E) none of these

24. From a piece of tin in the shape of a square 6 inches on a side, the largest possible circle is cut out. Of the following, the ratio of the area of the circle to the area of the original square is closest in value to

(A) ⅘      (B) ⅔
(C) ⅗      (D) ½
       (E) ¾

25. The approximate distance, s, in feet that an object falls in t seconds when dropped from a height is obtained by use of the formula $s = 16\ t^2$. In 8 seconds the object will fall

    (A) 15,384 feet
    (B) 1,024 feet
    (C) 256 feet
    (D) 2,048 feet
    (E) none of these

26. In the figure, AB = BC and angles BAD and BCD are right angles. Which one of the following conclusions may be drawn?

    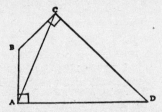

    (A) angle BCA=angle CAD
    (B) angle B is greater than angle D
    (C) AC=CD
    (D) AD = CD
    (E) BC is shorter than CD.

    *Questions 27-30 are to be answered with reference to the following explanatory paragraph:*

    Suppose in the place of a number system a symbol system were instituted which had digits □, ∧, Z, ≤, ▷, 5, ∂, ᢗ, × and ⊖ corresponding respectively to the digits 0, 1, 2, 3, 4, 5, 6, 7, 8 and 9. The digit □ is used in the same fashion as the 0 in the decimal system, e.g., ∧□ = 10.

27. Which is equal to $10^2$?

    (A) ∧□□
    (B) ∂▷
    (C) ∧□∧
    (D) 5≤
    (E) ×□∧

28. What is the sum of ▷ + ∂ + ≤ ?

    (A) Z∧
    (B) ∧≤
    (C) ≤▷
    (D) ∧∂
    (E) ∧∧

29. Which of the following indicates three-quarters of an inch?

    (A) $\dfrac{5}{∧□}$ inches

    (B) $\dfrac{∂}{×}$ inches

    (C) $\dfrac{ᢗ}{∧□}$ inches

    (D) $\dfrac{ᢗ}{∧□□}$ inches

    (E) $\dfrac{∂5}{□□}$ inches

30. What is the value of

    $$∧Z∂ - ▷ᢗ + \dfrac{∧□}{Z}\ ?$$

    (A) ▷∂
    (B) 5ᢗ
    (C) ×▷
    (D) ᢗ□
    (E) ⊖Z

31. A pound of water is evaporated from 6 pounds of sea water containing 4% salt. The percentage of salt in the remaining solution is

    (A) $3\frac{1}{3}$
    (B) 4
    (C) $4\frac{4}{5}$
    (D) 5
    (E) none of these

32. The product of $75^3$ and $75^7$ is

    (A) $(75)^{10}$
    (B) $(150)^{10}$
    (C) $(75)^{21}$
    (D) $(5625)^{10}$
    (E) $(75)^5$

33. The scale of a map is: ¾ of an inch = 10 miles. If the distance on the map between two towns is 6 inches, the actual distance is

    (A) 45 miles
    (B) 60 miles
    (C) 80 miles
    (D) 75 miles
    (E) none of these

34. If $d = m - \dfrac{50}{m}$, and m is a positive number which increases in value, d

 (A) increases in value
 (B) decreases in value
 (C) remains unchanged
 (D) increases, then decreases
 (E) decreases, then increases

35. If a cubic inch of a metal weighs 2 pounds, a cubic foot of the same metal weighs

 (A) 8 pounds
 (B) 24 pounds
 (C) 288 pounds
 (D) 96 pounds
 (E) none of these

*Questions 36-38 are to be answered with reference to the following illustrations:*

Here are three views of a single cube:

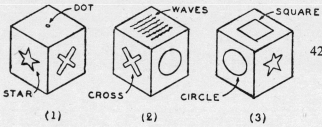

(1)         (2)         (3)

36. What symbol is opposite the dot?

 (A) circle
 (B) cross
 (C) square
 (D) waves
 (E) star

37. What symbol is opposite the cross?

 (A) circle
 (B) dot
 (C) square
 (D) waves
 (E) star

38. What symbol is on the bottom of figure 3?

 (A) cross
 (B) dot
 (C) star
 (D) waves
 (E) none of these

39. If the number of square inches in the area of a circle is equal to the number of inches in its circumference, the diameter of the circle is

 (A) 4 inches
 (B) 2 inches
 (C) 1 inch
 (D) $\pi$ inches
 (E) none of these

40. The least common multiple of 20, 24, 32 is

 (A) 960
 (B) 1920
 (C) 15,360
 (D) 240
 (E) none of these

41. Six quarts of a 20% solution of alcohol in water are mixed with 4 quarts of a 60% solution of alcohol in water. The alcoholic strength of the mixture is

 (A) 80%
 (B) 40%
 (C) 36%
 (D) 48%
 (E) none of these

42. To find the radius of a circle whose circumference is 60 inches

 (A) multiply 60 by $\pi$
 (B) divide 60 by $2\pi$
 (C) divide 30 by $2\pi$
 (D) divide 60 by $\pi$ and extract the square root of the result
 (E) multiply 60 by $\dfrac{\pi}{2}$

*Questions 43-45 are to be answered with reference to the following diagram:*

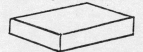

A unit block for construction is $1 \times 2 \times 3$ inches. Each of the three questions below refers to this unit block.

43. What is the maximum number of whole blocks required to cover an area 1 foot long by $1\frac{1}{4}$ feet wide with *one layer* of blocks?

 (A) 30 blocks
 (B) 72 blocks
 (C) 90 blocks
 (D) 60 blocks
 (E) 180 blocks

44. How many whole blocks will be needed to construct a solid cube of minimum size?

    (A) 6
    (B) 18
    (C) 36
    (D) 48
    (E) 215

45. How many blocks, arranged as shown in the diagram below, and including half blocks, would be required to build a wall 1 yard long, 2 inches wide, and ½ foot high?

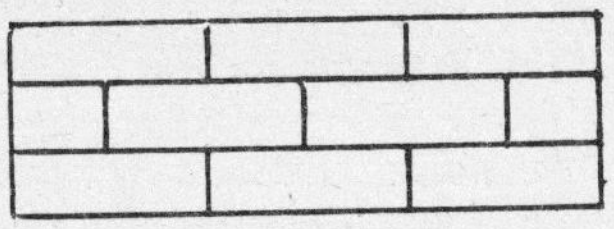

    (A) 72
    (B) 144
    (C) 216
    (D) 432
    (E) not determinable from given information

46. A micromillimeter is defined as one millionth of a millimeter. A length of 17 micromillimeters may be represented as

    (A) .00017 mm.
    (B) .0000017 mm.
    (C) .000017 mm.
    (D) .00000017 mm.
    (E) .000000017 mm.

47. If $9x + 5 = 23$, the numerical value of $18x + 5$ is

    (A) 46
    (B) 41
    (C) 32
    (D) 36
    (E) not determinable from given information

48. When the fractions ⅔, 5/7, 8/11 and 9/13 are arranged in ascending order of size, the result is

    (A) 8/11, 5/7, 9/13, ⅔
    (B) 5/7, 8/11, ⅔, 9/13
    (C) ⅔, 8/11, 5/7, 9/13
    (D) ⅔, 9/13, 5/7, 8/11
    (E) 9/13, ⅔, 8/11, 5/7

49. If the outer diameter of a metal pipe is 2.84 inches and the inner diameter is 1.94 inches, the thickness of the metal is

    (A) .45 of an inch
    (B) .90 of an inch
    (C) 1.94 inches
    (D) 2.39 inches
    (E) 1.42 inches

50. If one-half of the female students in a certain college eat in the cafeteria and one-third of the male students eat there, what fractional part of the student body eats in the cafeteria?

    (A) ⅚
    (B) 5/12
    (C) ¾
    (D) ⅖
    (E) cannot be determined

51. In a certain boys' camp, 30% of the boys are from New York State and 20% of these are from New York City. What percent of the boys in the camp are from New York City?

    (A) 50%
    (B) 33⅓%
    (C) 10%
    (D) 6%
    (E) 60%

*Questions 52-54 are to be answered with reference to the following diagram:*

A 2½ inch cube, as shown in the diagram, is made of half-inch cubes. Any one cube may be located in terms of a coordinate system. For example, cube *a* is in the fifth layer from the left, the fourth layer from the bottom, and the second from the front. It is, therefore, located in the position 5,4,2.

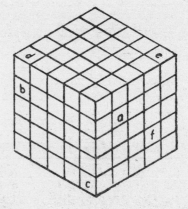

52. If the entire exterior surface is painted blue, what is the largest cube which can be built from the unpainted cubes?

    (A) ½ inch cube
    (B) 1 inch cube
    (C) 1½ inch cube
    (D) 2 inch cube
    (E) 2½ inch cube

53. The coordinates of the cube nearest the center of the cube shown in the diagram are

    (A) 1,1,1
    (B) 2,2,2

    (C) 3,3,3
    (D) 5,5,5
    (E) 4,4,4

54. A line drawn from the center of cube 1,2,1 through the center of cube 2,3,3 will also pass through the center of cube

    (A) 3,2,1
    (B) 5,5,5
    (C) 1,2,3
    (D) 3,4,5
    (E) 4,3,2

DIRECTIONS: Read each test question carefully. Each one refers to the following graph, and is to be answered solely on that basis. Select the best answer among the given choices and blacken the proper space on the answer sheet.

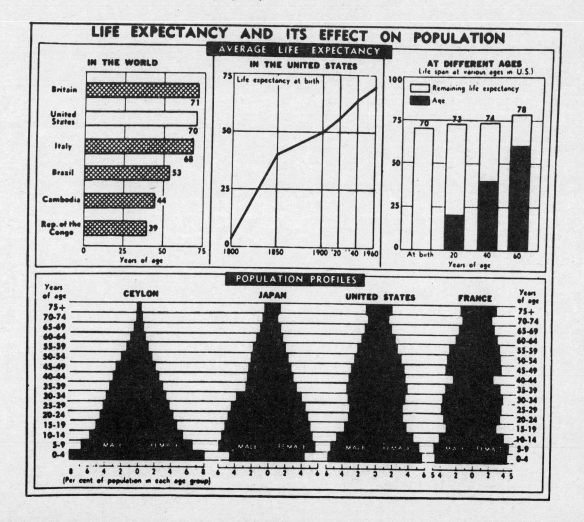

55. The country which has the highest per cent in the "75 and over" group among the countries listed is

    (A) Ceylon
    (B) Japan
    (C) United States
    (D) France
    (E) not determinable from chart

56. Among the countries of Ceylon, Japan, the United States, and France, there are as many females as males, or more females than males, in all of these countries in this age group:
    (A) 0-4
    (B) 30-34
    (C) 45-49
    (D) 55-59
    (E) 75+

57. The life expectancy in the United States in 1925 was about what percent of the average life expectancy in 1825?

    (A) 150
    (B) 175
    (C) 200
    (D) 250
    (E) 300

58. A person of 20 in this country, according to life expectancy findings, has lived about what per cent of his life?

    (A) 15%
    (B) 25%
    (C) 35%
    (D) 40%
    (E) 45%

59. The average life expectancy of people in the Republic of the Congo is about the same as that of a United States citizen in

    (A) 1830
    (B) 1850
    (C) 1900
    (D) 1920
    (E) 1940

60. In Japan, there are more people in which age group than in any other age group?

    (A) 0-4
    (B) 5-9
    (C) 10-14
    (D) 15-19
    (E) 20-24

## Correct Answers For The Foregoing Questions

*(Check your answers with these that we provide. You should find considerable correspondence between them. If not, you'd better go back and find out why. On the next page we have provided concise clarifications of basic points behind the key answers. Please go over them carefully because they may be quite useful in helping you pick up extra points on the exam.)*

| | | | | | | | |
|---|---|---|---|---|---|---|---|
| 1. E | 9. A | 17. C | 24. A | 31. C | 38. A | 45. A | 53. C |
| 2. C | 10. C | 18. E | 25. B | 32. A | 39. B | 46. C | 54. D |
| 3. B | 11. B | 19. D | 26. D | 33. C | 40. E | 47. B | 55. D |
| 4. B | 12. D | 20. B | 27. A | 34. A | 41. C | 48. D | 56. E |
| 5. A | 13. C | 21. A | 28. B | 35. E | 42. B | 49. A | 57. E |
| 6. C | 14. B | 22. C | 29. B | 36. A | 43. C | 50. E | 58. B |
| 7. A | 15. B | 23. B | 30. C | 37. C | 44. C | 51. D | 59. B |
| 8. C | 16. A | | | | | 52. C | 60. B |

# EXPLANATORY ANSWERS

*Elucidation, clarification, explication and a little help with the fundamental facts covered in the Previous Test. These are the points and principles likely to crop up in the form of questions on future tests.*

1. **(E)** Every hour, the minute hand of a clock goes around once, or 360°. In two hours, it rotates 720°.

2. **(C)** $^{15}/_{45}$ would be $\frac{1}{3}$. With a larger denominator, the fraction $^{15}/_{46}$ is less than $\frac{1}{3}$.

3. **(B)** Since the perimeter of a square is four times the length of a side, it is
$$4x\left(\frac{2x}{3} + 1\right), \text{ or } \frac{8x + 12}{3}$$

4. **(B)** IQ is 100 times this result: the mental age of a person divided by his chronological age. This is $100 \times 160 \div 128$, which equals 125.

5. **(A)** Time does not vary with latitude (distance from the equator), but only with longitude (distance from the prime meridian).

6. **(C)** ABD forms a right triangle with both legs equal to 1 inch. By the Pythagorean Theorem, $AD = \sqrt{2}$.

7. **(A)** Imagine the triangle ACH rotated 180° about AH. C will be lower than the present position of the ABEF plane.

8. **(C)** AX must be shorter than AH, which is $\sqrt{3}$, and longer than AB, which is 1.

9. **(A)** The first rotation puts X where ACGE was. The second leaves X in the same plane. The third rotation returns X to its original position.

10. **(C)** The carpenter needs a total of 33 inches for each board. The total length is 132 inches, or 11 feet.

11. **(B)** CM equals $1000 - 100$, or 900.
XL equals $50 - 10$, or 40.
IX equals $10 - 1$, or 9.
Their sum is 949.

12. **(D)** The line in the top graph is almost horizontal between 1957 and 1958. In the other years, the line is rising.

13. **(C)** In 1955, there were 1.2 deaths per 100 million passenger-miles, and 20 billion passenger-miles, which means there were 240 deaths. In 1956, there were 0.6 deaths per 100 million passenger-miles, and about 24 billion passenger-miles, which means there were about 144 deaths.

14. **(B)** In 1954, there were only 18 deaths, and in 1960, there were 300.

15. **(B)** See calculations for #13.

16. **(A)** In the period from 1951-1952, the death rate dropped to about $\frac{1}{3}$ of its previous level.

The answers to 17-21 can be readily seen from the diagram below.

17. C

18. E

19. D

20. B

21. A

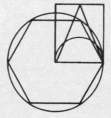

22. **(C)** In the first trip, the motorist travels 120 miles at 60 m.p.h., which takes 2 hours. On the way back, he travels the same distance at

40 m.p.h., which takes 3 hours. His average rate is the total distance (240 miles) divided by the total time (5 hours), which yields 48 m.p.h.

23. **(B)** The proportion to be solved is $2\frac{1}{2}:4 = 1\frac{7}{8}:x$, where x is the length of the shorter dimension of the enlargement. Solving, $x=3$.

24. **(A)** The area of the circle is $\pi$ times the square of the radius, or $9\pi$. The area of the square is 36. Thus, the ratio is $\frac{9\pi}{36}$, or $\frac{\pi}{4}$. Approximating $\pi$ as 3.14, we divide and obtain .785, which is closest to $\frac{4}{5}$.

25. **(B)** By simple substitutions, $s=16\times8\times8$, or 1024.

26. **(D)** If angles BAD and BCD are right angles, they are equal. Angle BAC equals angle BCA, since they are base angles of an isosceles triangle. Subtracting equals from equals, angle DAC equals angle DCA. Therefore, ACD is an isosceles triangle, and $AD=CD$.

27. **(A)** $10^2=100$, or $\wedge\square\square$

28. **(B)** $\triangleright+\beth+\leqslant=4+6+3=13=\wedge\leqslant$

29. **(B)** $\dfrac{\beth}{\times}=\dfrac{6}{8}=\dfrac{3}{4}$

30. **(C)** $\wedge Z\beth-\triangleright\triangledown+\dfrac{\wedge\square}{Z}=126-47+1\frac{0}{2}=$ $84=\times\triangleright$

31. **(C)** The original 6 pounds contained .24 pounds of salt. Now, the same .24 pounds are in 5 pounds of solution, so the percentage is $^{24}\!/_{5}$, or $4\frac{4}{5}$.

32. **(A)** By the Law of Exponents, $(75)^3\times(75)^7=(75)^{3+7}=(75)^{10}$.

33. **(C)** This is a proportion→ $\frac{3}{4}$ in.:6 in.=10 mi.:x. Solving, $x=80$ miles.

34. **(A)** If h is any positive quantity, then letting $d' = (m+h)-\left(\dfrac{50}{m+h}\right)$, we can see that d' is

greater than d, since h is greater than zero, and $\dfrac{50}{m}$ is greater than $\dfrac{50}{m+h}$. Therefore, d increases as m does.

35. **(E)** One cubic foot equals $12^3$ cubic inches, or 1728. Thus, one cubic foot of the metal would weigh 3456 pounds.

This is an unfolded view of the cube in questions 36-38:

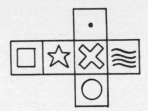

36. **(A)**

37. **(C)**

38. **(A)**

39. **(B)** The area of the circle is $\pi r^2$, and the circumference is $2\pi r$. If the area equals the circumference, solve the equation $\pi r^2=2\pi r$, so $r=2$. The diameter is 2r, or 4 inches.

40. **(E)** $20 = 2\times2\times5$; $24 = 2\times2\times2\times3$; $32 = 2\times2\times2\times2\times2$. The least common multiple is found by taking the highest power of each factor, and multiplying the results. The highest power of 2 is $2^5$, the highest power of 3 is $3^1$, and the highest power of 5 is $5^1$. The answer is $2^5\times3^1\times5^1$, or 480.

41. **(C)** The total volume is ten quarts. In the first solution, there are 20% of 6 quarts of alcohol, or 1.2. In the second solution, there are 60% of 4 quarts, or 2.4. Thus, there are 3.6 quarts of alcohol in 10 quarts of solution, and the percentage is 36%.

42. **(B)** If the circumference is 60 inches, since $C=2\pi r$, substitute $C=60$; therefore, $r=\dfrac{60}{2\pi}$

43. **(C)** The maximum number requires that the $1 \times 2$ faces be on the floor, so that each block will cover an area of only 2 inches. For an area of 1¼ square feet, or 180 square inches, 90 blocks will be needed.

44. **(C)** One edge of the minimum cube must be 6 inches, the lowest common multiple of 1, 2, and 3. Thus, it will have a volume of 216 cubic in., which is equal to 36 blocks.

45. **(A)** One block has a volume of 6 cubic inches. The volume of the wall is $36 \times 2 \times 6$ cubic inches, or 432, so 72 blocks will be used.

46. **(C)** 17 micromillimeters equals $\dfrac{17}{1,000,000}$ mm., or .000017 mm.

47. **(B)** If $9x + 5 = 23$, $9x = 18$, or $x = 2$. Thus $18x + 5 = 36 + 5 = 41$.

48. **(D)** Converting to decimals, $2/3 = .666 \ldots$, $5/7 = .7142 \ldots$, $8/11 = .7373 \ldots$, and $9/13 = .6923 \ldots$, so the order is 2/3, 9/13, 5/7, 8/11.

49. **(A)** The radii of the pipe are 1.42 in. and 0.97 in. The thickness is their difference, or .45 in.

50. **(E)** There is no indication as to the exact percentage of students who eat in the cafeteria, since we do not know how many boys or girls there are.

51. **(D)** The percent of boys from New York City is 20% of 30%, or 6%.

52. **(C)** By removing the outer layer of cubes, we have a cube three units on each side, or 1½ inches.

53. **(C)** The center of each face has the coordinate 3, so 3,3,3, is the center of the cube.

54. **(D)** The line follows the double equation $2x = 2y - 2 = z + 1$. This is also satisfied by 3,4,5.

55. **(D)** France has the widest line in the 75 + row of "Population Profiles"—over 5%.

56. **(E)** In the 75 + rows of the "Population Profiles" of all these nations, the sections labeled "Female" are longer than those labeled "Male."

57. **(E)** In 1925, the life expectancy was almost 60 years, while in 1825, it was just about 20 years. 60 is 300% of 20.

58. **(B)** A person of 20 has a life expectancy of 73, according to the chart. 20 is about 27% of 73, which is closest to 25%.

59. **(B)** In 1850, an American had an average life expectancy of 40 years, the closest to 39 in the Republic of the Congo.

60. **(B)** In Japan's "Population Profile," the widest band is in the 5-9 row.

# Trial Examination On Miscellaneous Problems

1. Assuming that the series will continue in the same pattern, the next number in the series 3, 5, 11, 29 . . . is:
   (A) 41      (B) 47
   (C) 65      (D) 83

2. DCCXLIX in Roman numerals represents the number:
   (A) 749      (B) 764
   (C) 1249      (D) 1264

3. If the total area of a picture measuring 10 inches by 12 inches plus a matting of uniform width surrounding the picture is 224 square inches, the width of the matting is:
   (A) 2 inches      (B) 2 $\frac{4}{11}$ inches
   (C) 3 inches      (D) 4 inches

4. The net price of a $25 item after successive discounts of 20% and 30% is:
   (A) $11.00      (B) $12.50
   (C) $14.00      (D) $19.00

5. The cost of 63 inches of ribbon at $.12 per yard is:
   (A) $.20      (B) $.21
   (C) $.22      (D) $.23

6. If 1½ cups of cereal are used with 4½ cups of water, the amount of water needed with ¾ of a cup of cereal is:
   (A) 2 cups      (B) 2⅛ cups
   (C) 2¼ cups      (D) 2½ cups

7. Under certain conditions, sound travels at about 1100 ft. per second. If 88 ft. per second is approximately equivalent to 60 miles per hour, the speed of sound, under the above conditions, is, of the following, closest to:
   (A) 730 miles per hour
   (B) 740 miles per hour
   (C) 750 miles per hour
   (D) 760 miles per hour

8. If one angle of a triangle is three times a second angle and the third angle is 20 degrees more than the second angle, the second angle is (in degrees):
   (A) 32      (B) 34
   (C) 40      (D) 50

9. Assuming that on a blueprint ¼ inch equals 12 inches, the actual length in feet of a steel bar represented on the blueprint by a line 3⅜ inches long is:
   (A) 3⅜      (B) 6¾
   (C) 12½      (D) 13½

10. If Mrs. Jones bought 3¾ yards of dacron at $1.16 per yard and 4⅔ yards of velvet at $3.87 per yard, the amount of change she receives from $25 is:
    (A) $2.12      (B) $2.28
    (C) $2.59      (D) $2.63

11. The water level of a swimming pool, 75 feet by 42 feet, is to be raised four inches. The number of gallons of water needed for this is:
    (A) 140      (B) 7,854.5
    (C) 31,500      (D) 94,500

12. If shipping charges to a certain point are 62 cents for the first five ounces and 8 cents for each additional ounce, the weight of a package for which the charges are $1.66 is:
    (A) 13 ounces      (B) 1⅛ pounds
    (C) 1¼ pounds      (D) 1½ pounds

13. If 15 cans of food are needed for seven men for two days, the number of cans needed for four men for seven days is:
    (A) 15      (B) 20
    (C) 25      (D) 30

14. The total saving in purchasing 30 13-cent ice cream pops for a class party at a reduced rate of $1.38 per dozen is:
    (A) $.35      (B) $.40
    (C) $.45      (D) $.50

15. A candy recipe calls for, among other things, 1½ cups of sugar and ¾ of a cup of boiling water. Mary wants to use this recipe, but has only one cup of sugar. How much boiling water should she use?
    (A) ¼ cup      (B) ⅓ cup
    (C) ½ cup      (D) ⅝ cup

16. In a 3-hour examination of 350 questions, there are 50 mathematics problems. If twice as much time should be allowed for each problem as for each of the other questions, how many minutes should be spent on the mathematical problems?
    (A) 45 minutes      (B) 52 minutes
    (C) 60 minutes      (D) 72 minutes

17. A rectangular picture measures 4½" by 6¾". If the picture is proportionally enlarged so that the shorter side is 7½", what will be the length of the longer side?
    (A) 9¾"      (B) 11¼"
    (C) 13½"      (D) 20¼"

18. A typewriter was listed at $120.00 and was bought for $96.00. What was the rate of discount?
    - (A) 16⅔%
    - (B) 20%
    - (C) 24%
    - (D) 25%

19. In two hours, the minute hand of a clock rotates through an angle of
    - (A) 90°
    - (B) 180°
    - (C) 360°
    - (D) 720°

20. Assuming that the following series will continue in the same pattern, the next number in the series 2, 6, 14, 30, 62, ........ is
    - (A) 96
    - (B) 126
    - (C) 186
    - (D) 216

21. An individual intelligence test is administered to John A when he is 10 years 8 months old. His recorded M.A. is 160 months. What I.Q. should be recorded?
    - (A) 80
    - (B) 125
    - (C) 128
    - (D) 160

22. When it is noon at prime meridian on the equator, what time is it at 75° north latitude on this meridian?
    - (A) 12M.
    - (B) 3 P.M.
    - (C) 5 P.M.
    - (D) 7 A.M.

23. A carpenter needs boards for 4 shelves, each 2'9" long, and ½" thick. How many feet of board should he buy?
    - (A) 11
    - (B) 11⅛
    - (C) 13
    - (D) 15½

24. CMXLIX in Roman numerals is the equivalent of
    - (A) 449
    - (B) 949
    - (C) 969
    - (D) 1149

25. If you subtract —1 from +1 the result will be
    - (A) —2
    - (B) 0
    - (C) 1
    - (D) 2

26. Of the following, the one which is the equivalent of 2⅓ is
    - (A) ⅓ of 2
    - (B) 2 and ⅓ of 1
    - (C) ⅔ of 1
    - (D) 2 and ⅓ of

27. A man bought a TV set that was listed at $160. He was given successive discounts of 20% and 10%. The price he paid was
    - (A) $112.00
    - (B) $115.20
    - (C) $119.60
    - (D) $129.60

28. The total length of fencing needed to enclose a rectangular area 46 feet by 34 feet is
    - (A) 26 yards 1 foot
    - (B) 26⅔ yards
    - (C) 52 yards 2 feet
    - (D) 53⅓ yards

29. Mr. Jones' income for a year is $15,000. He pays $2250 for income taxes. The percent of his income that he pays for income taxes is
    - (A) 9
    - (B) 12
    - (C) 15
    - (D) 22

30. Of the following, the one that is NOT a meaning of ⅔ is
    - (A) 1 of the 3 equal parts of 2
    - (B) 2 of the 3 equal parts of 1
    - (C) 2 divided by 3
    - (D) a ratio of 3 to 2

31. If the average weight of boys of John's age and height is 105 lbs. and if John weighs 110% of average, then John weighs
    - (A) 110 lbs.
    - (B) 110.5 lbs.
    - (C) 115½ lbs.
    - (D) 126 lbs.

32. On a house plan on which 2 inches represents 5 feet, the length of a room measures 7½ inches. The actual length of the room is
    - (A) 12½ feet
    - (B) 15¾ feet
    - (C) 17½ feet
    - (D) 18¾ feet

33. If pencils are bought at 35 cents per dozen and sold at 3 for 10 cents, the total profit on 5½ dozen is
    - (A) 25 cents
    - (B) 27½ cents
    - (C) 28½ cents
    - (D) 31½ cents

34. It costs 31 cents a square foot to lay linoleum. To lay 20 square yards of linoleum it will cost
    - (A) $16.20
    - (B) $18.60
    - (C) $55.80
    - (D) $62.00

35. The total number of eighths in two wholes and three-fourths is
    - (A) 11
    - (B) 14
    - (C) 19
    - (D) 22

36. The difference between one hundred five thousand eighty-four and ninety-three thousand seven hundred nine is
    - (A) 11,375
    - (B) 12,131
    - (C) 56,294
    - (D) 56,375

37. If a recipe for a cake calls for 2½ cups of flour and you wish to make three such cakes, the number of cups of flour you would have to use is
    - (A) 6½
    - (B) 7½
    - (C) 9
    - (D) 9½

38. A piece of wood 35 feet, 6 inches long was used to make 4 shelves of equal length. The length of each shelf was
    - (A) 8.9 inches
    - (B) 8 feet, 9 inches
    - (C) 8 feet, 9½ in.
    - (D) 8 feet, 10½ in.

39. If n and m are both positive integers greater than one, the largest fraction in the following group would be
    - (A) $\dfrac{2n}{m}$
    - (B) $\dfrac{2n}{m+1}$
    - (C) $\dfrac{2n+1}{m-1}$
    - (D) $\dfrac{2(n-1)}{m}$

40. John's father received a bonus of $450, which was 5% of his annual salary. His annual salary was
    (A) $9500　　　　(C) $800
    (B) $9000　　　　(D) $7500

41. The ratio of ¼ to ⅗ is
    (A) 1 to 3　　　　(C) 5 to 12
    (B) 3 to 20　　　(D) 3 to 4

42. Of the following, the fraction that is equal to ⅚ is

    (A) $\dfrac{5+2}{6+2}$　　　　(C) $\dfrac{5\times5}{6\times6}$

    (B) $\dfrac{5\times2}{6\times2}$　　　　(D) $\dfrac{5-2}{6-2}$

43. Jane has two pieces of ribbon. One piece is 2¾ yards; the other, 2⅔ yards. To make the two pieces equal she must cut off from the longer piece
    (A) 9 inches　　　(C) 6 inches
    (B) 8 inches　　　(D) 3 inches

44. The Mayflower sailed from Plymouth, England to Plymouth Rock, a distance of approximately 2800 miles, in 63 days. The average speed in miles per hour was closest to which one of the following?
    (A) ½　　　　　　(C) 2
    (B) 1　　　　　　(D) 3

45. Dividing the numerator of a fraction by 2 always
    (A) leaves the value of the fraction unchanged
    (B) makes the value of the fraction twice as great
    (C) makes the value of the fraction half as great
    (D) makes the denominator equal to the numerator

46. The scholarship board of a certain college loaned a student $200 at an annual rate of 6% from September 30 until December 15. To repay the loan and accumulated interest the student must give the college an amount closest to which one of the following?
    (A) $202.50　　　(C) $203.50
    (B) $203　　　　(D) $212

47. Pren and Wright invested $8000 and $6000, respectively, in a hardware business. At the end of the year, the profits were $3800. Each partner received 6% on his investment and the remainder was shared equally. What was the total that Pren received?
    (A) $2380　　　　(C) $1960
    (B) $2260　　　　(D) $1840

48. Assuming that 2.54 centimeters = 1 inch, a metal rod that measures 1½ feet would most nearly equal which one of the following?
    (A) 380 centimeters
    (B) 46 centimeters
    (C) 30 centimeters
    (D) none of these

49. Of the following, the number whose value is 1½% is
    (A) .0015　　　　(C) .0150
    (B) .012　　　　(D) .105

50. The regular price of a TV set that sold for $118.80 at a 20% reduction sale is
    (A) $148.50　　　(C) $138.84
    (B) $142.60　　　(D) $95.04

51. Of the following, the number which is nearest in value to 5 is
    (A) 4.985　　　　(C) 5.01
    (B) 5.005　　　　(D) 5.1

52. Successive discounts of 10% and 10% are equivalent to a single discount of
    (A) 15%　　　　(C) 19%
    (B) 18%　　　　(D) 20%

53. A governmental agency made 768 investigations in 1958, 960 investigations in 1959, and 1200 investigations in 1960. If the rate of increase remains the same, how many investigations will be made in 1961?
    (A) 1600　　　　(C) 1440
    (B) 1500　　　　(D) 1416

54. The present size of a dollar bill in the United States is 2.61 inches by 6.14 inches. The number of square inches of paper used for one bill is closest to which one of the following?
    (A) 160 square inches
    (B) 17.8 square inches
    (C) 16.0 square inches
    (D) 1.78 square inches

55. To represent 10½% on a chart of 100 equal squares, one must
    (A) fiill in ten squares and one-half of an eleventh
    (B) fill in nine squares and one-half of a tenth
    (C) fill in fifteen squares
    (D) show ten squares each half filled in

56. If .098 is subtracted from 3, the remainder is
    (A) 2.002　　　　(C) 2.902
    (B) 2.098　　　　(D) 2.92

57. Assuming that on a blueprint ⅛ inch equals 12 inches of actual length, the actual length (in feet) of a steel bar represented on the blueprint by a line 3¾ inches long is
    (A) 3¾　　　　　(C) 45
    (B) 30　　　　　(D) 360

58. In a circle graph a segment of 108 degrees is shaded to indicate the overhead in doing $150,000 gross business. The overhead amounts to
    (A) $1,200      (C) $12,000
    (B) $4,500      (D) $45,000

59. In a song with $\frac{4}{4}$ time signatures, one may find within a bar any one of the following combinations of notes *except*
    (A) two quarter notes, two eighth notes, four sixteenth notes
    (B) two quarter notes, one eighth note, six sixteenth notes
    (C) two quarter notes, two eighth notes, two sixteenth notes
    (D) two quarter notes, three eighth notes, two sixteenth notes

60. The Baltimore Colts won 8 games and lost 3. The ratio of games won to games played is
    (A) 8 : 11 (B) 3 : 11 (C) 8 : 3 (D) 3 : 8

61. Of the following, an expression whose value decreases as x increases to 10 is
    (A) $\dfrac{2x+1}{3}$      (C) $\dfrac{2x-1}{3}$
    (B) $\dfrac{4}{15-x}$      (D) $\dfrac{6}{2x-1}$

62. The relationship between .01% and .1 is
    (A) 1 to 10    (B) 1 to 100    (C) 1 to 1000
    (D) 1 to 10,000

63. When the fractions 2/3, 5/7, 8/11 and 9/13 are arranged in ascending order of size, the result is
    (A) 8/11, 5/7, 9/13, 2/3
    (B) 5/7, 8/11, 2/3, 9/13
    (C) 2/3, 8/11, 5/7, 9/13
    (D) 2/3, 9/13, 5/7, 8/11

64. If the outer diameter of a metal pipe is 2.84 inches and the inner diameter is 1.94 inches, the thickness of the metal is
    (A) .45 of an inch    (B) .90 of an inch
    (C) 1.94 inches    (D) 2.39 inches

65. An office manager employs 3 typists at $45 per week, 2 general clerks at $40 per week, and a messenger at $32 per week. The average weekly wage of these employees is
    (A) $37.25
    (C) $41.17
    (B) $39.00
    (D) none of these

66. If x is less than 10, and y is less than 5, it follows that
    (A) x is greater than y
    (B) x—y=5
    (C) x = 2 y
    (D) x + y is less than 15

67. A rectangular bin 4 feet long, 3 feet wide, and 2 feet high is solidly packed with bricks whose dimensions are 8 inches, 4 inches, and 2 inches. The number of bricks in the bin is
    (A) 54      (B) 648
    (C) 1,296      (D) none of these

68. A dealer sells an article at a loss of 50% of the cost. Based on the selling price, the loss is
    (A) 25%
    (B) 50%
    (C) 100%
    (D) none of these

69. An autoist drives 60 miles to his destination at an average speed of 40 miles per hour and makes the return trip at an average rate of 30 miles per hour. His average speed per hour for the entire trip is (A) 35 miles (B) 34-2/7 miles (C) 43-1/3 miles (D) none of these

70. In the Fahrenheit scale, the temperature that is equivalent to 50° Centigrade is (A) 122° (B) 90° (C) 106° (D) none of these

71. If the base of a rectangle is increased by 30% and the altitude is decreased by 20% the area is increased by (A) 25% (B) 10% (C) 5% (D) 4%

72. Of the following sets of fractions, the set which is arranged in increasing order is (A) 7/12, 6/11, 3/5, 5/8 (B) 6/11, 7/12, 5/8, 3/5 (C) 6/11, 7/12, 3/5, 5/8 (D) none of these

73. If the price of an automobile, including a 3% sales tax, is $2729.50, the amount of the sales tax is (A) $79.50 (B) $129.50 (C) $81.89 (D) none of these

74. If the sum of the edges of a cube is 48 inches, the volume of the cube is (A) 512 inches (B) 96 cubic inches (C) 64 cubic inches (D) none of these

75. A rectangular flower bed whose dimensions are 16 yards by 12 yards is surrounded by a walk 3 yards wide. The area of the walk is (A) 93 square yards (B) 96 square yards (C) 204 square yards (D) none of these

76. If the radius of a circle is diminished by 20%, the area is diminished by (A) 20% (B) 400% (C) 40% (D) 36%

77. If a distance estimated at 150 feet is really 140 feet, the per cent of error in this estimate is (A) 6-2/3% (B) 7-1/7% (C) 10% (D) none of these

78. If an airplane flies 550 yards in 3 seconds, the speed of the airplane, expressed in miles per hour, is (A) 125 (B) 375 (C) 300 (D) none of these

79. If the numerator and the denominator of a fraction are increased by the same quantity, the resulting fraction is (A) always greater than the original fraction (B) always less than the original fraction (C) always equal to the original fraction (D) none of these

80. A merchant sold two radios for $120. each. One was sold at a loss of 25% of the cost and the other was sold at a gain of 25% of the cost. On both transactions combined the merchant lost (A) $64 (B) $36 (C) $16 (D) none of these

81. The number missing in the series 2, 6, 12, 20, ?, 42, 56, 72 is (A) 30 (B) 40 (C) 36 (D) none of these

82. If two angles of a triangle are acute angles, the third angle (A) is less than the sum of the two given angles (B) is an acute angle (C) is the largest angle of the triangle (D) may be an obtuse angle

83. If an automobile travels 80 miles at the rate of 20 miles per hour and then returns over the same route at the rate of 40 miles per hour, the average speed per hour for the entire trip (going and return) is (A) 30 miles (B) 26⅔ miles (C) 60 miles (D) 33⅓ miles

84. The difference between one-tenth of 2000 and one-tenth per cent of 2000 is (A) 0 (B) 18 (C) 180 (D) 198

85. If the radius of a circle is decreased by 5 inches, the resulting decrease in its circumference is (A) $10\pi$ inches (B) 5 inches (C) 12 inches (D) 16 inches

86. If one acute angle of a right triangle is 5 times the other, the number of degrees in the smallest angle of the triangle is (A) 18° (B) 30° (C) 75° (D) 15°

87. The single commercial discount which is equivalent to successive discounts of 10% and 10% is (A) 20% (B) 19% (C) 17% (D) 15%

88. The price of an article has been reduced 25%. In order to restore the original price the new price must be increased by (A) 20% (B) 25% (C) 33-1/3% (D) 40%

89. A mortgage on a house in the amount of $4000 provides for quarterly payments of $200 plus interest on the unpaid balance at 4½%. The total second payment to be made is (A) $371.00 (B) $285.50 (C) $242.75 (D) $240.00

90. If four triangles are constructed with sides of the length indicated below, the triangle which will not be a right triangle is (A) 5, 12, 13 (B) 3, 4, 5 (C) 8, 15, 17 (D) 12, 15, 18

91. The number of hours it takes the sun to move from a point 60° N latitude, 30° E longitude, to a point 30° N latitude, 120° W longitude, is (A) 10 (B) 14 (C) 6 (D) 2

92. A piece of cardboard in the shape of a 15-inch square is rolled so as to form a cylindrical surface, without overlapping. The number of inches in the diameter of the cylinder is approximately (A) 45 (B) 23 (C) 5 (D) 2.5

93. A stationer buys blankbooks at $.75 per dozen and sells them at 25 cents apiece. The gross profit based on the cost is (A) 50% (B) 300% (C) 200% (D) 100%

94. A room 27 feet by 32 feet is to be carpeted. The width of the carpet is 27 inches. The length, in yards, of the carpet needed for this floor is (A) 1188 (B) 648 (C) 384 (D) 128

95. A bird flying 400 miles covers the first 100 at the rate of 100 miles an hour, the second 100 at the rate of 200 miles an hour, the third 100 at the rate of 300 miles an hour, and the last 100 at the rate of 400 miles an hour. The average speed was (in miles per hour) (A) 192 (B) 212 (C) 250 (D) 150

### Answer Key to Trial Examination

| | | | |
|---|---|---|---|
| 1. D | 25. D | 49. C | 73. A |
| 2. A | 26. B | 50. A | 74. C |
| 3. A | 27. B | 51. B | 75. C |
| 4. C | 28. D | 52. C | 76. D |
| 5. B | 29. C | 53. B | 77. B |
| 6. C | 30. D | 54. C | 78. B |
| 7. C | 31. C | 55. A | 79. A |
| 8. A | 32. D | 56. C | 80. C |
| 9. D | 33. B | 57. B | 81. A |
| 10. C | 34. C | 58. D | 82. D |
| 11. B | 35. D | 59. C | 83. B |
| 12. B | 36. A | 60. A | 84. D |
| 13. D | 37. B | 61. D | 85. A |
| 14. C | 38. D | 62. C | 86. D |
| 15. C | 39. C | 63. D | 87. B |
| 16. A | 40. B | 64. A | 88. C |
| 17. B | 41. C | 65. C | 89. C |
| 18. B | 42. B | 66. D | 90. D |
| 19. D | 43. D | 67. B | 91. A |
| 20. B | 44. C | 68. C | 92. C |
| 21. B | 45. C | 69. B | 93. B |
| 22. A | 46. A | 70. A | 94. D |
| 23. A | 47. C | 71. D | 95. A |
| 24. B | 48. B | 72. C | |

# ARITHMETICAL COMPUTATIONS

*To add valuable points to your exam score you must master arithmetical computations. And by this we mean doing them quickly and with absolute accuracy. The computations themselves will be simple, although the form in which they are presented may rattle you if you're not prepared. In addition to calculation, they measure your ability to interpret and act on directions. Thus this chapter provides practice through a series of tests modeled on the different question types that have actually appeared on examinations. An important tip from our years of experience with the self-tutored test-taker: Study the Directions! We have included those you are most likely to meet on your exam. Control over them will gain precious minutes for you. This doesn't mean you can skip reading directions on your actual exam. It does mean that you will be ahead of the game for knowing the language examiners use. Then you can afford to play it cool. A misunderstood direction can lead to a run of incorrect answers. Avoid this costly carelessness.*

## TO SCORE HIGH ON MATH TESTS

1. SCHEDULE YOUR STUDY. Set a definite time, and stick to it, as explained in the chapter, STUDYING AND USING THIS BOOK. Enter Arithmetical Computations on your Study Schedule.

2. PLAN on taking different types of Computation Tests in each study period. Keep alert to the differences and complications. That will help keep you bright and interested.

3. DO YOUR BEST and work fast to complete each test before looking at our Correct Answers. Keep pushing yourself, and use the help this book provides, for checking purposes only.

4. RECORD YOUR TIME for each test next to your score. Your schedule may allow you to take the tests again. And you may want to see how your speed and accuracy have improved.

5. REVIEW YOUR ERRORS. This is a must for every study session. Allow time for redoing every incorrect answer. The good self-tutor is a good self-critic. He learns most from his mistakes. And never makes them again.

6. DON'T GUESS AT ANSWERS. Because each practice test, like the actual examination, requires a multiple-choice answer, you might be tempted to pick up speed by approximating the answers. This is fatal. Carefully work out your answer to each question. Then choose the right answer. Any other way is certain to create confusion, slow you down, lower your score.

7. CLARITY & ORDER. Write all your figures clearly, in neat rows and columns. And this includes the figures you have to carry over from one column to another. Don't make mistakes because of lack of space and cramped writing. Use scratch paper wherever necessary.

8. SKIP THE PUZZLERS. If a single question gives you an unusual amount of trouble, go on to the next question. Come back to the tough one after you have done all the others and still have time left over.

9. STUDY THE SAMPLE SOLUTIONS. Note how carefully we have worked out each step. Get into this habit in doing all the practice tests. You'll quickly find that it's a time-saver . . . a high-scoring habit.

## Sample Questions and Detailed Solutions

*DIRECTIONS: Each question has five suggested answers lettered A, B, C, D, and E. Suggested answer E is NONE OF THESE. Blacken space E only if your answer for a question does not exactly agree with any of the first four suggested answers. When you have finished all the questions, compare your answers with the correct answers at the end of the test.*

Sample 1. Divide:

$$4.6 \overline{)233.404}$$

(A) 50.74
(B) 52.24
(C) 57.30
(D) 58.24
(E) None of these

Sample II. Multiply:

$$\begin{array}{r} 2\,946 \\ \times\,7.007 \end{array}$$

(A) 21,642.622
(B) 20,642.622
(C) 41,244.001
(D) 20,641.622
(E) None of these

SOLUTION 1.

$$
\begin{array}{r}
5\,0.74 \\
4/6.\overline{)233/4.04} \\
230 \times\times\times \\
\hline
340 \\
322 \\
\hline
184 \\
184
\end{array}
$$

Since the answer is clearly 50.74, blacken A on the answer sheet. Do not mark any of the other letter choices. There is only one correct answer.

SOLUTION II.

$$
\begin{array}{r}
2\,946 \\
\times\,7.007 \\
\hline
20622 \\
0000 \\
0000 \\
20622 \\
\hline
20,642.622
\end{array}
$$

The answer is 20,642.622, which is answer choice B. This answer is similar to answer choices A and D, but it is not the same. So you must be careful not to let the A and D choices confuse you. Blacken only B on your answer sheet.

Now, push forward! Test yourself and practice for your test with the carefully constructed quizzes that follow. Each one presents the kind of question you may expect on your test. And each question is at just the level of difficulty that may be expected. Don't try to take all the tests at one time. Rather, schedule yourself so that you take a few at each session, and spend approximately the same time on them at each session. Score yourself honestly, and date each test. You should be able to detect improvement in your performance on successive sessions.

# ARITHMETIC SUMMATION TEST

### Time Allowed: 10 minutes

*DIRECTIONS: In this test you are asked to do two of the fundamental operations in arithmetic: addition and multiplication. They are closely related in that multiplication is really a succession of additions. For the multiplication problems, blacken the space under A if the given answer is correct. Blacken the space under B if the answer is incorrect. For the addition problems, blacken the space under D if the given answer is correct. Blacken the space under E if the answer is incorrect. We suggest that you do all of the multiplication problems before going on to addition. You should be able to work more accurately and quickly that way.*

## MULTIPLICATION

```
1)   16          2)   69
   ×  4             ×  8
   ─────          ─────
     64             552
```

```
3)   27          4)   46
   ×  3             ×  5
   ─────          ─────
     71             51
```

```
5)   79          6)   58
   ×  2             ×  4
   ─────          ─────
    158             222
```

```
7)   15          8)   28
   ×  3             ×  6
   ─────          ─────
     35             168
```

```
9)   49         10)   89
   ×  7             ×  9
   ─────          ─────
    343             801
```

### WORK SPACE

### Answer Sheet

|    | A | B | C | D | E |
|----|---|---|---|---|---|
| 1  | ∷ | ∷ | ∷ | ∷ | ∷ |
| 2  | ∷ | ∷ | ∷ | ∷ | ∷ |
| 3  | ∷ | ∷ | ∷ | ∷ | ∷ |
| 4  | ∷ | ∷ | ∷ | ∷ | ∷ |
| 5  | ∷ | ∷ | ∷ | ∷ | ∷ |
| 6  | ∷ | ∷ | ∷ | ∷ | ∷ |
| 7  | ∷ | ∷ | ∷ | ∷ | ∷ |
| 8  | ∷ | ∷ | ∷ | ∷ | ∷ |
| 9  | ∷ | ∷ | ∷ | ∷ | ∷ |
| 10 | ∷ | ∷ | ∷ | ∷ | ∷ |

## ADDITION

```
1)   68          2)   44
     30               57
     46               60
   + 52             + 32
   ─────          ─────
    206             193
```

```
3)   37          4)   24
     63               43
     12               72
   + 78             + 57
   ─────          ─────
    190             197
```

```
5)   20          6)   48
     59               42
     66               77
   + 81             + 16
   ─────          ─────
    236             184
```

```
7)   34          8)   94
     28               36
     65               89
   + 41             + 64
   ─────          ─────
    168             283
```

```
9)   25         10)   52
     40               17
     66               25
   + 31             + 64
   ─────          ─────
    152             158
```

## WORK SPACE

## MULTIPLICATION

11) 67
× 3
---
191

12) 54
× 7
---
378

13) 67
× 6
---
412

14) 29
× 8
---
222

15) 36
× 5
---
190

16) 78
× 4
---
312

17) 18
× 4
---
72

18) 25
× 7
---
165

19) 47
× 6
---
282

20) 88
× 4
---
352

21) 68
× 5
---
330

22) 53
× 8
---
414

23) 64
× 3
---
192

24) 28
× 9
---
242

25) 82
× 8
---
656

**WORK SPACE**

### Answer Sheet

| | A | B | C | D | E |
|---|---|---|---|---|---|
| 11 | | | | | |
| 12 | | | | | |
| 13 | | | | | |
| 14 | | | | | |
| 15 | | | | | |
| 16 | | | | | |
| 17 | | | | | |
| 18 | | | | | |
| 19 | | | | | |
| 20 | | | | | |
| 21 | | | | | |
| 22 | | | | | |
| 23 | | | | | |
| 24 | | | | | |
| 25 | | | | | |

SCORE
.......... %
NO. CORRECT
NO. OF QUESTIONS
ON THIS TEST

## ADDITION

11) 44
68
75
+ 38
---
225

12) 26
64
39
+ 24
---
163

13) 58
64
27
+ 67
---
216

14) 65
34
48
+ 92
---
249

15) 11
18
85
+ 42
---
156

16) 33
26
94
+ 35
---
178

17) 88
64
38
+ 46
---
226

18) 29
63
11
+ 84
---
187

19) 54
36
29
+ 63
---
182

20) 48
75
63
+ 68
---
254

21) 75
62
32
+ 64
---
223

22) 38
82
46
+ 54
---
220

23) 12
43
65
+ 57
---
187

24) 46
58
42
+ 23
---
179

25) 28
94
35
+ 32
---
199

**WORK SPACE**

## Correct Answers

*(You'll learn more by writing your own answers before comparing them with these.)*

| | | | |
|---|---|---|---|
| 1. A-E | 8. A-D | 15. B-D | 22. B-D |
| 2. A-D | 9. A-E | 16. A-E | 23. A-E |
| 3. B-D | 10. A-D | 17. A-E | 24. B-E |
| 4. B-E | 11. B-D | 18. B-D | 25. A-E |
| 5. A-E | 12. A-E | 19. A-D | |
| 6. B-E | 13. B-D | 20. A-D | |
| 7. B-D | 14. B-E | 21. B-E | |

# ARITHMETIC DIMINUTION TEST

### Time Allowed: 10 minutes

*DIRECTIONS: Subtraction and division are two of the basic operations in arithmetic. This test will help you gain proficiency in both these diminution processes, and thereby in many others. For the division problems, blacken the space under A if the given answer is correct. Blacken the space under B if the answer is incorrect. For the subtraction problems, blacken the space under D if the given answer is correct. Blacken the space under E if the answer is incorrect. For this test the space under C will not be blackened. We suggest that you do all the division problems before going on to subtraction. Although the processes are related, you should be able to work more accurately and quickly if you do the test this way.*

## SUBTRACTION

$$1)\ \begin{array}{r} 16 \\ -11 \\ \hline 5 \end{array} \qquad 2)\ \begin{array}{r} 23 \\ -18 \\ \hline 15 \end{array}$$

$$3)\ \begin{array}{r} 55 \\ -29 \\ \hline 16 \end{array} \qquad 4)\ \begin{array}{r} 61 \\ -32 \\ \hline 39 \end{array}$$

$$5)\ \begin{array}{r} 32 \\ -19 \\ \hline 13 \end{array} \qquad 6)\ \begin{array}{r} 77 \\ -51 \\ \hline 26 \end{array}$$

$$7)\ \begin{array}{r} 48 \\ -39 \\ \hline 9 \end{array} \qquad 8)\ \begin{array}{r} 53 \\ -25 \\ \hline 38 \end{array}$$

$$9)\ \begin{array}{r} 86 \\ -47 \\ \hline 49 \end{array} \qquad 10)\ \begin{array}{r} 66 \\ -52 \\ \hline 14 \end{array}$$

$$11)\ \begin{array}{r} 38 \\ -17 \\ \hline 21 \end{array} \qquad 12)\ \begin{array}{r} 94 \\ -43 \\ \hline 51 \end{array}$$

$$13)\ \begin{array}{r} 69 \\ -31 \\ \hline 38 \end{array} \qquad 14)\ \begin{array}{r} 99 \\ -19 \\ \hline 70 \end{array}$$

$$15)\ \begin{array}{r} 57 \\ -32 \\ \hline 15 \end{array} \qquad 16)\ \begin{array}{r} 35 \\ -14 \\ \hline 21 \end{array}$$

### Answer Sheet

| | A | B | C | D | E |
|---|---|---|---|---|---|
| 1 | ‖ | ‖ | ‖ | ‖ | ‖ |
| 2 | ‖ | ‖ | ‖ | ‖ | ‖ |
| 3 | ‖ | ‖ | ‖ | ‖ | ‖ |
| 4 | ‖ | ‖ | ‖ | ‖ | ‖ |
| 5 | ‖ | ‖ | ‖ | ‖ | ‖ |
| 6 | ‖ | ‖ | ‖ | ‖ | ‖ |
| 7 | ‖ | ‖ | ‖ | ‖ | ‖ |
| 8 | ‖ | ‖ | ‖ | ‖ | ‖ |
| 9 | ‖ | ‖ | ‖ | ‖ | ‖ |
| 10 | ‖ | ‖ | ‖ | ‖ | ‖ |
| 11 | ‖ | ‖ | ‖ | ‖ | ‖ |
| 12 | ‖ | ‖ | ‖ | ‖ | ‖ |
| 13 | ‖ | ‖ | ‖ | ‖ | ‖ |
| 14 | ‖ | ‖ | ‖ | ‖ | ‖ |
| 15 | ‖ | ‖ | ‖ | ‖ | ‖ |
| 16 | ‖ | ‖ | ‖ | ‖ | ‖ |

## DIVISION

1) $5\overline{)30}$ → 6  2) $2\overline{)18}$ → 8

3) $5\overline{)25}$ → 4  4) $7\overline{)35}$ → 5

5) $4\overline{)12}$ → 4  6) $8\overline{)24}$ → 4

7) $6\overline{)24}$ → 4  8) $7\overline{)49}$ → 7

9) $4\overline{)32}$ → 9  10) $5\overline{)35}$ → 7

11) $9\overline{)81}$ → 8  12) $7\overline{)42}$ → 7

13) $7\overline{)28}$ → 4  14) $5\overline{)40}$ → 8

15) $8\overline{)16}$ → 2  16) $4\overline{)16}$ → 3

## WORK SPACE

## SUBTRACTION

17) $\begin{array}{r} 61 \\ -19 \\ \hline 42 \end{array}$   18) $\begin{array}{r} 78 \\ -51 \\ \hline 26 \end{array}$   19) $\begin{array}{r} 64 \\ -28 \\ \hline 26 \end{array}$

20) $\begin{array}{r} 36 \\ -16 \\ \hline 20 \end{array}$   21) $\begin{array}{r} 83 \\ -38 \\ \hline 55 \end{array}$   22) $\begin{array}{r} 43 \\ -12 \\ \hline 31 \end{array}$

23) $\begin{array}{r} 87 \\ -79 \\ \hline 8 \end{array}$   24) $\begin{array}{r} 55 \\ -31 \\ \hline 23 \end{array}$   25) $\begin{array}{r} 80 \\ -14 \\ \hline 76 \end{array}$

26) $\begin{array}{r} 93 \\ -40 \\ \hline 53 \end{array}$   27) $\begin{array}{r} 79 \\ -64 \\ \hline 5 \end{array}$   28) $\begin{array}{r} 28 \\ -12 \\ \hline 16 \end{array}$

29) $\begin{array}{r} 70 \\ -34 \\ \hline 46 \end{array}$   30) $\begin{array}{r} 98 \\ -83 \\ \hline 15 \end{array}$   31) $\begin{array}{r} 69 \\ -37 \\ \hline 42 \end{array}$

32) $\begin{array}{r} 47 \\ -33 \\ \hline 14 \end{array}$   33) $\begin{array}{r} 60 \\ -49 \\ \hline 11 \end{array}$   34) $\begin{array}{r} 73 \\ -28 \\ \hline 45 \end{array}$

35) $\begin{array}{r} 21 \\ -16 \\ \hline 4 \end{array}$   36) $\begin{array}{r} 88 \\ -77 \\ \hline 11 \end{array}$   37) $\begin{array}{r} 97 \\ -59 \\ \hline 39 \end{array}$

38) $\begin{array}{r} 53 \\ -29 \\ \hline 25 \end{array}$   39) $\begin{array}{r} 31 \\ -19 \\ \hline 12 \end{array}$   40) $\begin{array}{r} 77 \\ -49 \\ \hline 28 \end{array}$

## DIVISION

17) $7\overline{)21}^{\,4}$   18) $2\overline{)14}^{\,7}$   19) $7\overline{)56}^{\,8}$

20) $5\overline{)45}^{\,8}$   21) $9\overline{)72}^{\,9}$   22) $7\overline{)14}^{\,2}$

23) $5\overline{)20}^{\,4}$   24) $7\overline{)63}^{\,9}$   25) $3\overline{)12}^{\,4}$

26) $5\overline{)15}^{\,2}$   27) $4\overline{)20}^{\,4}$   28) $9\overline{)63}^{\,7}$

29) $8\overline{)32}^{\,3}$   30) $8\overline{)56}^{\,7}$   31) $4\overline{)24}^{\,6}$

32) $9\overline{)54}^{\,5}$   33) $8\overline{)40}^{\,6}$   34) $4\overline{)28}^{\,7}$

35) $6\overline{)54}^{\,9}$   36) $6\overline{)18}^{\,4}$   37) $8\overline{)48}^{\,7}$

38) $3\overline{)18}^{\,6}$   39) $6\overline{)36}^{\,7}$   40) $9\overline{)27}^{\,4}$

## WORK SPACE

**Answer Sheet**

| | A | B | C | D | E |
|---|---|---|---|---|---|
| 17 | | | | | |
| 18 | | | | | |
| 19 | | | | | |
| 20 | | | | | |
| 21 | | | | | |
| 22 | | | | | |
| 23 | | | | | |
| 24 | | | | | |
| 25 | | | | | |
| 26 | | | | | |
| 27 | | | | | |
| 28 | | | | | |
| 29 | | | | | |
| 30 | | | | | |
| 31 | | | | | |
| 32 | | | | | |
| 33 | | | | | |
| 34 | | | | | |
| 35 | | | | | |
| 36 | | | | | |
| 37 | | | | | |
| 38 | | | | | |
| 39 | | | | | |
| 40 | | | | | |

SCORE

.................... %

NO. CORRECT

NO. OF QUESTIONS ON THIS TEST

## Correct Answers

*(You'll learn more by writing your own answers before comparing them with these.)*

| | | | | | | | |
|---|---|---|---|---|---|---|---|
| 1. A-D | 11. B-D | 21. B-E | 31. A-D |
| 2. B-E | 12. B-D | 22. A-D | 32. B-D |
| 3. B-E | 13. A-D | 23. A-D | 33. B-D |
| 4. A-E | 14. A-E | 24. A-E | 34. A-D |
| 5. B-D | 15. A-E | 25. A-E | 35. A-E |
| 6. B-D | 16. B-D | 26. B-D | 36. B-D |
| 7. A-D | 17. B-D | 27. B-E | 37. B-E |
| 8. A-E | 18. A-E | 28. A-D | 38. A-E |
| 9. B-E | 19. A-E | 29. B-E | 39. B-D |
| 10. A-D | 20. B-D | 30. A-D | 40. B-D |

# COMPUTATIONAL SPEED TEST

### Time Allowed: 10 minutes

*DIRECTIONS: Each question has five suggested answers lettered A, B, C, D, and E. Suggested answer E is NONE OF THESE. Blacken space E only if your answer for a question does not exactly agree with any of the first four suggested answers. When you have finished all the questions, compare your answers with the correct answers at the end of the test.*

**ANSWERS**

1) Multiply:

      896
    × 708

(A) 643,386
(B) 634,386
(C) 634,368
(D) 643,368
(E) None of these

2) Divide:

    9 / 4266

(A) 447
(B) 477
(C) 474
(D) 475
(E) None of these

3) Add:

    $125.25
        .50
      70.86
    +  6.07

(A) $201.68
(B) $202.69
(C) $200.68
(D) $202.68
(E) None of these

4) Subtract:

    $1,250.37
    —   48.98

(A) $1,201.39
(B) $1,201.49
(C) $1,200.39
(D) $1,201.38
(E) None of these

5) Divide:

    29 / 476.92

(A) 16.4445
(B) 17.4445
(C) 16.4555
(D) 17.4455
(E) None of these

**Answer Sheet**

```
    A   B   C   D   E
 1  ┆┆  ┆┆  ┆┆  ┆┆  ┆┆
    A   B   C   D   E
 2  ┆┆  ┆┆  ┆┆  ┆┆  ┆┆
    A   B   C   D   E
 3  ┆┆  ┆┆  ┆┆  ┆┆  ┆┆
    A   B   C   D   E
 4  ┆┆  ┆┆  ┆┆  ┆┆  ┆┆
    A   B   C   D   E
 5  ┆┆  ┆┆  ┆┆  ┆┆  ┆┆
    A   B   C   D   E
 6  ┆┆  ┆┆  ┆┆  ┆┆  ┆┆
    A   B   C   D   E
 7  ┆┆  ┆┆  ┆┆  ┆┆  ┆┆
    A   B   C   D   E
 8  ┆┆  ┆┆  ┆┆  ┆┆  ┆┆
    A   B   C   D   E
 9  ┆┆  ┆┆  ┆┆  ┆┆  ┆┆
    A   B   C   D   E
10  ┆┆  ┆┆  ┆┆  ┆┆  ┆┆
```

**ANSWERS**

6) Multiply:

    7962.27
    ×   .06

(A) 4777.362
(B) 477.6732
(C) 4787.632
(D) 477.7362
(E) None of these

7) Add:

       28
       19
       17
    + 24

(A) 87
(B) 88
(C) 90
(D) 89
(E) None of these

8) Divide:

    3.7 / 2339.86

(A) 632.4
(B) 62.34
(C) 642.3
(D) 63.24
(E) None of these

## WORK SPACE

9) Add:

       4 ½
       5 ¾
    + 3 ⅔

(A) 13 10/13
(B) 12 ¾
(C) 13 ⅔
(D) 12 ½
(E) None of these

10) Multiply:

      45,286
    ×  4 1/5

(A) 190,021 1/5
(B) 190,234
(C) 190,201 1/5
(D) 190,202 2/5
(E) None of these

## ANSWERS

11) Subtract:

$$8\ \tfrac{1}{6}$$
$$-\ 5\ \tfrac{2}{3}$$

(A) 3 ⅔
(B) 2 ⅓
(C) 3 ⅙
(D) 2 ½
(E) None of these

12) Multiply:
$1/9 \times \tfrac{2}{3} \times \tfrac{7}{8} =$

(A) 6/108
(B) 7/108
(C) 14/27
(D) 14/108
(E) None of these

13) Divide:
$4\ \tfrac{1}{3}\ /\ \tfrac{1}{4}$

(A) 3/52
(B) 5/52
(C) 17 ⅓
(D) 12/52
(E) None of these

14) Find 6 ⅔%
of $13.50.

(A) $.89
(B) $.91
(C) $.88
(D) $.95
(E) None of these

15) Reduce 11/16
to a decimal.

(A) .8675
(B) .6875
(C) .6785
(D) .6578
(E) None of these

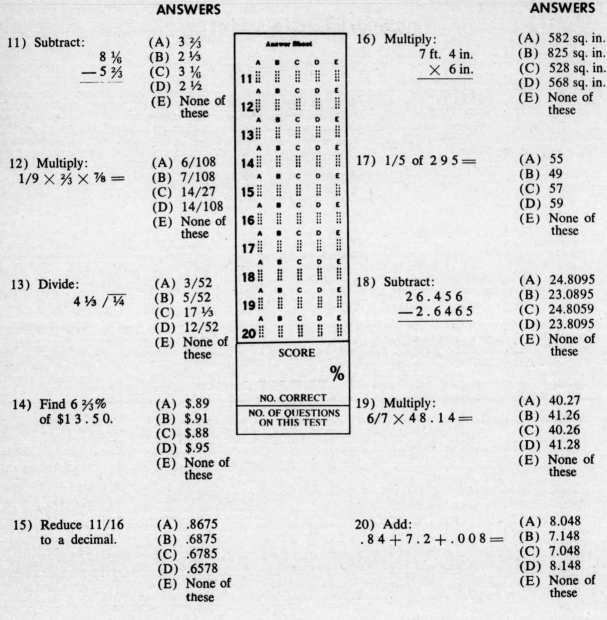

Answer Sheet

| | A | B | C | D | E |
|---|---|---|---|---|---|
| 11 | | | | | |
| 12 | | | | | |
| 13 | | | | | |
| 14 | | | | | |
| 15 | | | | | |
| 16 | | | | | |
| 17 | | | | | |
| 18 | | | | | |
| 19 | | | | | |
| 20 | | | | | |

SCORE

........... %

NO. CORRECT

NO. OF QUESTIONS ON THIS TEST

## ANSWERS

16) Multiply:

$$7\ \text{ft.}\ 4\ \text{in.}$$
$$\times\ 6\ \text{in.}$$

(A) 582 sq. in.
(B) 825 sq. in.
(C) 528 sq. in.
(D) 568 sq. in.
(E) None of these

17) 1/5 of 295 =

(A) 55
(B) 49
(C) 57
(D) 59
(E) None of these

18) Subtract:

$$26.456$$
$$-2.6465$$

(A) 24.8095
(B) 23.0895
(C) 24.8059
(D) 23.8095
(E) None of these

19) Multiply:
$6/7 \times 48.14 =$

(A) 40.27
(B) 41.26
(C) 40.26
(D) 41.28
(E) None of these

20) Add:
$.84 + 7.2 + .008 =$

(A) 8.048
(B) 7.148
(C) 7.048
(D) 8.148
(E) None of these

## WORK SPACE

## Correct Answers

*(You'll learn more by writing your own answers before comparing them with these.)*

| | | | |
|---|---|---|---|
| 1. C | 6. D | 11. D | 16. C |
| 2. C | 7. B | 12. B | 17. D |
| 3. D | 8. A | 13. A | 18. D |
| 4. A | 9. E | 14. E | 19. E |
| 5. E | 10. C | 15. B | 20. A |

# WORD PROBLEMS TEST

**Time Allowed: 10 minutes**

*DIRECTIONS: The following arithmetic word problems have been devised to make you think with numbers. In each question, the arithmetic is simple, but the objective is to comprehend what you have to do with the numbers and/or quantities. Read the problem carefully and choose the correct answer from the five choices that follow each question. Mark the answer on your answer sheet, and, when you have finished, check your answers with the correct answers at the end of the test.*

1. Add the following: 40¢, $2.75, $186.21, $24,865, $.74, $8.42, $2,475.28, $11,998.24.

   (A) $38,537.04    (B) $39,537.04
   (C) $38,533.40    (D) $39,573.40
   (E) None of these

2. Perform the indicated operations and express your answer in its simplest form: ⅝ divided by 20/3 times 7/19 divided by 63/38 times 16/21 divided by 1/14.

   (A) 2/9    (B) ½
   (C) ⅓    (D) 5/9
   (E) None of these

3. Perform the indicated operations: .020301 times 2.15 divided by .00000063.

   (A) 69218.19    (B) 69821.19
   (C) 69281.91    (D) 69281.19
   (E) None of these

4. Add the following fractions: 1½, 2 1/16, 9⅓, 2¼, 6 1/5.

   (A) 21 8/20    (B) 21½
   (C) 20    (D) 20 9/20
   (E) None of these

5. Perform the indicated operations and express your answer in inches: 12 feet, minus 7 inches, plus 2 feet 1 inch minus 7 feet, minus 1 yard, plus 2 yards 1 foot 3 inches.

   (A) 130 inches    (B) 128 inches
   (C) 129 inches    (D) 131 inches
   (E) None of these

6. Add:

   7 years,  3 months
   5 years,  6 months
   8 years, 11 months

   (A) 20 yrs.    (B) 20 yrs. 8 mos.
   (C) 21 yrs. 9 mos.    (D) 21 yrs. 8 mos.
   (E) None of these

7. Find the cost of 2 dozen boxes of pencils at $3.60 per ¼ dozen boxes.

   (A) $28.80    (B) $29.50
   (C) $20.88    (D) $28.08
   (E) None of these

8. When 5.1 is divided by 0.017 the quotient is

   (A) 30    (B) 300
   (C) 3,000    (D) 30,000
   (E) None of these

9. One percent of $23,000 is

   (A) $.023    (B) $2.30
   (C) $23    (D) $2300
   (E) None of these

10. The sum of $82.79; $103.06 and $697.88 is, most nearly,

    (A) $1628    (B) $791
    (C) $873    (D) $1395
    (E) None of these

11. The sum of 2345 and 4483 is

    (A) 6288    (B) 6828
    (C) 6882    (D) 8628
    (E) None of these

12. The difference between 2876 and 1453 is

   (A) 1342        (B) 1324
   (C) 1234        (D) 1423
        (E) None of these

13. If each of 5 sections has 15 cans, the total for all five sections is

   (A) 70        (B) 65
   (C) 60        (D) 80
        (E) None of these

14. The area of a street 100 yards long and 30 yards wide is

   (A) 3,000 sq. yds.   (B) 3,500 sq. yds.
   (C) 2,500 sq. yds.   (D) 130 sq. yds.
        (E) None of these

15. Five tons of snow will weigh how many pounds?

   (A) 1,000 lbs.     (B) 10,000 lbs.
   (C) 100 lbs.       (D) 5,000 lbs.
        (E) None of these

16. If a man earns $3000 a year, approximately how much is his weekly pay?

   (A) $45       (B) $50
   (C) $55       (D) $60
        (E) None of these

17. A man who works 8 hours a day for 6 days will work a total of how many hours?

   (A) 40 hrs.     (B) 45 hrs.
   (C) 50 hrs.     (D) 47 hrs.
        (E) None of these

18. If a load of snow contains 3 tons, it will weigh how many lbs.?

   (A) 3,000 lbs.     (B) 1,500 lbs.
   (C) 12,000 lbs.    (D) 6,000 lbs.
        (E) None of these

19. A section of pavement which is 10 feet long and 8 feet wide contains how many square feet?

   (A) 80 sq. ft.     (B) 92 sq. ft.
   (C) 800 sq. ft.    (D) 18 sq. ft.
        (E) None of these

20. If a man mops 13 halls each day for 15 days, he will have mopped a total of how many halls?

   (A) 165 halls    (B) 190 halls
   (C) 200 halls    (D) 175 halls
        (E) None of these

21. If you divided 56 pounds of soap powder equally among 8 men, each man would get how many pounds of soap powder?

   (A) 6 lbs.       (B) 7 lbs.
   (C) 8 lbs.       (D) 5 lbs.
        (E) None of these

22. The sum of 284.5, 3016.24, 8.9736, and 94.15 is, most nearly,

   (A) 3402.9     (B) 3403.0
   (C) 3403.9     (D) 4036.1
        (E) None of these

23. If 8394.6 is divided by 29.17, the result is most nearly

   (A) 288      (B) 347
   (C) 2880     (D) 3470
        (E) None of these

24. If two numbers are multiplied together, the result is 3752. If one of the two numbers is 56, the other number is

   (A) 41      (B) 15
   (C) 109     (D) 76
        (E) None of these

25. The sum of the fractions $\frac{1}{4}$, $\frac{2}{3}$, $\frac{3}{8}$, $\frac{5}{6}$, and $\frac{3}{4}$ is

   (A) 20/33     (B) 1 19/24
   (C) 2¼       (D) 2⅞
        (E) None of these

## Correct Answers

| | | | |
|---|---|---|---|
| 1. B | 8. B | 15. B | 22. C |
| 2. A | 9. E | 16. C | 23. A |
| 3. D | 10. C | 17. E | 24. E |
| 4. E | 11. B | 18. D | 25. D |
| 5. C | 12. D | 19. A | |
| 6. D | 13. E | 20. E | |
| 7. A | 14. A | 21. B | |

| SCORE |
|---|
| % |
| .................................. |
| NO. CORRECT ÷ |
| NO. OF QUESTIONS ON THIS TEST |

# GRAPH, CHART, AND TABLE INTERPRETATION

*The material in this chapter has appeared repeatedly on past examinations. It's all quite relevant, and well worth every minute of your valuable study time. Beginning with basic rules and a concise text, it proceeds to an illuminating presentation of a wide variety of questions and answers that exemplify the basic text while they strengthen your ability to answer actual test questions quickly and accurately.*

GRAPH and table interpretation forms an important part of your examination. Many jobs require the ability to read graphs and charts, or to make them up from a collection of data. You need a thorough understanding of their forms and meaning. Wherever a question is based on a map, chart, graph or table, remember that it is important to answer it solely on the basis of the information presented in the particular chart or table, without adding any ideas of your own. You are allowed to use scratch paper for computation while working on questions of this type.

## A SAMPLE QUESTION ANALYZED

Which one of the lines on the graph at the right most closely represents the data in these two columns?

Look at the two columns of data below:

| Time sec. | Velocity ft./sec. |
|-----------|-------------------|
| 0 | 2 |
| 2 | 3 |
| 4 | 4 |
| 6 | 5 |
| 8 | 6 |
| 10 | 7 |

CHART NO. I

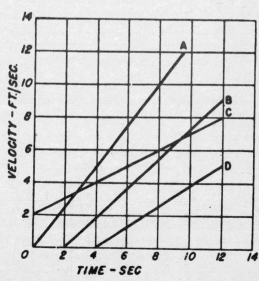

A B C D E

An examination of the graph shows that time values are indicated along the horizontal scale, and velocity values along the vertical scale. If we observe the velocity value at zero time, we see that the A line has a value of 0 velocity, and the C line a value of 2 ft./sec. No values are shown at 0 time for lines B and D. Hence line C is the only one which shows a velocity of 2 ft./sec. at 0 time.

Similarly at 2 sec. the velocity value for line B is 0, for line A is 2.5, and for line C, 3. Here again C is the only line which corresponds to the data in the table. At 4 sec. the velocity value for line D is 0, for line B is 1.9, for line C is 4, and for line A is 5. Here also line C is the only one that gives the value shown in the table. The same process can be repeated for time values 6, 8, and 10 sec., all of which show that line C is the only one corresponding to the values given in the table.

# TWO TEST-TYPE QUIZZES FOR PRACTICE

*The questions presented below on the interpretation of graphs and statistical tables have been compiled from various previous Civil Service examinations, and are designed to help you evaluate your reasoning and analytical ability.*

Now, push forward! Test yourself and practice for your test with the carefully constructed quizzes that follow. Each one presents the kind of question you may expect on your test. And each question is at just the level of difficulty that may be expected. Don't try to take all the tests at one time. Rather, schedule yourself so that you take a few at each session, and spend approximately the same time on them at each session. Score yourself honestly, and date each test. You should be able to detect improvement in your performance on successive sessions.

A portion of the standard answer sheet is provided after each test for marking your answers in the way you'll be required to do on the actual exam. At the right of this answer sheet, to make the scoring job simpler (after you have derived your own answers), you'll find our correct answers.

# INTERPRETATION TEST ONE

Questions 1 to 10 are to be answered solely on the basis of Chart II which relates to the Investigation Division of Department X. This chart contains four curves which connect the points that show for each year the variations in percentage deviation from normal in the number of investigators, the number of clerical employees, the cost of personnel, and the number of cases processed for the period 1942-1952 inclusive. The year 1942 was designated as the normal year. The personnel of the Investigation Division consists of investigators and clerical employees only.

## CHART NO. II

INVESTIGATION DIVISION, DEPARTMENT X
VARIATIONS IN NUMBER OF CASES PROCESSED, COST OF PERSONNEL
NUMBER OF CLERICAL EMPLOYEES, AND NUMBER OF INVESTI-
GATORS FOR EACH YEAR FROM 1942 TO 1952 INCLUSIVE
(IN PERCENTAGES FROM NORMAL)

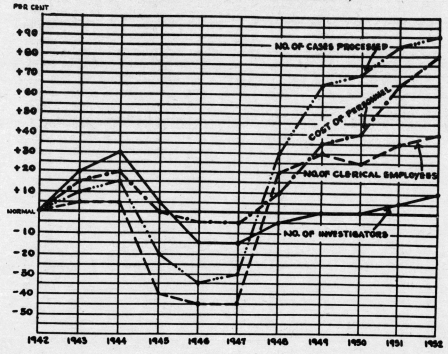

1. If 1300 cases were processed by the division in 1946, then the number of cases processed in 1942 was
   (A) 2000  (B) 1755
   (C) 2145  (D) 1650.

2. Of the following, the year in which there was no change in the size of the division's total staff from that of the preceding year is
   (A) 1945  (B) 1947
   (C) 1949  (D) 1951.

3. Of the following, the year in which the size of the division's total staff decreased most sharply from that of the preceding year is

(A) 1945          (B) 1946
(C) 1947          (D) 1948.

4. An inspection of the chart discloses that the curve that fluctuated *least*, as determined by the average deviation from normal, is the curve for the
(A) number of cases processed
(B) cost of personnel
(C) number of clerical employees
(D) number of investigators.

5. A comparison of 1946 with 1942 reveals an increase in 1946 in the
(A) cost of personnel for the division
(B) number of cases processed per investigator
(C) number of cases processed per clerical employee
(D) number of clerical employees per investigator.

6. If the personnel cost per case processed in 1942 was $12.30, then the personnel cost per case processed in 1952 was most nearly
(A) $ 9.85          (B) $10.95
(C) $11.65          (D) $13.85.

7. Suppose that there was a total of 108 employees in the division in 1942 and a total of 125 employees in 1950. On the basis of these figures, it is most accurate to state that the number of investigators employed in the division in 1950 was

(A) 40          (B) 57
(C) 68          (D) 85.

8. It is predicted that the number of cases processed in 1953 will exceed the number processed in 1952 by exactly the same quantity that the number processed in 1952 exceeded that processed in 1951. It is also predicted that the personnel cost in 1953 will exceed the personnel cost in 1952 by exactly the same amount that that the 1952 personnel cost exceeded that for 1951. On the basis ot these predictions, it is most accurate to state that the personnel cost per case in 1953 will be
(A) ten per cent less than the personnel cost in 1952
(B) exactly the same as the personnel cost per case in 1952
(C) twice as much as the personnel cost per case in 1942
(D) exactly the same as the personnel cost per case in 1942.

9. The variation between the per cent of cases processed and the number of investigators of Department X was greatest in
(A) 1949          (B) 1951
(C) 1952          (D) 1944.

10. In 1950, the difference between two categories in Department X is equal to a third. The third is the
(A) number of investigators
(B) cost of personnel
(C) number of clerical employees
(D) number of cases processed.

## Correct Answers

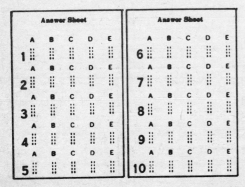

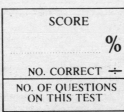

SCORE

................................. %

NO. CORRECT ÷

NO. OF QUESTIONS ON THIS TEST

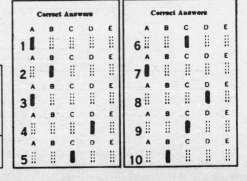

# INTERPRETATION TEST TWO

*DIRECTIONS: Read each test question carefully. Each one refers to the following graph, and is to be answered solely on that basis. Select the best answer among the given choices and blacken the proper space on the answer sheet.*

In the following graph the heavy curve represents postal receipts at St. Louis from 1930 to 1939.

The light curve represents postal receipts at Detroit from 1930 to 1939.

## CHART NO. III

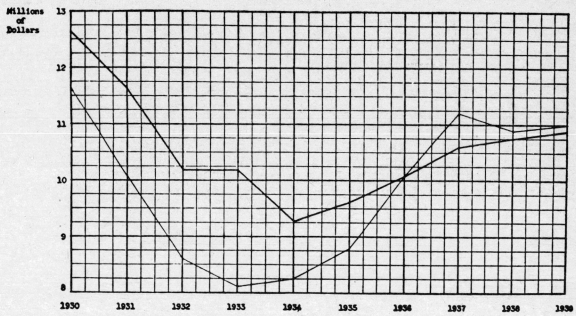

1. In 1937 the value of receipts in St. Louis was
   (A) 10,300,000    (B) 10,600,000
   (C) 11,100,000    (D) 11,200,000

2. Receipts were greatest in Detroit in
   (A) 1930    (B) 1933
   (C) 1937    (D) 1939

3. Detroit's and St. Louis' receipts were equal in
   (A) 1930     (B) 1933     (C) 1936

4. Receipts in St. Louis were least in
   (A) 1932    (B) 1933
   (C) 1934    (D) 1937

5. In 1935 the ratio of the receipts in St. Louis to those in Detroit was
   (A) 2 to 1    (B) 5 to 3
   (C) 10 to 9    (D) 12 to 11

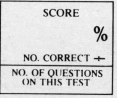

# Practice Using Answer Sheets

Alter numbers to match the practice and drill questions in each part of the book.
Make only ONE mark for each answer. Additional and stray marks may be counted as mistakes.
In making corrections, erase errors COMPLETELY. Make glossy black marks.

# PART FOUR

## *Perceptual Motor Ability*

## *Final Model Exam and Some Final Advice*

4

# Practice Using Answer Sheets

Alter numbers to match the practice and drill questions in each part of the book.
Make only ONE mark for each answer. Additional and stray marks may be counted as mistakes.
In making corrections, erase errors COMPLETELY. Make glossy black marks.

270

# THE TEST IN CARVING

ONE of the most important phases of the Dental Aptitude Test is that part of the examination which tests your manual dexterity. This section of the test, usually given first of all in the morning session, requires you to carve out of chalk two different figures. You are provided with a pencil and a six-inch ruler for planning the work, and with a knife for the actual carving of the figures. You are advised to do the neatest job possible.

## HOW THE CARVING TEST IS RATED

In this manual dexterity test you are rated for the following:

1. the extent to which your angles are sharply cut.

2. the extent to which your surfaces are symmetrical and well-rounded.

3. the extent to which your surfaces are smooth and flat.

4. the extent to which your finished carving is similar to the drawing (with its given dimensions) that you are to follow.

## WHAT THE CARVING TEST IS ABOUT

At the beginning of this carving test, you are given three pieces of chalk. Each piece is about 3 1/4 inches long and about 5/8 of an inch in diameter. The knife provided is much like the one that is used at home to pare potatoes.*

With the first of the three pieces of chalk that you are given, you are directed to practice carving for ten minutes. What you do with this piece of chalk does not count.

Then you are asked to do the first of the two carvings that count. This first carving is easier to do than the second. You are allowed 40 minutes for this carving. Below you will find an illustration of a typical "first carving" model that you are to follow:

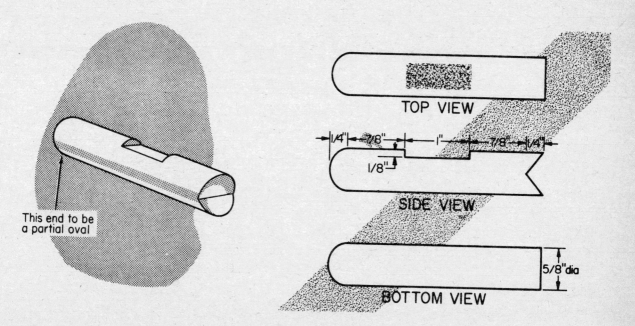

This end to be a partial oval

TOP VIEW

1/4" 7/8" 1" 7/8" 1/4"

1/8"

SIDE VIEW

5/8"dia

BOTTOM VIEW

* You are strongly advised to buy such chalk (often called "Alpha" type) which many art supply stores carry. The knife can be purchased in a hardware or "dime" store. Devote plenty of pre-exam preparation to practice in carving the chalk.

The time allowance for the second carving is 50 minutes. Here is a typical "second carving" situation:

Under no circumstances are you permitted to rub the chalk on any surface or to use sandpaper.

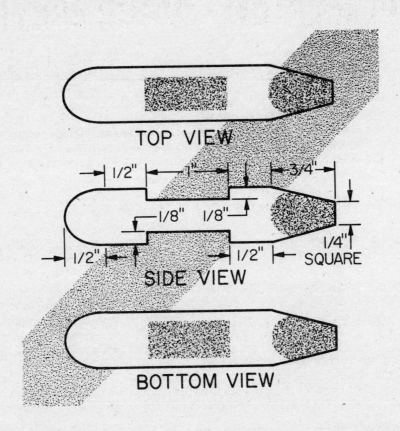

TOP VIEW

SIDE VIEW

BOTTOM VIEW

## HELPFUL HINTS IN CARVING

1. *Handle your knife properly.* If you hold the knife at a good angle, you will be able to remove the chalk better. With this procedure, you will also get a smooth and shiny surface.

2. *Check often to see that you are getting a flat surface.* The best way to check is to place your ruler on the surface in various positions. If the ruler remains smack on the surface, you're all right.

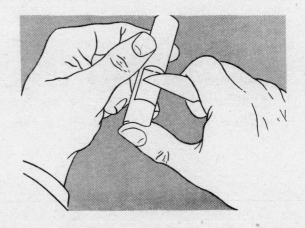

# PERCEPTUAL-MOTOR ABILITY

*The spatial relations problems in this chapter are designed by the test-makers to measure your reasoning ability without depending on educational background. The answers do not depend on your vocabulary, your reading ability, or your other verbal skills. They do depend on how well you understand the task and the directions. That's why, to afford plenty of practice, we've constructed a large number of these items, and have arranged them as a series of tests. Each test is just about as long and as difficult as the sub-test you will encounter. Observe the time limits; space and schedule your test-taking; record your progress.*

## FIGURE CLASSIFICATION QUESTIONS EXPLAINED

*DIRECTIONS: In this type of test, each problem consists of two groups of figures labeled 1 and 2. These two groups are followed by five answer figures, lettered A, B, C, D, and E. For each problem you must decide what characteristic each of the figures in Group 1 has that none of the figures in Group 2 has. Then select the lettered answer figure that has this characteristic.*

*Now look at the sample problems and the explanations we have provided. That should make the DIRECTIONS quite clear.*

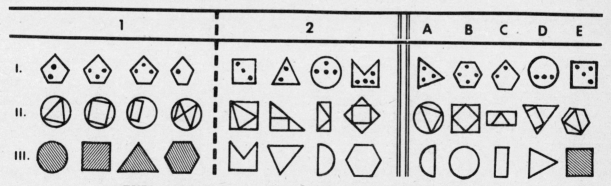

*EXPLANATION: In Sample problem 1 all the figures in Group 1 are pentagons, but none of the figures in Group 2 is a pentagon, so C is the answer.*

*In Sample problem II, all the figures in Group 1 include a circle, but none of the figures in Group 2 include a circle; so A is the answer.*

*In Sample problem III, all the figures in Group I are shaded figures, but none in Group 2 is a shaded figure. So the correct lettered answer figure is E.*

**Correct Answers To Each Test Are Given After Each Test**

# FIGURE CLASSIFICATION TEST ONE

## 20 Minutes

DIRECTIONS: *In this type of test, each problem consists of two groups of figures labeled 1 and 2. These two groups are followed by five answer figures, lettered A, B, C, D, and E. For each problem you must decide what characteristic each of the figures in Group 1 has that none of the figures in Group 2 has. Then select the lettered answer figure that has this characteristic.*

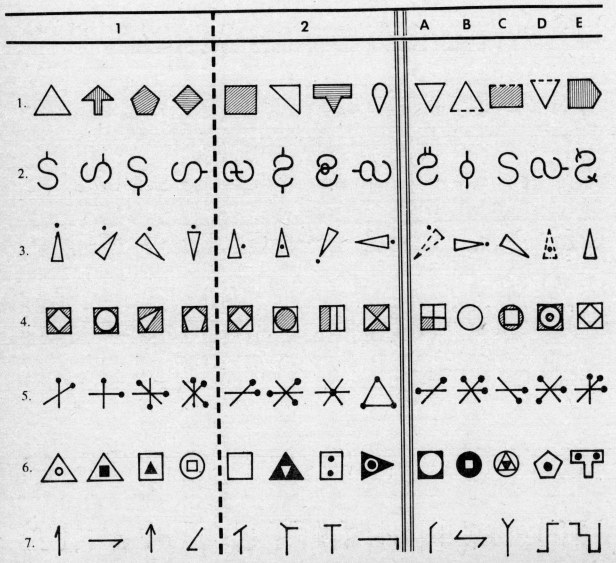

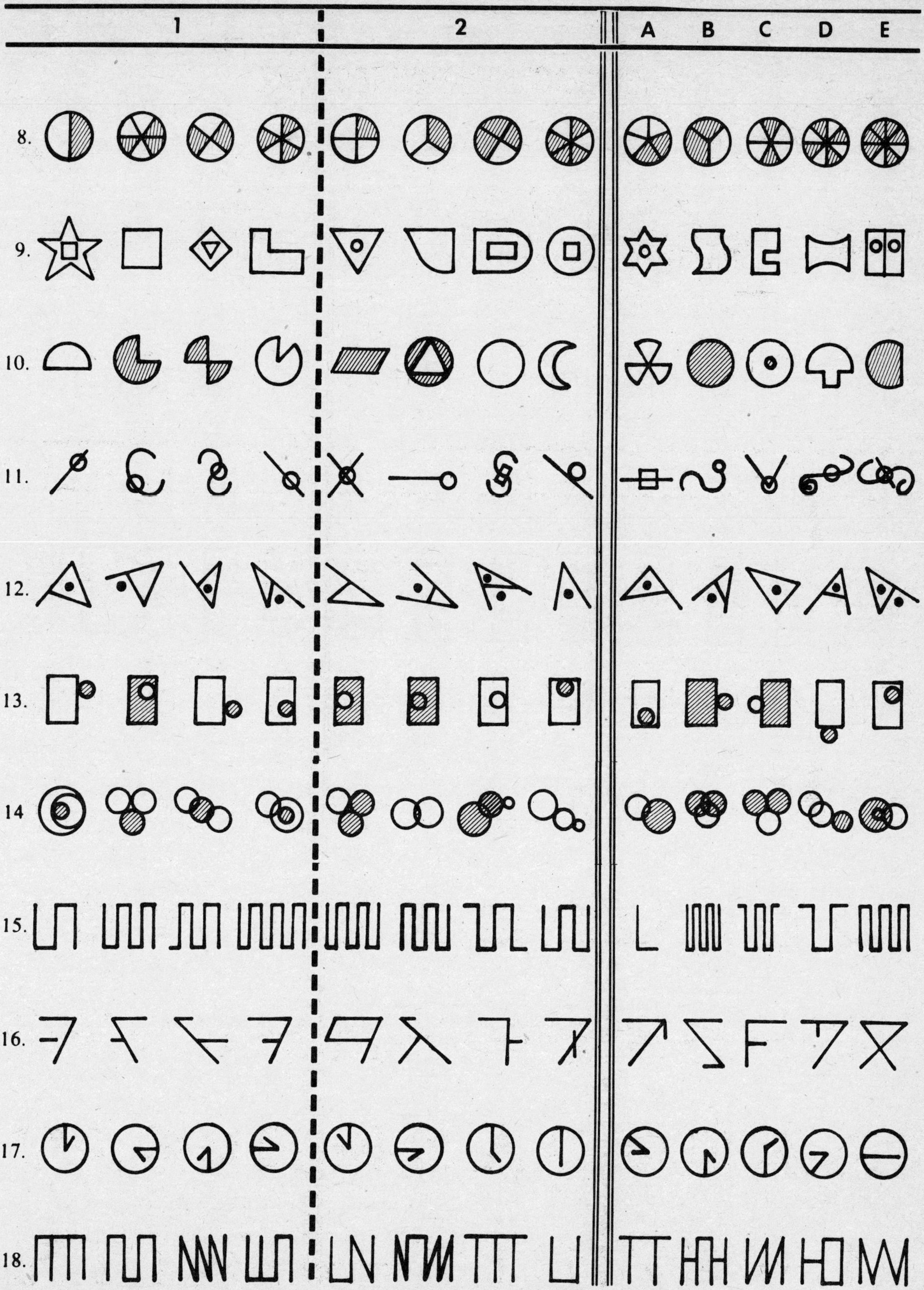
1
2
A B C D E
8.
9.
10.
11.
12.
13.
14
15.
16.
17.
18.

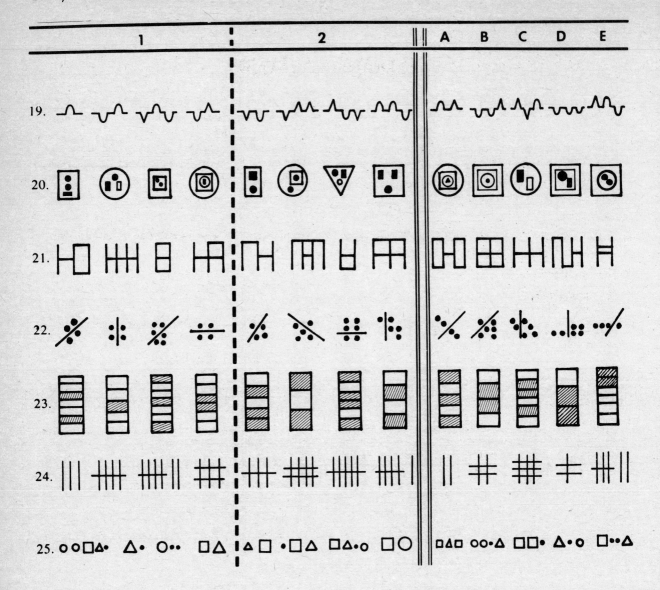

**END OF SECTION**

*If you finish before the allotted time is up, check your work on this section only. When time is up, proceed directly to the next section and do not return to this section.*

# EXPLANATORY ANSWERS

*Every figure in Group I, but no figure in Group II...*

1. **(B)**...has a point on top.
2. **(C)**...contains a forward "S" (which may be on its side, but not a mirror image).
3. **(A)**...has a dot above.
4. **(C)**...consists of a single white figure in the center of a shaded figure.
5. **(E)**...includes one vertical line.
6. **(D)**...is a *single* figure (of any color or shape) on a white background.
7. **(B)**...includes no right or obtuse angles (only acute angles).
8. **(D)**...is divided equally between white and black area.
9. **(C)**...includes only straight lines.
10. **(A)**...is a circle with "pie-shaped" sector(s) removed.
11. **(D)**...is a circle with a line or curve running completely through it.
12. **(A)**...is a triangle with one side extended, and one dot anywhere.
13. **(E)**...is a rectangle with a different-colored circle attached to its rightmost side.
14. **(D)**...consists of two white circles and one shaded circle.
15. **(E)**...ends on a down stroke: ⌐ (at the rightmost end).
16. **(B)**...consists of two horizontal lines and one diagonal line.
17. **(D)**...has an acute angle going *clockwise* from the long "hand" to the short one.
18. **(B)**...includes four (and only four) vertical lines.
19. **(C)**...has no two adjacent protrusions on the same side of the line.
20. **(B)**...consists of two circles and two rectangles (only).
21. **(D)**...has three horizontal lengths (between verticals).
22. **(A)**...has the same number of dots on each side of the line.
23. **(E)**...has more white boxes than shaded ones.
24. **(D)**...has an odd number of lines.
25. **(C)**...has the parts arranged so that all circles come to the left of everything else, all squares come to the left of triangles and dots, and all triangles precede dots.

| SCORE |
|---|
| .......................... **%** |
| NO. CORRECT |
| NO. OF QUESTIONS |

# FIGURE CLASSIFICATION TEST TWO

**20 minutes**

*DIRECTIONS: Each of these problems consists of two groups of figures, labeled 1 and 2. These are followed by five lettered answer figures. For each problem you are to decide what characteristic each of the figures in group 1 has that none of the figures in group 2 has. Then select the lettered answer figure that has this characteristic.*

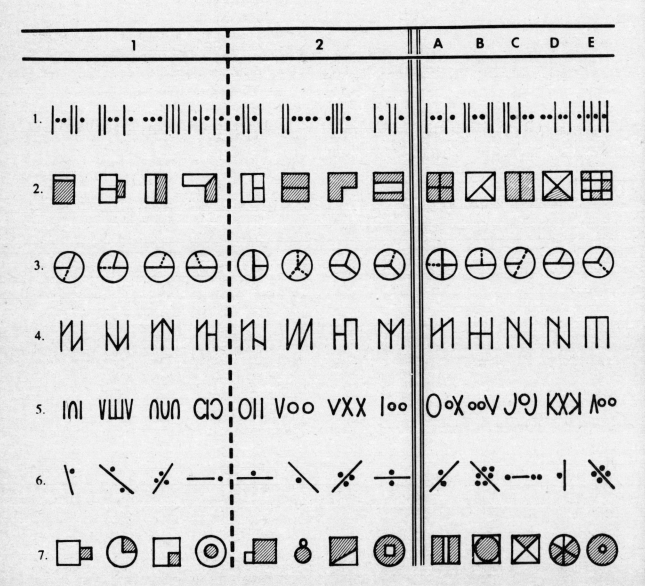

S1207

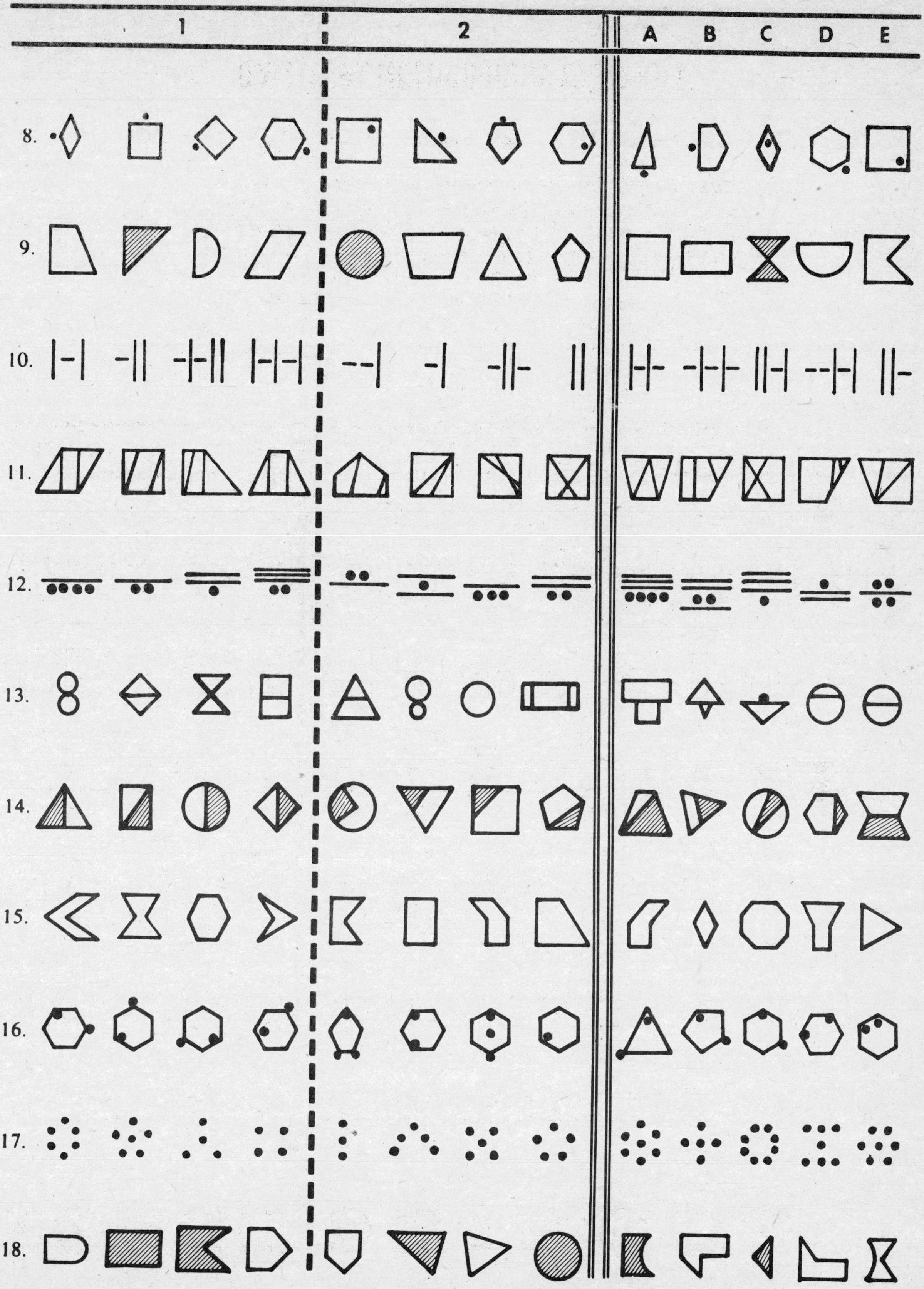
1
2
A B C D E
8.
9.
10.
11.
12.
13.
14.
15.
16.
17.
18.

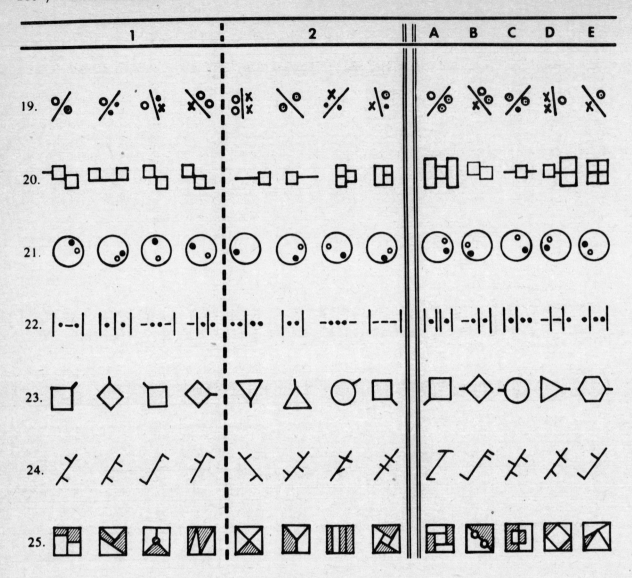

## END OF SECTION

*If you finish before the allotted time is up, check your work on this section only. When time is up, proceed directly to the next section and do not return to this section.*

# EXPLANATORY ANSWERS

*Every figure in Group I, but no figure in Group II...*

1. **(C)** consists of three lines and three dots.

2. **(D)** consists of a single undivided shaded region touching any number of white regions.

3. **(B)** is a circle with three radii, two solid and one dotted such that two angles are formed totaling 180°

4. **(B)** contains intersections in the middle of its leftmost and rightmost vertical lines.

5. **(D)** has three elements, the first and third being mirror images.

6. **(A)** has exactly one dot to the right of the line.

7. **(C)** has more white area than shaded area.

8. **(D)** has an even number of sides, with the dot outside the figure.

9. **(E)** is *a*symmetrical if a vertical line is drawn through the center.

10. **(E)** has one more vertical line than the number of horizontal lines.

11. **(D)** consists of one quadrilateral inscribed inside another quadrilateral.

12. **(A)** has an odd number of elements, with no dot above any line.

13. **(E)** consists of two congruent parts.

14. **(E)** has equal areas of white and shaded territory.

15. **(B)** has no vertical lines.

16. **(C)** is a hexagon with one dot inside and one dot outside.

17. **(C)** has an even number of dots.

18. **(A)** has ⌐ at its leftmost end.

19. **(E)** has two elements to the right of the line and one to the left of it (a dot in a circle together count as two elements).

20. **(B)** has two rectangles.

21. **(E)** has the black dot above the white dot.

22. **(B)** contains five parts, two of which are dots.

23. **(B)** is a quadrilateral with a line attached to it and extending horizontally, straight up, or diagonally up.

24. **(E)** is a line slanted like this  /  , with two perpendicular lines attached to it.

25. **(C)** consists of two shaded regions and two white ones.

| SCORE |
|:---:|
| ............................ **%** |
| NO. CORRECT |
| NO. OF QUESTIONS ON THIS TEST |

# FIGURE CLASSIFICATION TEST THREE

### 20 Minutes

DIRECTIONS: *Each of these problems consists of two groups of figures, labeled 1 and 2. These are followed by five lettered answer figures. For each problem you are to decide what characteristic each of the figures in group 1 has that none of the figures in group 2 has. Then select the lettered answer figure that has this characteristic.*

S1207

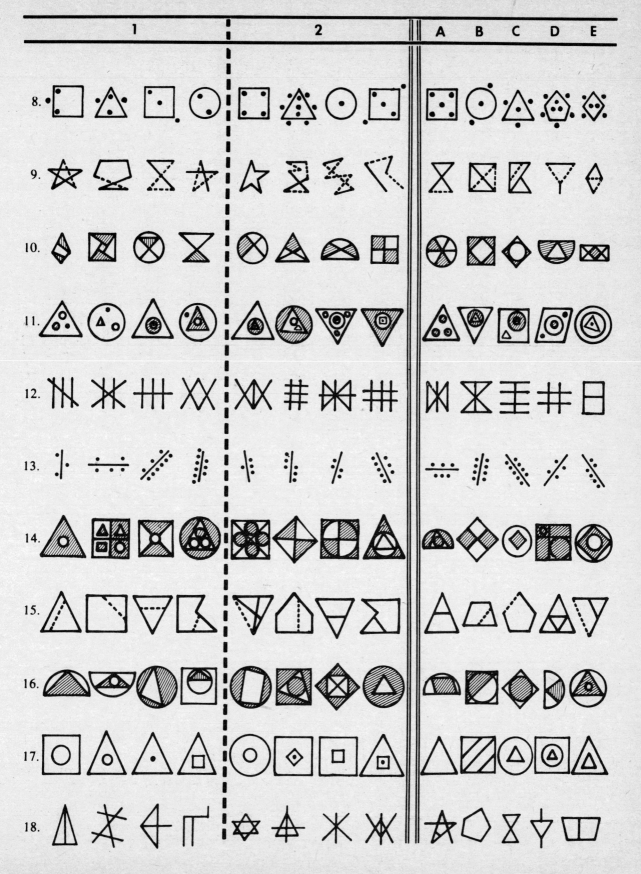

| | 1 | 2 | A B C D E |

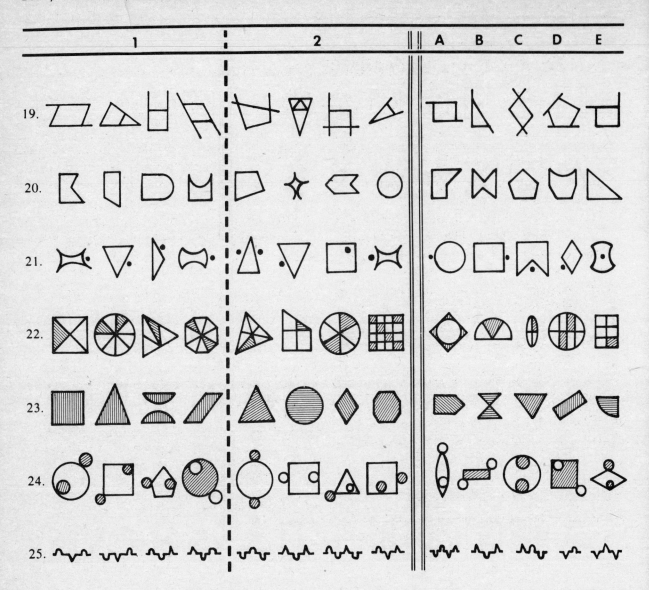

19.

20.

21.

22.

23.

24.

25.

*END OF SECTION*

# EXPLANATORY ANSWERS

*Every figure in Group I, but no figure in Group II...*

1. (**D**)...includes an upward angle made by a solid line and a dotted line.

2. (**A**)...has the dot on the right side when the V is rotated clockwise.

3. (**D**)...has three different figures, one inside the other without touching.

4. (**B**)...has four white regions, two shaded ones, two black ones.

5. (**C**)...has an equal number of white and/or black dots on either side of the line.

6. (**A**)...has three horizontal lines.

7. (**E**)...has two lines attached inside and one line outside.

8. (**E**)...has two two dots inside the figure.

9. (**B**)...has a dotted line crossing over a solid line.

10. (**B**)...includes at least one shaded triangle.

11. (**E**)...consists of a triangle, two circles, and a dot.

12. (**D**)...has four lines.

13. (**C**)...has an odd number of dots.

14. (**E**)...contains at least one empty white circle.

15. (**B**)...is a solid figure with one triangular piece cut off by a dotted line.

16. (**B**)...includes a semicircle (with its diameter) and a triangle.

17. (**C**)...has a figure, inside of which is one different type of figure (consider a dot a figure).

18. (**C**)...can be drawn with only four straight lines.

19. (**A**)...is a quadrilateral with only two opposite sides extended.

20. (**A**)...includes three sides of a rectangle.

21. (**B**)...has only one dot which is to the right of the main figure.

22. (**C**)...is one-quarter shaded in area.

23. (**D**)...has vertical shading.

24. (**D**)...has one circle inside, and one outside attached at opposite ends of the main figure; circles must be of a color different from the main figure.

25. (**C**)...has two curved humps and one pointed one.

| SCORE |
| --- |
| .......................... **%** |
| NO. CORRECT |
| NO. OF QUESTIONS ON THIS TEST |

# Practice Using Answer Sheets

DIRECTIONS: Read each question and its lettered answers. When you have decided which answer is correct, blacken the corresponding space on this sheet with a No. 2 pencil. Make your mark as long as the pair of lines, and completely fill the area between the pair of lines. If you change your mind, erase your first mark COMPLETELY. Make no stray marks; they may count against you.

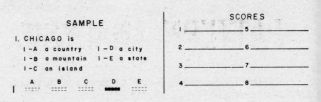

SAMPLE

1. CHICAGO is
   1-A a country
   1-B a mountain
   1-C an island
   1-D a city
   1-E a state

1 A B C D E

SCORES

1 ________ 5 ________
2 ________ 6 ________
3 ________ 7 ________
4 ________ 8 ________

| | | | | | | | |
|---|---|---|---|---|---|---|---|
| 1 | A B C D E | 2 | A B C D E | 3 | A B C D E | 4 | A B C D E |
| 5 | A B C D E | 6 | A B C D E | 7 | A B C D E | 8 | A B C D E |
| 9 | A B C D E | 10 | A B C D E | 11 | A B C D E | 12 | A B C D E |
| 13 | A B C D E | 14 | A B C D E | 15 | A B C D E | 16 | A B C D E |
| 17 | A B C D E | 18 | A B C D E | 19 | A B C D E | 20 | A B C D E |
| 21 | A B C D E | 22 | A B C D E | 23 | A B C D E | 24 | A B C D E |
| 25 | A B C D E | 26 | A B C D E | 27 | A B C D E | 28 | A B C D E |
| 29 | A B C D E | 30 | A B C D E | 31 | A B C D E | 32 | A B C D E |
| 33 | A B C D E | 34 | A B C D E | 35 | A B C D E | 36 | A B C D E |
| 37 | A B C D E | 38 | A B C D E | 39 | A B C D E | 40 | A B C D E |
| 41 | A B C D E | 42 | A B C D E | 43 | A B C D E | 44 | A B C D E |
| 45 | A B C D E | 46 | A B C D E | 47 | A B C D E | 48 | A B C D E |
| 49 | A B C D E | 50 | A B C D E | 51 | A B C D E | 52 | A B C D E |
| 53 | A B C D E | 54 | A B C D E | 55 | A B C D E | 56 | A B C D E |
| 57 | A B C D E | 58 | A B C D E | 59 | A B C D E | 60 | A B C D E |
| 61 | A B C D E | 62 | A B C D E | 63 | A B C D E | 64 | A B C D E |
| 65 | A B C D E | 66 | A B C D E | 67 | A B C D E | 68 | A B C D E |
| 69 | A B C D E | 70 | A B C D E | 71 | A B C D E | 72 | A B C D E |
| 73 | A B C D E | 74 | A B C D E | 75 | A B C D E | 76 | A B C D E |
| 77 | A B C D E | 78 | A B C D E | 79 | A B C D E | 80 | A B C D E |
| 81 | A B C D E | 82 | A B C D E | 83 | A B C D E | 84 | A B C D E |
| 85 | A B C D E | 86 | A B C D E | 87 | A B C D E | 88 | A B C D E |
| 89 | A B C D E | 90 | A B C D E | 91 | A B C D E | 92 | A B C D E |
| 93 | A B C D E | 94 | A B C D E | 95 | A B C D E | 96 | A B C D E |
| 97 | A B C D E | 98 | A B C D E | 99 | A B C D E | 100 | A B C D E |
| 101 | A B C D E | 102 | A B C D E | 103 | A B C D E | 104 | A B C D E |
| 105 | A B C D E | 106 | A B C D E | 107 | A B C D E | 108 | A B C D E |
| 109 | A B C D E | 110 | A B C D E | 111 | A B C D E | 112 | A B C D E |
| 113 | A B C D E | 114 | A B C D E | 115 | A B C D E | 116 | A B C D E |
| 117 | A B C D E | 118 | A B C D E | 119 | A B C D E | 120 | A B C D E |
| 121 | A B C D E | 122 | A B C D E | 123 | A B C D E | 124 | A B C D E |
| 125 | A B C D E | 126 | A B C D E | 127 | A B C D E | 128 | A B C D E |
| 129 | A B C D E | 130 | A B C D E | 131 | A B C D E | 132 | A B C D E |
| 133 | A B C D E | 134 | A B C D E | 135 | A B C D E | 136 | A B C D E |
| 137 | A B C D E | 138 | A B C D E | 139 | A B C D E | 140 | A B C D E |
| 141 | A B C D E | 142 | A B C D E | 143 | A B C D E | 144 | A B C D E |
| 145 | A B C D E | 146 | A B C D E | 147 | A B C D E | 148 | A B C D E |
| 149 | A B C D E | 150 | A B C D E | | | | |

# PATTERN ANALYSIS AND COMPREHENSION

*Practice exercises. Important variations
on a significant test theme in spatial relations and
aptitude exams.*

## Visualizing Figures

IN questions like these, which are given on tests like yours, you are required to select one of the drawings of objects (A), (B), (C), or (D) below, that could be made from the flat piece drawn at the left, if this flat piece were folded on the dotted lines shown in the drawing.

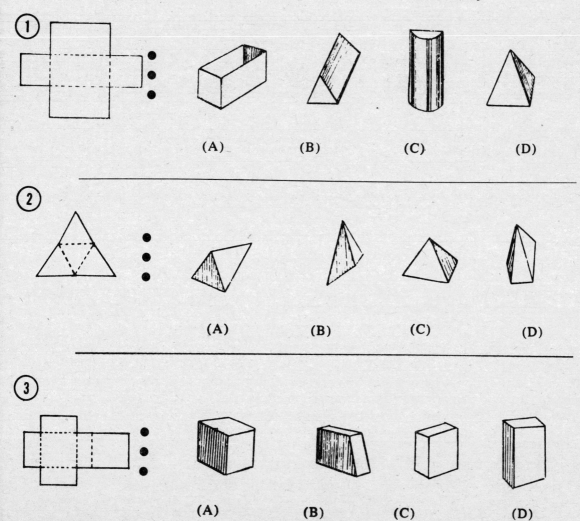

(1)

      (A)      (B)      (C)      (D)

(2)

      (A)      (B)      (C)      (D)

(3)

      (A)      (B)      (C)      (D)

S719

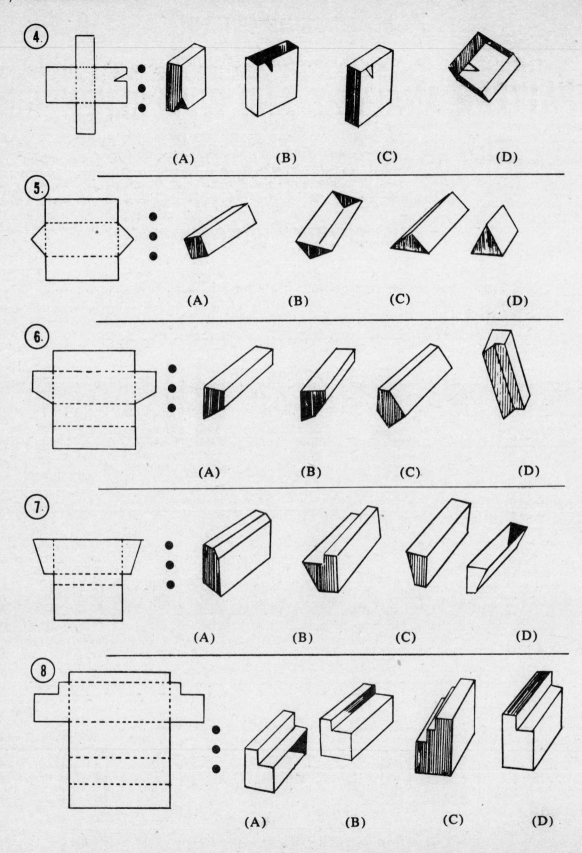

**4.**

(A)    (B)    (C)    (D)

**5.**

(A)    (B)    (C)    (D)

**6.**

(A)    (B)    (C)    (D)

**7.**

(A)    (B)    (C)    (D)

**8.**

(A)    (B)    (C)    (D)

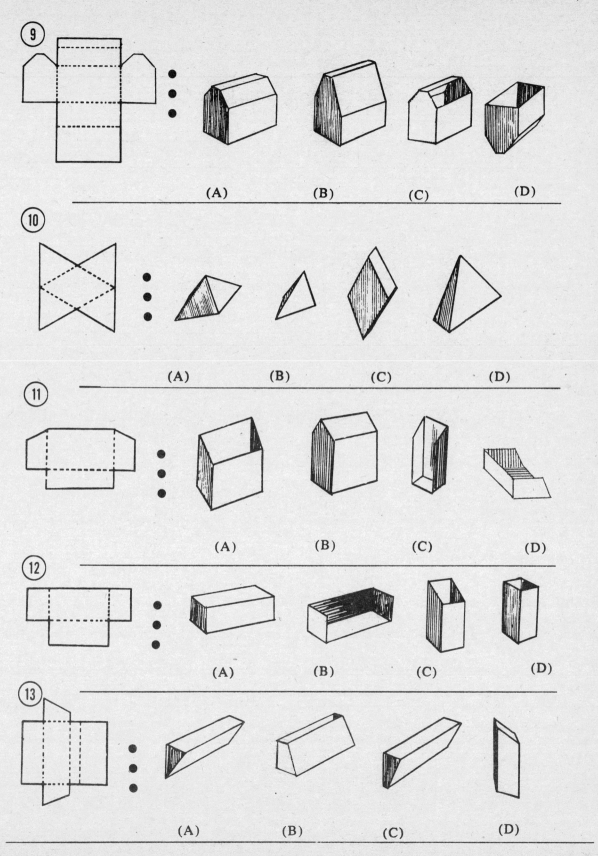

9

(A)    (B)    (C)    (D)

10

(A)    (B)    (C)    (D)

11

(A)    (B)    (C)    (D)

12

(A)    (B)    (C)    (D)

13

(A)    (B)    (C)    (D)

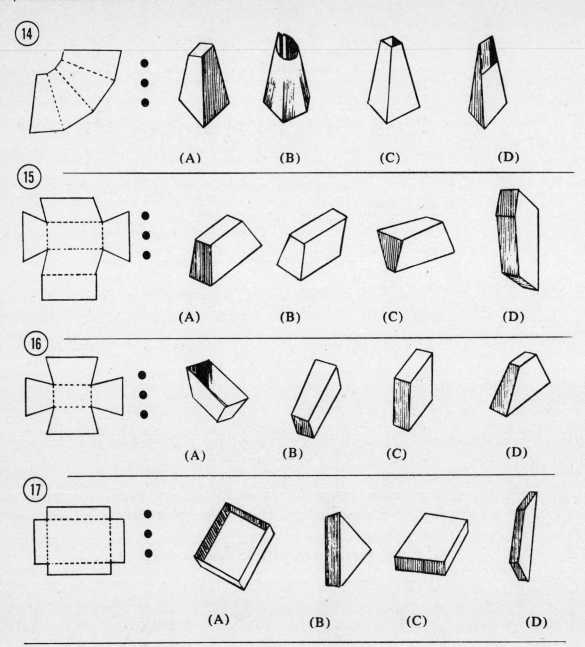

## Correct Answers

*(You'll learn more by writing your own answers before comparing them with these.)*

| | | | |
|---|---|---|---|
| 1. A | 5. C | 9. C | 13. C |
| 2. C | 6. A | 10. A | 14. C |
| 3. C | 7. D | 11. D | 15. B |
| 4. B | 8. B | 12. B | 16. A |
| | | | 17. A |

# PRACTICE FOR VIEW QUESTIONS

*In View Questions, you are faced again with fairly simple questions which any intelligent person can answer, given sufficient time. But on your test, you probably won't be given sufficient time. That causes you to rush along faster than you should, and as a result, you make errors. By practicing with the scientific selection of questions in this chapter, you will noticeably, increase your speed, your skill and your accuracy in answering questions of this type. On your test, you will find that you are familiar with them and that they offer you little difficulty.*

## DIRECTIONS

In these View Questions, you are asked to select one of the drawings of objects lettered (A), (B), (C), or (D), which would have the top, front and side views as shown in the drawing at the left. For each of the 18 questions that follow, work as quickly and accurately as you can in choosing your answers. Then compare them with those given at the end of the chapter.

## EIGHTEEN EXERCISES IN ANALYSIS AND COMPREHENSION

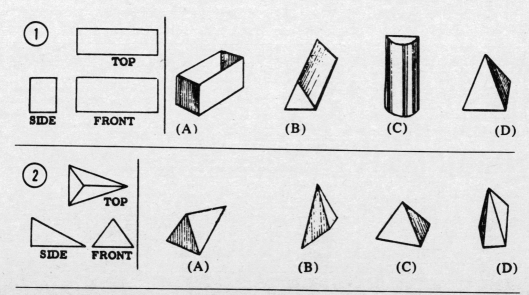

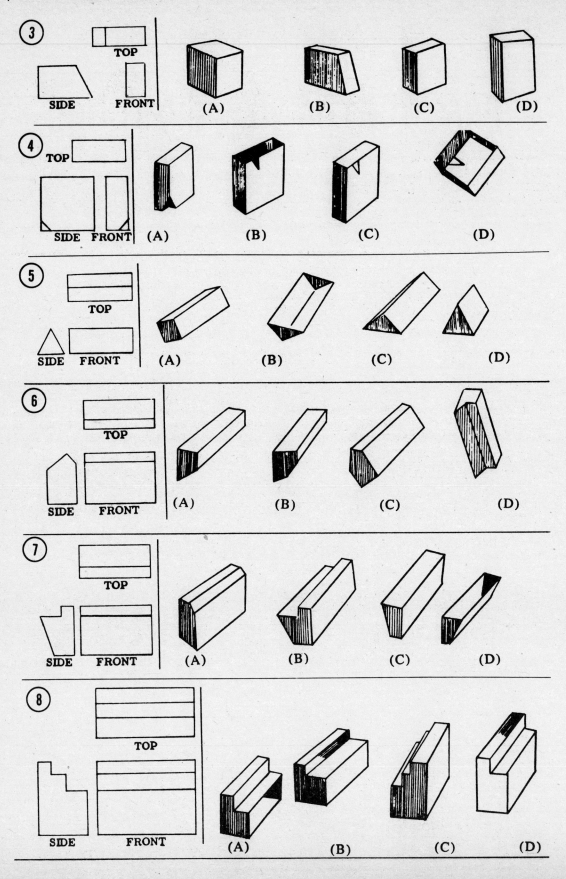

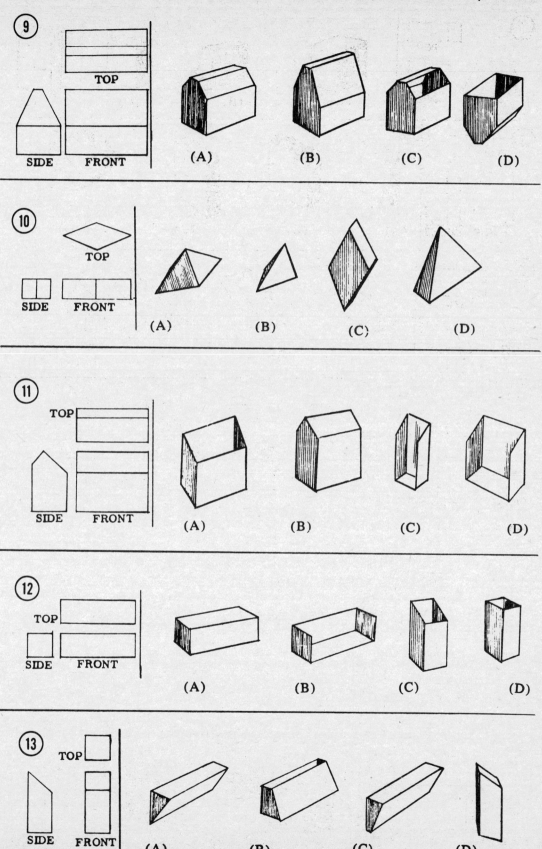

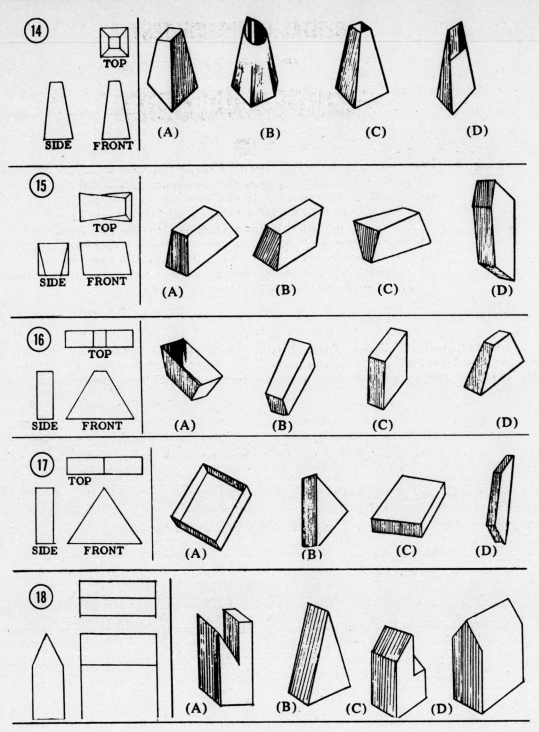

## Correct Answers

| | | | | |
|---|---|---|---|---|
| 1. A | 5. C | 9. B | 13. D | 17. B |
| 2. A | 6. C | 10. C | 14. C | 18. D |
| 3. B | 7. B | 11. B | 15. C | |
| 4. A | 8. C | 12. A | 16. D | |

# FIGURE ANALOGIES

*Your ability to see the differences between, and the relationship between various abstract symbols is one indication of your ability to learn. It is a measure of your ability to meet new situations and evaluate them. The following practice questions will help to familiarize you with this type of question. As in other analogy problems—verbal analogies and numerical series—the best approach is to translate into words the exact relationship between the key figures. Be sure to avoid the traps of similar figures which do not have the same relationship.*

IN the following problems, the symbols in columns 1 and 2 have a relationship to each other. Select from the symbols in columns A, B, C, D and E the symbol which has the same relationship to the symbol in column 3, as the symbol in column 2 has to the symbol in column 1:

1 : 2 : : 3 : ? (A) (B) (C) (D) (E)

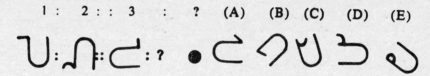

The correct answer is (D)

## TEST QUESTIONS FOR PRACTICE

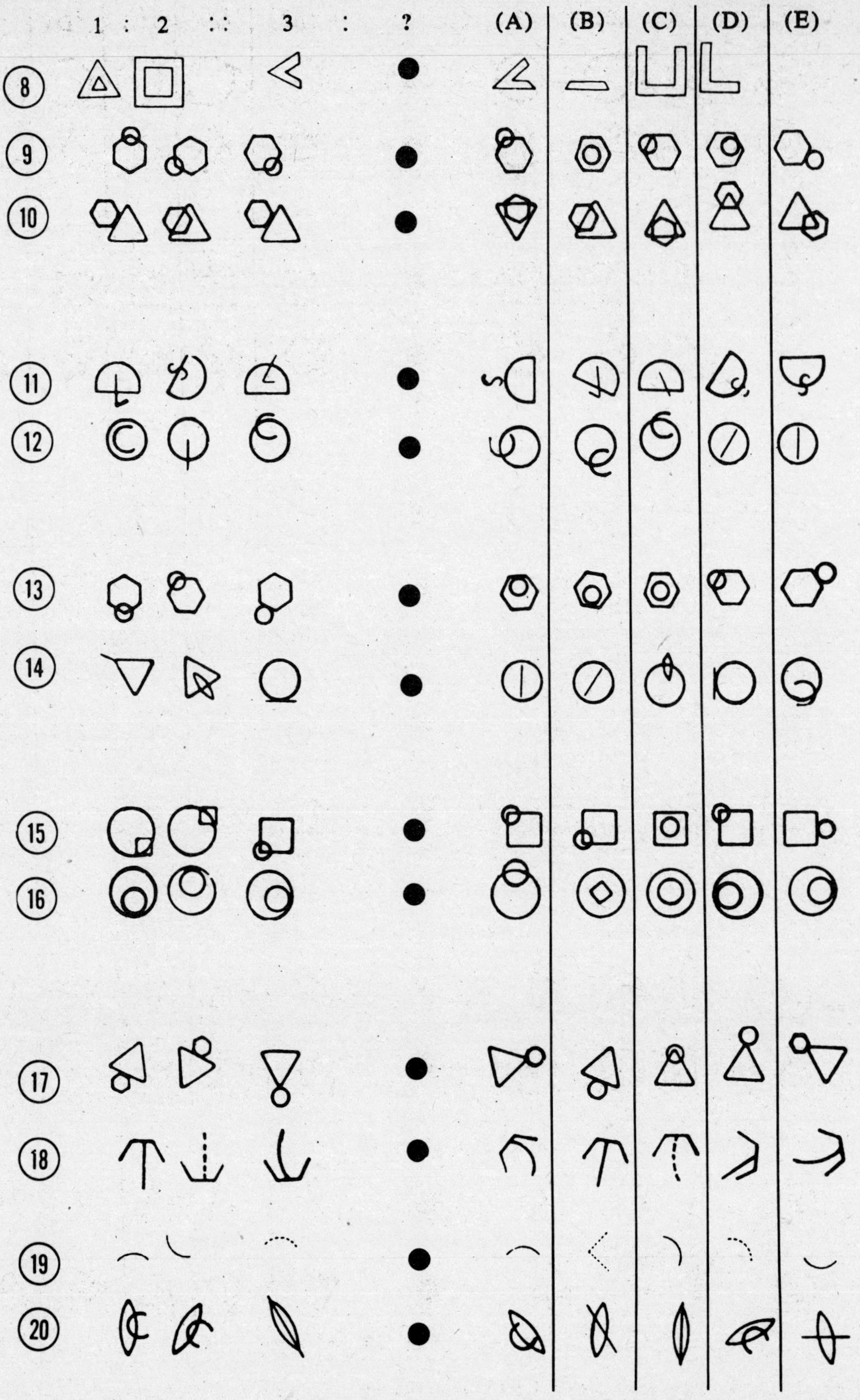
1 : 2 :: 3 : ?
(A)
(B)
(C)
(D)
(E)
8
9
10
11
12
13
14
15
16
17
18
19
20

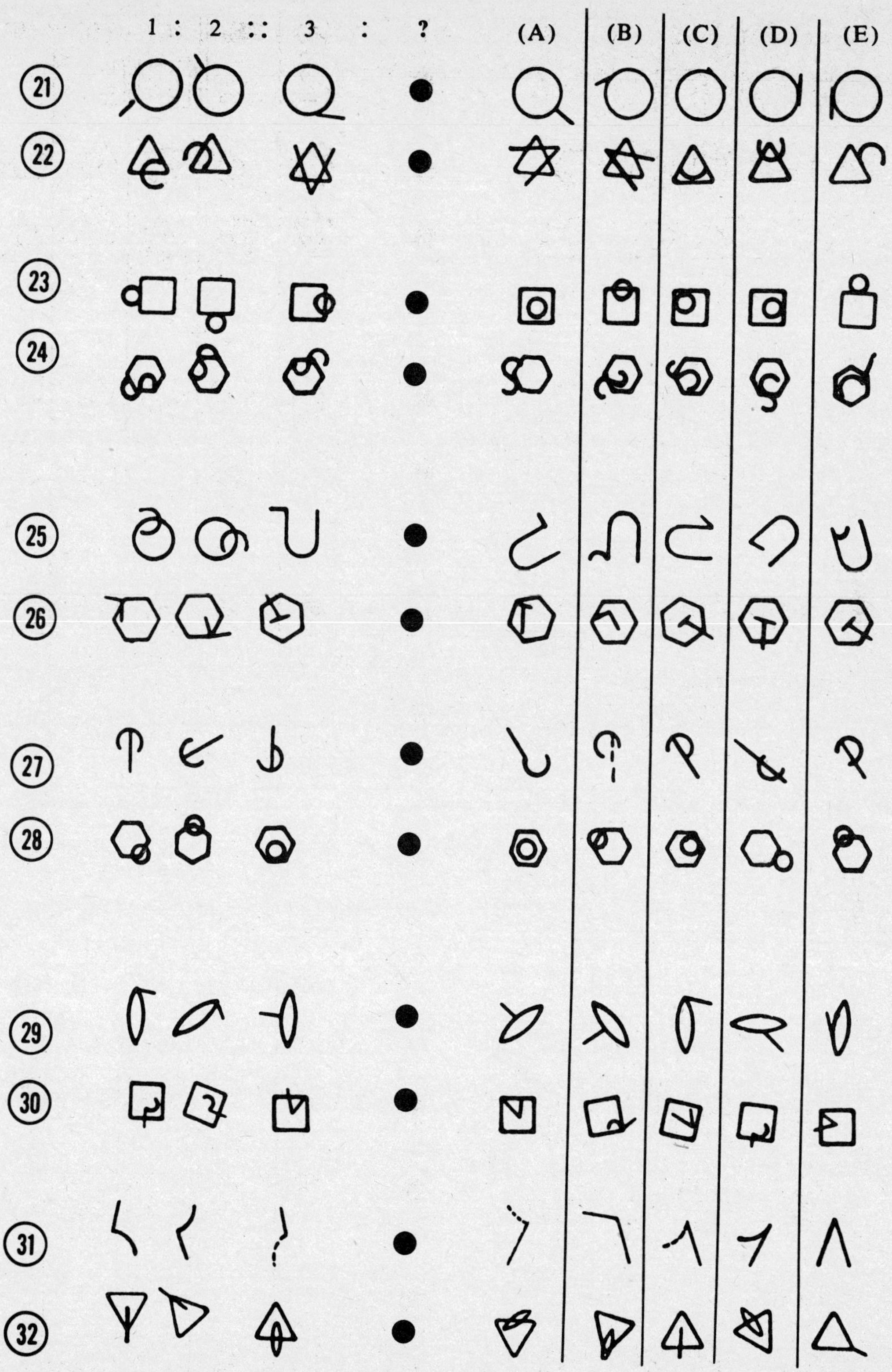
1 : 2 :: 3 : ?
(A)
(B)
(C)
(D)
(E)
21
22
23
24
25
26
27
28
29
30
31
32

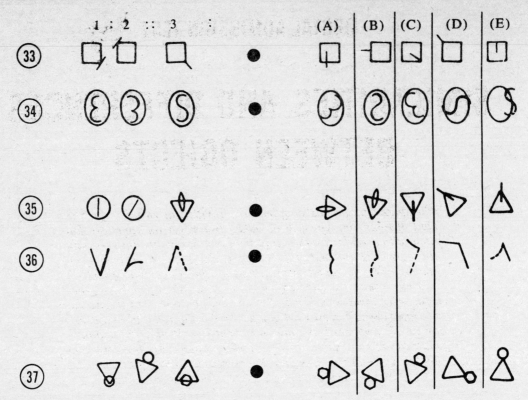

## Correct Answers For The Foregoing Questions

*(Please make every effort to answer the questions on your own before looking at these answers. You'll make faster progress by following this rule.)*

| | | | | |
|---|---|---|---|---|
| 1. C | 9. A | 17. D | 25. A | 33. D |
| 2. B | 10. B | 18. C | 26. E | 34. B |
| 3. D | 11. D | 19. D | 27. C | 35. B |
| 4. A | 12. E | 20. C | 28. C | 36. E |
| 5. A | 13. E | 21. D | 29. A | 37. D |
| 6. A | 14. D | 22. B | 30. E | |
| 7. B | 15. A | 23. B | 31. A | |
| 8. C | 16. D | 24. C | 32. A | |

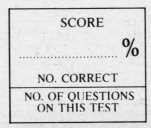

SCORE

............................ %

NO. CORRECT

NO. OF QUESTIONS
ON THIS TEST

# SIMILARITIES AND DIFFERENCES BETWEEN OBJECTS

*The questions in this chapter are provided as practice for the kind of questions you will be asked to answer on your test. Do them all carefully yourself and then compare your answers with those given at the end of the chapter. These questions have been scientifically designed to bring out all the tricks and difficulties you may expect to encounter on your test. When you have practiced with them you will be better able to cope with the actual test questions. Try to work quickly and accurately. If your score on the first trial is less than 70% right you should plan to do the chapter over at some later date. And when you do it over you should expect to note an improvement in your score. Let at least two weeks elapse before trying it for the second time.*

IN each question there is a series of five drawings lettered A, B, C, D, and E. Four of the drawings are alike. Find the one drawing that is different from the other four, and indicate the letter of the answer you have chosen on your answer sheet.

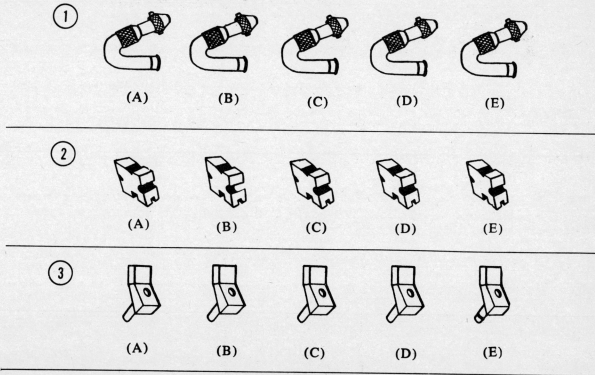

① (A)    (B)    (C)    (D)    (E)

② (A)    (B)    (C)    (D)    (E)

③ (A)    (B)    (C)    (D)    (E)

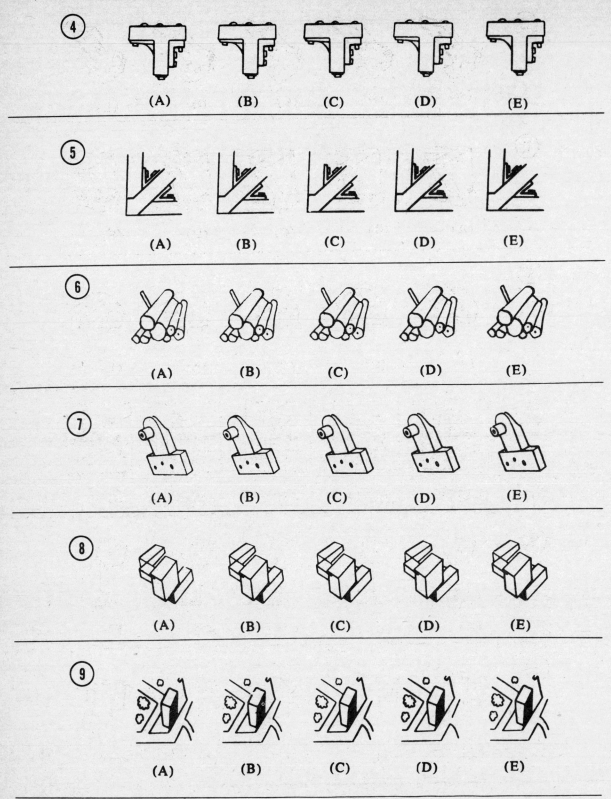

4.

(A)        (B)        (C)        (D)        (E)

5.

(A)        (B)        (C)        (D)        (E)

6.

(A)        (B)        (C)        (D)        (E)

7.

(A)        (B)        (C)        (D)        (E)

8.

(A)        (B)        (C)        (D)        (E)

9.

(A)        (B)        (C)        (D)        (E)

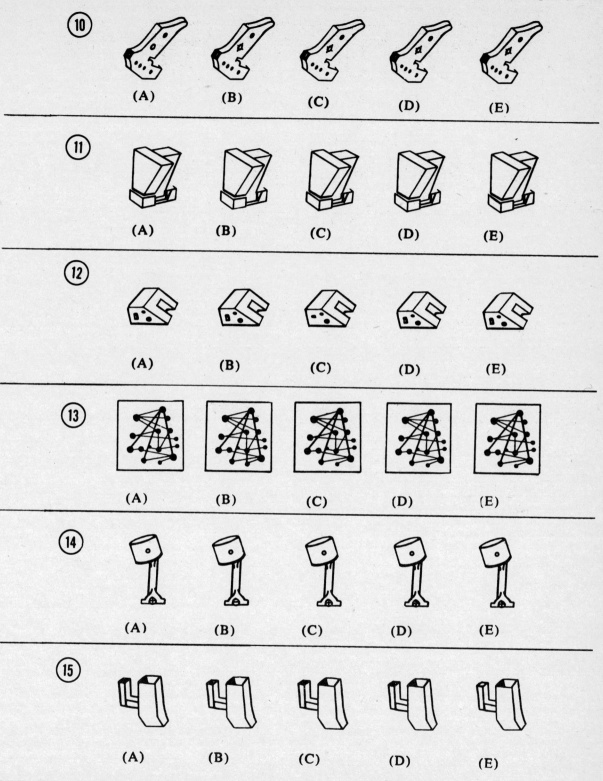

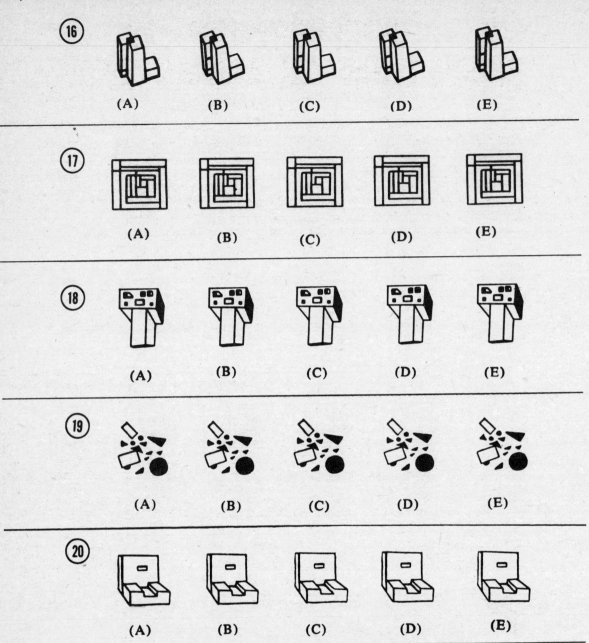

16 (A) (B) (C) (D) (E)

17 (A) (B) (C) (D) (E)

18 (A) (B) (C) (D) (E)

19 (A) (B) (C) (D) (E)

20 (A) (B) (C) (D) (E)

## Correct Answers For The Foregoing Questions

*(Please make every effort to answer the questions on your own before looking at these answers. You'll make faster progress by following this rule.)*

| | | | |
|---|---|---|---|
| 1. D | 6. D | 11. B | 16. A |
| 2. B | 7. B | 12. C | 17. C |
| 3. E | 8. A | 13. B | 18. D |
| 4. E | 9. D | 14. B | 19. E |
| 5. C | 10. A | 15. E | 20. C |

# BLOCK COUNTING AND ANALYSIS

*COUNTING, Turning, Visualizing and Analyzing them in different arrangements, positions and groupings. Variations on an important test theme in spatial relations and aptitude exams.*

ABOUT this type of question there is little to be explained. In fact, the more we say, the more difficult will the task appear. You should examine each diagram critically, count the number of horizontal and vertical rows of blocks and be sure you're not leaving any out in figuring the total number of blocks in the pile.

Each pile of blocks will present a different problem and therefore should be attacked without any preconceptions. For instance, you might have a figure with four apparently identical parts. Under no circumstances should you count the number of blocks in one part and multiply by four to find the number of blocks in the whole figure. Count each part separately.

If you're hasty, you'll fall into a similar trap by counting the same column or row of blocks twice.

One other difficulty arises when dealing with this type of test question. If you stare too fixedly at one portion of the block pile it may seem to change shape. If it does, you should shift your gaze and approach the figure from a different angle.

In the 33 block-counting items that follow, blocks rest upon blocks immediately beneath them with the exception of the arches in items 4, 11 and 17, and with the exception of six upper blocks in item 13, which are presumably kept in place by a very strong cement.

The answer given for item 9 assumes there is no block in the northern corner. And for item 24 you will get the correct answer if you realize that there is at least one block in every column.

## CUBE COUNTING ITEMS

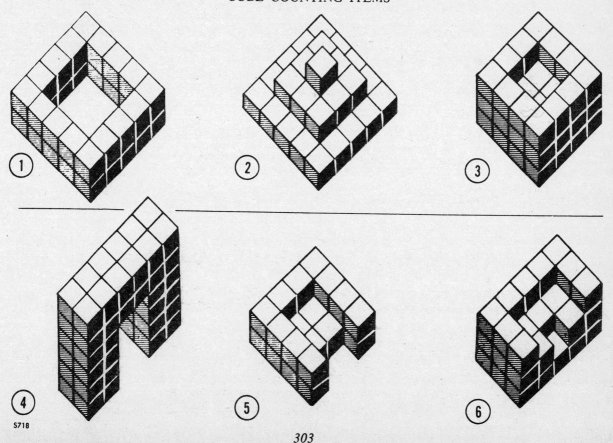

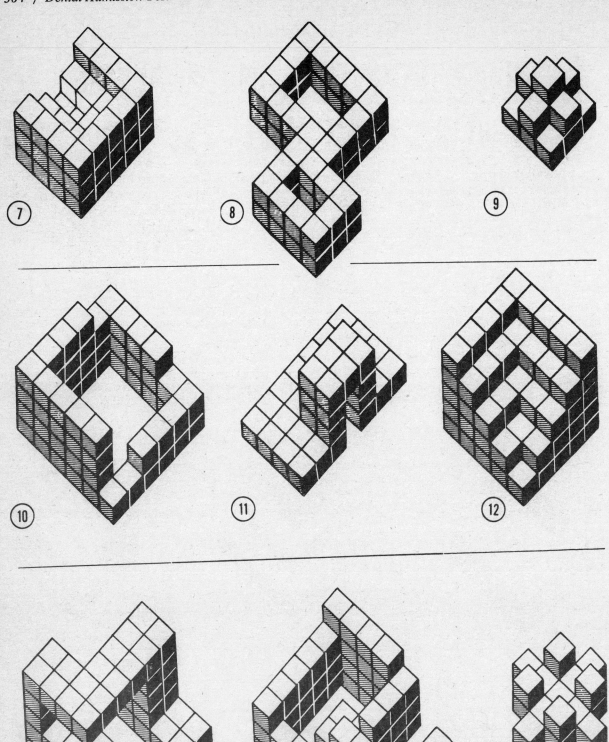

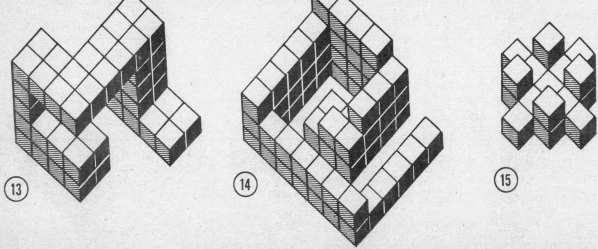

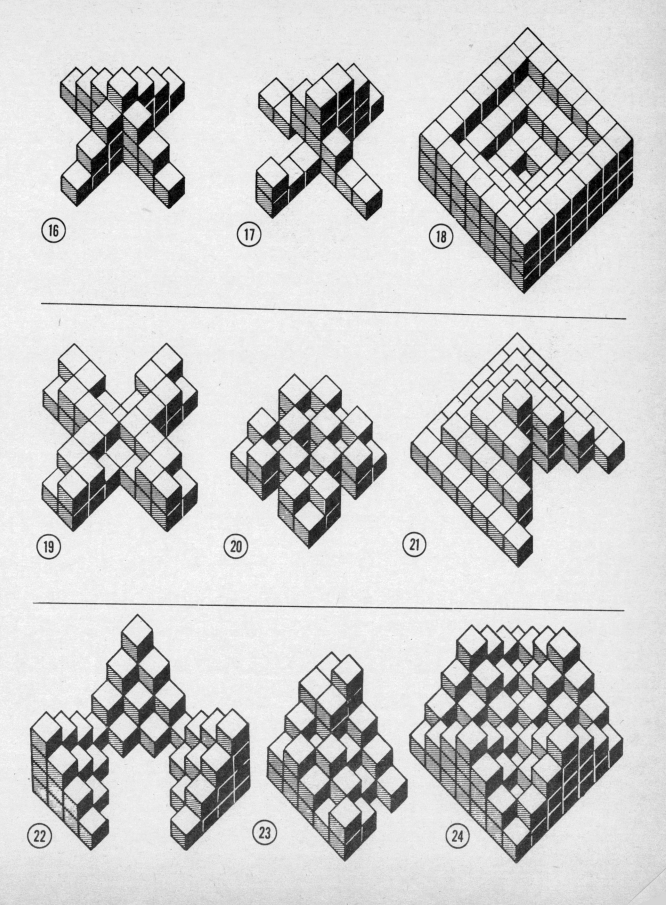

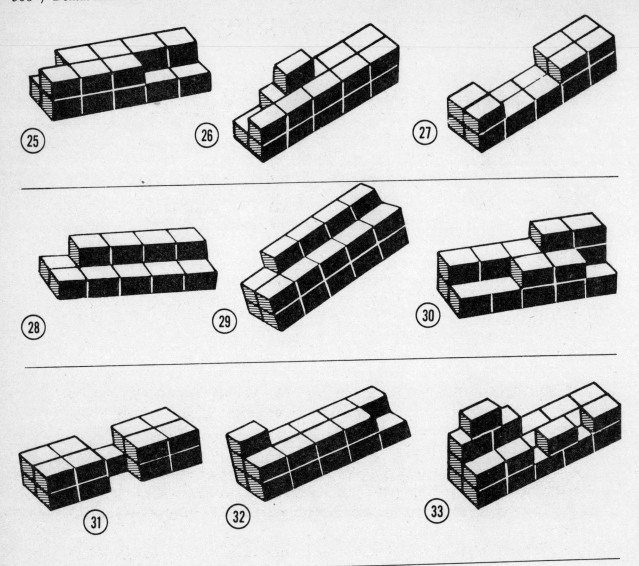

## Correct Answers For The Foregoing Questions

*(Please make every effort to answer the questions on your own before look-ing at these answers. You'll make faster progress by following this rule.)*

| | | | | |
|---|---|---|---|---|
| 1. 32 | 8. 48 | 15. 17 | 22. 58 | 29. 24 |
| 2. 35 | 9. 14 | 16. 28 | 23. 47 | 30. 19 |
| 3. 44 | 10. 59 | 17. 24 | 24. 105 | 31. 17 |
| 4. 56 | 11. 40 | 18. 112 | 25. 17 | 32. 20 |
| 5. 24 | 12. 95 | 19. 46 | 26. 20 | 33. 22 |
| 6. 38 | 13. 56 | 20. 32. | 27. 16 | |
| 7. 49 | 14. 63 or 64 | 21. 70 | 28. 14 | |

# IV. FINAL PREDICTIVE EXAMINATION

*Testing your assimilation of the contents of this book. Hopefully, we are also proving your new-found ability to score high on the exam to come. Each of the included subjects is, in our judgment, likely to appear on your exam. You should be able to do equally well on all of them.*

**The time allowed for the entire examination is 4 hours 30 minutes. In order to create the climate of the test to come, that's precisely what you should allow yourself . . . no more, no less. Use a watch and keep a record of your time, especially since you may find it convenient to take the test in several sittings.**

In constructing this Examination we tried to visualize the questions you are *likely* to face on your actual exam. We included those subjects on which they are *probably* going to test you.

In making up the Tests we predict for your exam, great care was exercised to prepare questions having just the difficulty level you'll encounter on your exam. Not easier; not harder, but just what you may expect.

The various subjects expected on your exam are represented by separate Tests.

The questions on each Test are represented exactly on the special Answer Sheet provided. Mark your answers on this sheet.

Proceed through the entire exam without pausing after each Test. Remember that you are taking this Exam under actual battle conditions, and therefore you do not stop until told to do so by the proctor.

Correct answers for all the questions in all the Tests of this Exam appear at the end of the Exam.

308 / Dental Admission Test

# IV. FINAL PREDICTIVE EXAMINATION

| ANALYSIS AND TIMETABLE: PREDICTIVE PRACTICE EXAMINATION | |
|---|---|
| *Since the number of questions for each test may vary on different forms of the actual examination, the time allotments below are flexible.* | |
| *SUBJECT TESTED* | *Time Allowed* |
| TEST I. BIOMEDICAL SCIENCE | 65 Minutes |
| TEST II. INTERPRETATION OF SCIENCE READINGS | 75 Minutes |
| TEST III. VOCABULARY | 20 Minutes |
| TEST IV. VERBAL ANALOGIES | 20 Minutes |
| TEST V. SENTENCE COMPLETIONS | 15 Minutes |
| TEST VI. QUANTITATIVE ABILITY | 60 Minutes |
| TEST VII. PERCEPTUAL MOTOR ABILITY | 20 Minutes |

# ANSWER SHEET FOR PREDICTIVE EXAMINATION IV.

## TEST I. BIOMEDICAL SCIENCE

An answer grid with numbered questions 1–50, each with answer options 1 2 3 4 5.

## TEST II. INTERPRETATION OF SCIENCE READINGS

An answer grid with numbered questions 1–11, each with answer options A B C D E.

## TEST III. VOCABULARY

An answer grid with numbered questions 1–30, each with answer options A B C D E.

## TEST IV. VERBAL ANALOGIES

An answer grid with numbered questions 1–20, each with answer options A B C D E.

# TEST V. SENTENCE COMPLETIONS

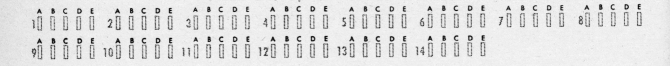

# TEST VI. QUANTITATIVE ABILITY

# TEST VII. PERCEPTUAL MOTOR ABILITY

# TEST I. BIOMEDICAL SCIENCE

## TIME: 65 Minutes

DIRECTIONS: *For each of the following questions, select the choice which best answers the question or completes the statement.*

1. Hemophilia is a hereditary disorder characterized by
   1. delayed clotting of the blood
   2. rapid increase in the white cell count
   3. severe anemia
   4. too rapid clotting of the blood

2. Tornadoes occur most commonly between
   1. midnight and 6 a.m.
   2. 6 a.m. and 12 noon
   3. 12 noon and 6 p.m.
   4. 6 p.m. and midnight

3. A *faraday* is a unit of quantity of electricity the flow of which results in
   1. analyzing the constituents of an eutectic mixture
   2. depositing one gram-atomic weight of metal on an electrode
   3. determining the isotopic structure of a compound
   4. performing catalytic hydrogenation of organic compounds

4. The disease *hepatitis* is on the increase in the U.S.A. This disease, caused by viruses in the blood stream, is most likely to cause damage to the
   1. gall bladder
   2. heart
   3. liver
   4. pancreas

5. Recently it was reported that a radar signal had been sent from the earth to the sun and back. About how long would such a signal take to go from the earth to the sun and return?
   1. 17 seconds
   2. 17 minutes
   3. 17 hours
   4. 17 days

6. Fasciae are
   1. connected with astronomy
   2. devices for counting ionizing events
   3. layers of connective tissue
   4. missile terms

7. *Infrasonic* waves are
   1. produced only by tornadoes
   2. too low in amplitude to be heard
   3. too low in frequency to be heard
   4. too slow in speed to be heard

8. The incidence of type A blood increases with increase of latitude in North America. Which of the following statements is in best agreement with our understanding of this problem?
   1. The incidence of persons of North European descent increases with latitude in North America.
   2. The incidence of type A blood is influenced by temperature during pregnancy.
   3. The incidence is related to the percentage of Indian blood in the population.
   4. At present there is no explanation for the observation.

9. $\frac{\partial p}{\partial x}$ is
   1. an index showing the altitude of the "jet stream"
   2. a partial derivative
   3. a statement of dosage for medicine
   4. used to describe acceleration in outer space

10. Which of the following statements is *true* for our solar system?
    1. The planetary orbits are pretty well in the same plane.
    2. The planets all travel around the sun with about the same speed.
    3. The planets are practically alike in their physical characteristics except for size.
    4. There are just seven planets rotating about the sun.

11. "Blood-typing of dairy cattle may soon be as effective in identifying cows as fingerprints are in identifying humans." Upon which of the following is this based?
    1. Cattle have the same antigenic factors as do humans.
    2. Percent of solids in the blood provides a basis for unique identification.
    3. Plasma of the blood of cattle contains globules of fat.
    4. Some fifty antigenic factors are the basis for blood types in cattle.

12. An area 600 miles wide and 800 miles long received a snowstorm averaging the equivalent of one inch of rain. If this moisture were all drained into a lake 50 feet deep, about how many square miles would the lake cover?
    1. 500 square miles
    2. 800 square miles
    3. 1,100 square miles
    4. 1,400 square miles

13. A *maxwell* is
    1. a cgs unit of magnetic flux
    2. equal to one BTU per hour
    3. equal to one newton per square meter
    4. a dosage unit used for antibiotics

14. Which one of the following is *not* a stage in the development of the crab?
    1. egg
    2. megalops
    3. pupa
    4. zoca

15. An *optical maser* is
    1. a device for greatly amplifying light
    2. a device for producing polarization
    3. the link between mass and light
    4. the smallest amount of light which can be recognized

16. Gallium-68, useful in the study of uses of coal, is made from
    1. germanium-68
    2. nitrogen
    3. tin
    4. titanium

17. Which of the following animals is a ruminant?
    1. elephant
    2. giraffe
    3. hippopotamus
    4. zebra

18. *Hexadecanol,* in a monomolecular layer, on a reservoir does *not*
    1. diminish wave action
    2. help water to dissolve oxygen
    3. kill microscopic plant life
    4. reduce evaporation

19. Which of the following is *not* an amino acid?
    1. aspartic acid      3. glutamic acid
    2. gibberellic acid   4. methionine

20. A *nephoscope* is used to measure
    1. direction and velocity of clouds
    2. frequency of wing movements in insects
    3. movement of very small organisms
    4. wind velocities

21. At what time of year does the Perseid meteor shower occur?
    1. autumn
    2. spring
    3. summer
    4. winter

22. *Homo neanderthalensis* lived
    1. less than 4,000 years ago
    2. between 5,000 and 10,000 years ago
    3. between 40,000 and 80,000 years ago
    4. not less than 200,000 years ago

23. *Tsunami* is the technical term for
    1. a marine plant
    2. a warm wind in the South Pacific
    3. magnetic phenomena in the Antarctic
    4. seismic sea waves

24. The terms *strophoid* and *cardioid* would most likely be encountered in a book on
    1. botany        3. mathematics
    2. herpetology   4. physiology

25. Which of the following materials are used in producing magnets of *greatest* permanence?
    1. cobalt and zinc
    2. copper and aluminum
    3. iron and nickel
    4. manganese and bismuth

26. Which of the following is *not* used in classifying the "personality" of a hurricane?
    1. amount of rain about the center
    2. horizontal and vertical cloud distribution
    3. prevailing winds
    4. size of the relatively calm "eyes" of the storm

27. What is the total number of "rare earth" elements?
    1. 6          3. 12
    2. 9          4. 15

28. Which of the following offers the *greatest* difficulty in predicting the paths of hurricanes?
    1. inadequate knowledge of tropical and semi-tropical weather structure
    2. lack of detailed knowledge of high altitude winds
    3. lack of observation stations in the areas in which hurricanes start
    4. slowness with which weather data are processed

29. "Most of the sea birds have precocial young." This means that their chicks
    1. are able to assume adult living patterns quite rapidly
    2. are able to learn rapidly
    3. are relatively well developed on hatching
    4. feather out very rapidly

30. Seasonal color changes have been observed on the planet Mars and the dark areas appear to contain hydrocarbon-like materials. Such evidence
    1. demonstrates that the minimum conditions for life on Mars are present
    2. does not disprove the possibility that there is life on Mars
    3. means there is life on Mars
    4. shows there has been life on Mars

## SECTION A

It may seem paradoxical to equate energy with the property, mass, that measures inertia, but remember that in Newtonian mechanics the bullet penetrates because of its inertia, which makes it continue in its state of motion. However, mass is only one property of matter and perhaps not even the most important. The study of the many curious particles which have been found in cosmic rays and later produced in the giant so-called "atom-smashers" has shown the persistence of certain features in spite of the bewildering number of spontaneous changes which these particles undergo. Two groups of these particles have appeared such that the net number in each group remains always the same, and this in contrast to a third group for which there is no such constancy. By the phrase *net number* is meant the difference, in each case, between the numbers of the "ordinary" particles and of the antiparticles. Thus electrons are a member of one group called "leptons," to which neutrinos also belong. In reckoning the net number of electrons one subtracts the number of positrons from the number of ordinary electrons. Thus the creation of an electron-positron pair does not alter the net number. The rule states that no interaction between particles of any kind, including the photons of radiant energy and the mesons of the cosmic rays, can alter the *sum* of the *net numbers* of the three kinds of particles — electrons, neutrinos, and $\mu$ mesons — which count as leptons. A similar rule holds for the class of particles — protons, neutrons, and some others — which rank as "baryons." Leptons can never change into baryons, or reversely.

## QUESTIONS ON SECTION A

31. In the section the author asserts that mass may not be the most important property of matter. What may be inferred with regard to his belief about the importance to matter of the following combination of properties?
    1. Energy and inertia are the most important.
    2. Energy and mass are the most important.
    3. Inertia and mass are the most important.
    4. The author is inconclusive in this regard.

32. Genus or family is to species as
    1. baryons are to leptons
    2. electrons are to positrons
    3. leptons are to baryons
    4. leptons are to electrons

33. What characteristics do the two groups of particles discussed have in common?
    1. All their particles are positively charged.
    2. All their particles are negatively charged.
    3. In each group of particles, the difference between the number of ordinary particles and the number of antiparticles is invariant.
    4. In each group of particles, the difference between the number of ordinary particles and the number of antiparticles is variable.

34. From this section it would not be unreasonable to assume that one kind of antiparticle is
    1. the electron    3. —1 times any baryon
    2. the positron    4. —1 times any lepton

35. The first sentence of this section notwithstanding, it may not be paradoxical or strange to equate energy with mass when one recalls the basic relationship between energy (E) and mass (M), in which a third variable c is involved. c
    1. equals E/M
    2. is Planck's constant
    3. is the velocity of light
    4. varies directly with the value of M

## SECTION B

"Photographic developers are chemical solutions containing a number of different compounds so proportioned as to produce the controlled reduction of exposed silver halide grains. During reduction the exposed silver halides are reduced to metallic silver, the invisible latent image formed by exposure being converted into a silver deposit or visible image. Developing solutions normally contain components which can be classified according to their functions into the following heads:

> Developing agents.
> Preservatives.
> Activators.
> Restrainers.

Occasionally, developers are encountered which contain less than four components. In these cases, one of the components exhibits more than one function. In other cases additional components are added according to the result desired."

## QUESTIONS ON SECTION B

36. We may see the image on exposed photographic film by
    1. holding it up to a light
    2. reducing all the silver halides
    3. reducing silver halides struck by light
    4. reducing some of the silver halides

37. All photographic developers
    1. are virtually identical
    2. have at least 3 components
    3. have separate developing components
    4. produce a metallic image

## SECTION C

Here are three views of a single cube:

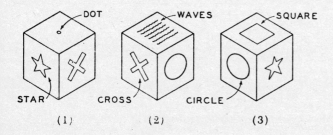

## QUESTIONS ON SECTION C

38. What symbol is opposite the dot?
    1. circle      3. square
    2. dot         4. waves

39. What symbol is opposite the cross?
    1. circle      3. square
    2. dot         4. waves

40. What symbol is on the bottom of figure 3?
    1. cross
    2. dot
    3. star
    4. waves

## SECTION D

There are a large number of implications and uses of animal sensing devices. The use of ultrasonic cries for echolocation by the bat is well known, if not yet fully understood. Its precision, speed, and freedom from interference make this a profitable system for study by the physicist, not only for military purposes but as an aid to the blind. The sensitivity of the moth's ear in intercepting hostile bat sounds is of great value.

The sonar system of porpoises and whales has been little studied, but evidence indicates that they have a highly developed and accurate location sense combined with a high degree of intelligence and ability to communicate. An institute is now being formed in the Virgin Islands dedicated to the study of these animals.

Other animal sensing devices are perhaps less well known but appear to the practical-minded to have equal potentialities. Many fish have electro-receptors which they use to detect obstacles. These fish emit pulses of low voltage with frequencies characteristic for each species. The frequencies may range from 50 to 1600 cycles per second. The alteration of the pattern of the electric field as a result of objects, apertures, or other fish in the surrounding water can be detected. So sensitive is this response that the fish will respond to the movement of electrostatic charge produced by waving a comb (that has been run through one's hair) in front of the aquarium. They can differentiate between a conductor and a nonconductor or respond to the presence of a stationary magnet outside the aquarium.

The rattlesnake is equipped with exquisitely sensitive temperature receptors. These receptors will respond to an increase or decrease of $10^{-11}$ calorie (small) in 0.1 second, which represents a change in tissue temperature of 0.001°C. Expressed in terms of a temperature quotient of $Q_{10}$, the frequency of nerve impulses in a single fiber is $10^{30}$. When two balls of equal size differing minutely in temperature are presented to the snake, it will invariably and unhesitatingly strike at the warmer.

## QUESTIONS ON SECTION D

41. Certain fish can be expected to differentiate between the two items in which one of the following groups?
    1. glass and copper      3. rubber and wood
    2. gold and aluminum      4. wool and leather

42. The sensitivity of tne moth's ear in intercepting hostile bat sounds would be most related to the area of
    1. computer development   3. microphonics
    2. electronics            4. missile detection

43. The highly effective sonar system of porpoises and whales result from the
    1. disturbing effects produced by atmospheric electric phenomena in the surroundings
    2. high-frequency vibrations which are reflected back from objects
    3. rapid chemical decomposition of their environs by the action of electric currents
    4. wave properties of electrons in passing from a point of low potential to a point higher in potential

44. The receptors of the rattlesnake respond to an increase or decrease of $10^{-11}$ small calorie (amount of heat required to raise one gram of water 1°C) in 0.1 second. If one were interested in the increase or decrease of the large caloric (the amount of heat required to raise one kilogram of water 1°C), it would be necessary to multiply by
    1. 1,000,000    3. 100
    2. 1,000        4. 10

## SECTION E

The first representatives of the Osteichthyes appeared in the middle Devonian, soon after the earliest sharks. As the fossils are known, these bony fishes are separated at the outset into the three types of lobe-finned fishes, ray-finned fishes, and lung-fishes, which means that their differentiation from a common ancestry was well advanced. The lobe-fins in turn can be identified as including forms that were forerunners of the first land vertebrates.

Surprising as it may seem, a lung or lungs appear to have been present in many, if not all, of these early bony fishes, perhaps as an adaptation to life in stagnant pools that may have been formed recurrently in the watercourses under the climatic conditions of the Devonian. Apparently the swim bladder of modern bony fishes, which is homologous with the lungs of tetrapod vertebrates is not the organ from which lungs arose but a modification of the primitive lung in the early ancestors of these fishes. After making a beginning of air-breathing it seems that one line, the lobe-finned fishes, gave rise to the Amphibia and so to the land vertebrates . . ., while another line, the ray-finned fishes, gave rise to the bony fishes of the present day, in which the primitive lung was transformed into a hydrostatic organ, the swim bladder.

It is significant in this connection that in the most primitive of existing ray-finned fishes, such as the "bichir" of the Nile, *Polypterus,* the lung still persists in its original function; another and independent survival of the primitive lung appears in the three genera of lung-fishes (Dipnoi) *Ceratodus, Protopterus,* and *Lepidosiren.* In North America the sturgeon, *Acipenser,* the paddle fish, *Polyodon,* the gar pike, *Lepisosteus,* and the bow-fin, *Amia,* are ray-fins of primitive type although they do not have lungs as does the more primitive *Polypterus.* The more specialized ray-fins include all the most familiar fishes of fresh and salt water, such as the trout, salmon, carp, bass, perch, catfish, cod, herring, mackerel, and many others that are highly specialized.

## QUESTIONS ON SECTION E

45. The word "homologous" as used in the section means
    1. compatible
    2. having the same function
    3. having the same origin
    4. having the same structure

46. Which of the following belongs to the most primitive type
    1. catfish
    2. codfish
    3. frog
    4. sturgeon

47. The mammals are derived from
    1. fish with swim bladders
    2. the Dipnoi
    3. the lobe-fins
    4. the ray-fins

48. The Devonian is a
    1. climatic region
    2. geological period
    3. region infested with sharks
    4. sunken continent

49. *Osteichthyes* are
    1. algae
    2. amphibians
    3. fish
    4. sharks

50. The gar pike, found in midwestern U.S.A. is a
    1. lobe-finned fish
    2. lung-fish
    3. ray-finned fish
    4. tetrapod vertebrate

## SECTION F

Consider the planetary system in the figure where planet X, rotating on its axis, is the center. Planet Y, while rotating on its axis, revolves around planet X. P is an observer situated on planet X. The entire system moves through space in a straight line.

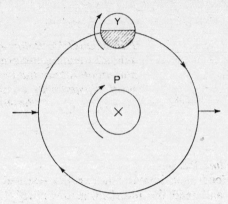

## QUESTIONS ON SECTION F

51. If the period of rotation of Y is 3 times greater than its period of revolution, and the rotation of X is equal to the period of revolution of Y, the observer on P, in one revolution of Y, will see
    1. both the shaded and light surfaces intermittently
    2. only the light surface except when in its original position
    3. only the shaded surface of Y
    4. none of the above

52. When the system moves a distance through space equal to the circumference of the orbit of Y, and the planet completes one revolution each time this distance is covered, a fixed observer outside the system should describe the path of Y as
    1. a circle
    2. a cycloid
    3. an ellipse
    4. a straight line

53. When the period of rotation of X is equal to the period of revolution of Y, an observer at P should describe the path of Y as
    1. a circle
    2. a cycloid
    3. a point
    4. none of the above

# TEST II. INTERPRETATION OF SCIENCE READINGS

## TIME: 75 Minutes

*DIRECTIONS: Below each of the following passages of natural science reading material you will find one or more incomplete statements about the passage. Select the words or expressions that most satisfactorily complete each statement in accordance with the meaning of the paragraph.*

*Reading Passage*

Woodsmen, hunters and trackers learned to follow and read the information unwittingly left behind by animals, men, nature and time. Their ability to survive depended on their skill in reading these signs. Soon they reasoned that if signs left behind accidentally had so much meaning, they could leave signs deliberately for their own future use or for the benefit of friends following them. Thus trail signs and symbols came into being and soon became more or less standardized. A trail blazer in new territory hacked pieces of bark off some of the trees in his path so that he could find his way back or so that others could follow him. Indians frequently made a cut on both sides of the tree so that the trail could be seen from either direction and from either side of the tree. The white men chipped from one side only, and then trails were harder to follow.

1. The title below that best expresses the ideas of this passage is
   (A) Early trail markers
   (B) Needs for trail markers in the woods
   (C) Blazing new trails
   (D) Differences between the Indians' and the white men's trail markers
   (E) Historic trails.

2. The author implies that the earliest trail signs may have been left
   (A) by nature
   (B) deliberately by animals, white men or time
   (C) intentionally by the Indians
   (D) in written codes
   (E) to benefit friends.

3. White men marked one side of a tree to
   (A) indicate where the trail turned
   (B) help in following the trail

(C) save time in camp
(D) make following the trail a test of skill
(E) make the trail difficult.

*Reading Passage*

Land that has lost its productivity keeps its people poor, but that is only the surface story. More important is this: the soil did not work from the fertile Alabama fields into the tidal marshes while an alert, energetic, and solvent class of farmers tried determinedly to hold it. If the soil had been guarded by farmers answering this description, it could have been held, for we have the knowledge to hold topsoil and maintain fertility, but the economic and social climate made good farming a matter of secondary importance. The ideals of the farming people eroded first. The land simply followed to the infertile marshes.

4. The title below that best expresses the ideas of this passage is
   (A) Causes of rural poverty in Alabama
   (B) The only reason for farmers' difficulties
   (C) A losing battle in Alabama's marshes
   (D) Results of erosion in southern Alabama
   (E) Topsoil and productivity.

5. The writer states that farm land became unproductive because
   (A) there was no knowledge of how to keep topsoil from washing away
   (B) the fields sloped to marsh areas
   (C) the climate was unfavorable
   (D) the farmers were not interested in efficient farming
   (E) the land owners were poor.

6. The author implies that he considers Alabama farmers

(A) hardworking    (D) dishonest
(B) unthrifty    (E) alert.
(C) discouraged

*Reading Passage*

To stop science would create more problems than solutions. Aside from military considerations, it would be disastrous to freeze culture at its present high point. The highly technical civilization of the 20th century is like an airplane in flight, supported by its forward motion. It can not stop without falling. If all the world's inhabitants, for instance, learn to use natural resources as fast as Americans do now, many necessary substances will be exhausted. Scientists confidently count on improvements, including atomic energy, to provide ample substitutes. Present techniques won't do.

Where will man's curve of scientific progress take him ultimately? The surprises since 1900 have made scientists humble. They know that as science grows, it only penetrates deeper into mystery. Human knowledge may be visualized as an expanding sphere whose volume grows larger as its diameter increases. But the area of the sphere's surface, its frontier with the unknown, increases as the square of the diameter. Beyond that frontier—nobody can know, until the frontier advances.

7. The title below that best expresses the ideas in this passage is
   (A) The future of science
   (B) New frontiers
   (C) Progress unlimited
   (D) The 20th century
   (E) Our technical civilization.

8. Scientists feel that improvements which can provide substitutes are required to
   (A) prevent useless loss of life
   (B) keep culture advancing
   (C) advance scientific knowledge

(D) prevent exhaustion of basic materials
(E) improve techniques of aviation.

9. Scientists regard expanding scientific knowledge with
   (A) enthusiasm    (D) pride
   (B) despair    (E) disgust.
   (C) humility

*Reading Passage*

Like all insects, it wears its skeleton on the outside—a marvelous chemical compound called chitin which sheathes the whole of its body. This flexible armor is tremendously tough, light and shatterproof, and resistant to alkali and acid compounds which would eat the clothing, flesh and bones of man. To it are attached muscles so arranged around catapult-like hind legs as to enable the 'hopper to hop, if so diminutive a term can describe so prodigious a leap as ten or twelve feet—about 150 times the length of the one-inch or so long insect. The equivalent feat for a man would be a casual jump, from a standing position, over the Washington Monument.

10. The title below that best expresses the ideas of this passage is
    (A) The grasshopper vs. alkali and acid
    (B) The champion jumper
    (C) A marvelous insect
    (D) Man meets his conqueror
    (E) Chitin, muscles, and catapult.

11. The passage suggests that
    (A) a man should be able to jump over the Washington Monument
    (B) the 'hopper is an enemy of man
    (C) the word *hop* as a term is prodigious
    (D) insects are protected by their skeletons
    (E) chitin is easily destroyed by certain chemicals.

# TEST III. VOCABULARY

## TIME: 20 Minutes

*DIRECTIONS: For each question in this test, select the appropriate letter preceding the word which is most nearly the same in meaning as the italicized word in each sentence.*

1. calcareous
   - (A) corpse-like
   - (B) heat-producing
   - (C) chalky
   - (D) gourd-shaped.

2. capstan
   - (A) quarter-deck of a ship
   - (B) anchor
   - (C) ship's funnel
   - (D) device for raising weights.

3. carapace
   - (A) shell covering all or part of an animal
   - (B) gargoyle
   - (C) playful leap or skip
   - (D) panoply.

4. catamaran
   - (A) raised structure on which a body is carried in state
   - (B) craft with twin parallel hulls
   - (C) monument in memory of a person whose body is elsewhere
   - (D) food fish found in the Indian Ocean.

5. chalice
   - (A) necklace
   - (B) goblet
   - (C) ecclesiastical garment
   - (D) mountain hut

6. champ
   - (A) paw nervously
   - (B) ram down
   - (C) chew noisily
   - (D) restrain forcefully.

7. condign
   - (A) pretentious
   - (B) patronizing
   - (C) pungent
   - (D) suitable.

8. crass
   - (A) ostentatious
   - (B) avaricious
   - (C) alluringly deceitful
   - (D) coarse.

9. dado
   - (A) grotesque ornamentation
   - (B) musical composition in which a theme is repeated and varied
   - (C) prank or antic
   - (D) covering for the lower part of a wall.

10. denizen
    - (A) criminal
    - (B) frequenter of squalid retreats
    - (C) inhabitant
    - (D) deep-water fish.

11. monad
    - (A) single-voiced melody
    - (B) bacchante
    - (C) generative tissue
    - (D) simple organism.

12. motley
    - (A) vulgar
    - (B) heterogeneous
    - (C) crowded
    - (D) forest green.

13. necromancy
    - (A) obituary notice
    - (B) magic
    - (C) fanciful medieval tale
    - (D) servility.

14. nugatory
    - (A) debatable
    - (B) chewy
    - (C) changeable
    - (D) worthless.

15. obfuscate
    - (A) block
    - (B) make unnecessary
    - (C) bewilder
    - (D) penetrate.

16. palanquin
    - (A) litter borne by poles on men's shoulders
    - (B) knightly champion
    - (C) buffoon
    - (D) pyramidal building.

17. parlous
    - (A) loquacious
    - (B) debatable
    - (C) merry
    - (D) shocking.

18. **Parthian shaft**
    (A) last retort
    (B) adjunct to a Persian chariot
    (C) ancient Near-Eastern tunnel
    (D) vigorous onslaught.

19. patina
    (A) local dialect
    (B) base metal
    (C) Italian folk-dance
    (D) chemical coating.

20. peignoir
    (A) dressing gown
    (B) knot formed by twisting and pinning up long hair
    (C) inclination or desire
    (D) fur collar.

21. heinous
    (A) atrocious          (B) unbelievable
    (C) secretive          (D) dangerous.

22. incipient
    (A) passive
    (B) unbelievable
    (C) infected
    (D) initial.

23. jettison
    (A) anchor          (B) cast off
    (C) swagger        (D) support.

24. mundane
    (A) spiritual          (B) sophisticated
    (C) lasting            (D) worldly.

25. nemesis
    (A) nightmare
    (B) one who bears the same title
    (C) retributive justice
    (D) climax of a story.

26. obtuse
    (A) blunt              (B) obscure
    (C) complicated     (D) elephantine.

27. pecuniary
    (A) miserly            (B) monetary
    (C) unusual           (D) small.

28. picaresque
    (A) type of prose fiction
    (B) Mexican sport
    (C) Spanish dance
    (D) school of painting.

29. plangent
    (A) reverberating
    (B) pertaining to marine organisms
    (C) clamoring
    (D) pertaining to the coast.

30. plethora
    (A) bloodiness       (B) base of a column
    (C) waste             (D) superabundance.

# TEST IV. VERBAL ANALOGIES
### TIME: 15 Minutes

*DIRECTIONS: In these test questions each of the two CAPI-*
*TALIZED words have a certain relationship to each other.*
*Following the capitalized words are other pairs of words, each*
*designated by a letter. Select the lettered pair wherein the words*
*are related in the same way as the two CAPITALIZED words are*
*related to each other.*

## EXPLANATIONS OF KEY POINTS BEHIND THESE QUESTIONS ARE GIVEN WITH THE ANSWERS

1. ARGUMENT : DEBATE ::

 (A) philosophy : psychology
 (B) challenge : opponent
 (C) violence : peace
 (D) individual : group
 (E) fight : contest

2. GRASS : LETTUCE ::

 (A) truck : station wagon
 (B) onion : flower
 (C) snow : milk
 (D) farm : garden
 (E) agriculture : planter

3. SODIUM : SALT ::

 (A) soda : solution
 (B) molecule : atom
 (C) oxygen : water
 (D) chemistry : biochemistry
 (E) analysis : synthesis

4. DAM : WATER ::

 (A) over : under
 (B) embargo : trade
 (C) curse : $H_2O$
 (D) beaver : fish
 (E) river : stream

5. ALLAY : PAIN ::

 (A) damp : noise
 (B) retard : progress
 (C) regain : consciousness
 (D) fray : edge
 (E) soothe : nerves

6. LATENT : LATE ::

 (A) crude : callous
 (B) potential : tardy
 (C) natty : nettled
 (D) obvious : concealed
 (E) decorous : deceased

7. CALIBER : RIFLE ::

 (A) reputation : blast
 (B) compass : bore
 (C) army : navy
 (D) gauge : rails
 (E) cavalry : infantry

8. CHOP : MINCE ::

 (A) fry : bake
 (B) meat : cake
 (C) axe : mallet
 (D) Washington : Lincoln
 (E) stir : beat

9. PECCADILLO : CRIME ::

 (A) district attorney : criminal
 (B) David : Goliath
 (C) armadillo : bone
 (D) bushel : peck
 (E) sheriff : jail

10. WOOD : PAPER ::

 (A) iron : steel
 (B) chair : wall
 (C) cut : clip
 (D) fireplace : lighter
 (E) forest : fire

11. LIMP : CANE ::

   (A) machete : sugar
   (B) walk : crutch
   (C) cold : tissue
   (D) corset : stiffness
   (E) lump : sugar

12. CONCRETE : ADOBE ::

   (A) brick : building
   (B) paper : papyrus
   (C) American : Mexican
   (D) pour : spill
   (E) contractor : purchaser

13. LEGS : MORPHEUS ::

   (A) feet : destiny
   (B) body : Venus
   (C) eyes : sleep
   (D) torso : beauty
   (E) limbs : head

14. PUBLICATION : LIBEL ::

   (A) newspaper : editorial
   (B) radio : television
   (C) information : liability
   (D) journalism : attack
   (E) speech : slander

15. CANAL : PANAMA ::

   (A) water : country
   (B) ships : commerce
   (C) diameter : circle
   (D) locks : waterway
   (E) country : continent

16. ALLEVIATE : AGGRAVATE ::

   (A) joke : worry
   (B) elevate : agree
   (C) level : grade
   (D) plastic : rigorous
   (E) alluvial : gravelly

17. BEHAVIOR : IMPROPRIETY ::

   (A) honesty : morality
   (B) freedom : servitude
   (C) response : stimulus
   (D) word : malapropism
   (E) grammar : usage

18. ELM : TREE ::

   (A) dollar : dime
   (B) currency : dime
   (C) map : leaves
   (D) oak : maple
   (E) dollar : money

19. DOCTOR : DISEASE ::

   (A) miser : money
   (B) illness : prescription
   (C) sheriff : crime
   (D) theft : punishment
   (E) intern : hospital

20. EXAMINATION : CHEAT ::

   (A) lawyer : defendant
   (B) compromise : principles
   (C) army : gripe
   (D) swindle : business
   (E) politics : graft

# TEST V. SENTENCE COMPLETIONS

### TIME: 15 Minutes

*DIRECTIONS: Each of the completion questions in this test consists of an incomplete sentence. Each sentence is followed by a series of lettered words, one of which best completes the sentence. Select the word that best completes the meaning of each sentence, and mark the letter of that word opposite that sentence.*

1. The admiration the Senator earns is _____ by his _____ instinct for getting onto the front pages.
   - (A) concocted . . . proverbial
   - (B) evolved . . . haughty
   - (C) belied . . . aggressive
   - (D) engendered . . . unerring
   - (E) transcended . . . dogged

2. The accelerated growth of public employment _____ the dramatic expansion of budgets and programs.
   - (A) parallels
   - (B) contains
   - (C) revolves
   - (D) escapes
   - (E) populates

3. So great is the intensity of Shakespeare's dramatic language that the audience becomes _____ and sees messages and equivocations everywhere, until the play becomes an apocalypse of _____ and fall.
   - (A) stunned . . . rise
   - (B) hallucinated . . . temptation
   - (C) aroused . . . doubt
   - (D) dulled . . . zeal
   - (E) weary . . . disgust

4. Not every _____ mansion, church, battle site, theater, or other public hall can be preserved.
   - (A) novel
   - (B) structured
   - (C) comparative
   - (D) unknown
   - (E) venerable

5. Man is still a _____ in the labor market.
   - (A) glut
   - (B) possibility
   - (C) commodity
   - (D) resumption
   - (E) provision

6. As we moved on to Melford shortly after noon on Saturday, the clear air and the rolling _____ made one wonder whether this festival would lead all others, at least in altitude.
   - (A) stones
   - (B) hovels
   - (C) skyline
   - (D) oaks
   - (E) terrain

7. Witness the long waiting list for the overworked psychiatrists and psychologists and the twentieth-century _____ for lying on the couch talking about oneself and the neuroses that have resulted from a too intense _____ with oneself.
   - (A) wish . . . inspection
   - (B) process . . . tirade
   - (C) plan . . . understanding
   - (D) fad . . . preoccupation
   - (E) garb . . . implication

8. The book will be _____ by every Western student of the USSR, and it will be a thrilling adventure for any reader.
   - (A) skimmed
   - (B) perused
   - (C) rejected
   - (D) blasphemed
   - (E) borrowed

9. With this realization, the people suddenly found themselves left with _____ moral values and little ethical _____.

(A) obsolete . . . perspective
(B) established . . . grasp
(C) portentous . . . insinuation
(D) extreme . . . judgment
(E) continued . . . pronouncement

10. There is a notion abroad that history has gotten away from us; that our lives are beyond control; that there are no points of _____ which mean anything any more.

(A) conference       (B) inference
(C) prudence         (D) incidence
          (E) reference

11. I cannot honestly number myself among the pious and I have frequently had the experience of being _____ among the unholy.

(A) regenerated       (B) deteriorated
(C) compiled          (D) consigned
          (E) inflamed

12. These avant-garde thinkers believe that the major peace movements are ineffective because the thinking that underlies these movements is old-fashioned, confused, _____, and out-of-step with the findings of _____ science.

(A) stimulating . . . natural
(B) delusionary . . . behavioral
(C) loaded . . . true
(D) uncertain . . . physical
(E) blatant . . . scholastic

13. Today, we who read Latin return far more often to the exuberance of Apuleius than to the carefully molded _____ of Cicero.

(A) literature        (B) redundancies
(C) objects           (D) piracies
          (E) platitudes

14. If the process of decision-making was _____ a half-century or more ago, consider how it has become _____ since.

(A) dedicated . . . simplified
(B) complicated . . . compounded
(C) revived . . . encouraged
(D) imbedded . . . obvious
(E) enhanced . . . improved

15. Scientists should have choice as to what areas they explore, and certainly have the _____ right and obligations as _____ to influence what use is made of their discoveries.

(A) impeccable . . . teachers
(B) inescapable . . . philosophers
(C) definitive . . . recorders
(D) divine . . . lecturers
(E) ethical . . . humanists

16. Under the contest rules, the award goes to an undergraduate college student who has collected a _____ personal library.

(A) distinguished      (B) well-managed
(C) modified           (D) precise
          (E) stocked

17. The consequences of the establishment of the colonies were a rapid and careless _____ of natural resources, and _____ human suffering.

(A) depletion . . . appalling
(B) cancellation . . . remarkable
(C) disappearance . . . planned
(D) development . . . unfailing
(E) disintegration . . . compelled

18. The Crusades can be seen as the first great collective military _____ in which all Europe participated.

(A) embarrassment     (B) compilation
(C) review            (D) drawing board
          (E) enterprise

19. The first essential in building a missile submarine is the _____ of literally millions of parts.

(A) application
(B) reassembling
(C) integration
(D) infiltration
(E) assignment

20. The _____ researchers had heard that kind of talk often before, but what came next _____ them.

(A) avid . . . encouraged
(B) asinine . . . revived
(C) studious . . . involved
(D) assembled . . . jolted
(E) fatigued . . . enervated

# TEST VI. QUANTITATIVE ABILITY

### TIME: 60 Minutes

*This test covers topics taught at both the elementary and high school level. Some topics which may be covered are definitions, ratios, percent, decimals, fractions, mathematical symbols, indirect measurement, interpretation of graphs and tables, scale drawings, approximate computation, and units of measurement. Some questions are based on techniques taught in elementary algebra and plane geometry courses. Questions frequently test knowledge of mathematical principles and stress their applications through the performance of mathematical operations and manipulations. The ability to express practical problems in mathematical terms is frequently tested. The test may also include one or two questions based on the concepts of modern mathematics.*

*DIRECTIONS: Study each of the following problems and work out your answers in the blank space at the right. Below each problem you will find a number of suggested answers. Select the one that you have figured out to be right and mark its letter on the answer sheet. In the sample questions provided, the correct answers are: S1 = A; S2 = C.*

*Samples:*

S1. If the area of a square is 62 square inches, find to the nearest tenth of an inch the length of one side.
A. 7.9
B. 9.7
C. 6.2
D. 2.6.

S2. Solve the following equation for a:
$5a + 3b = 14$
A. $14 - 3b + 5$
B. $3b - 14 \times 5$
C. $\dfrac{14 - 3b}{5}$
D. $3b - 14$.

## DO YOUR FIGURING HERE

1. Solve for x and y.

$$5x - 2y = 19$$
$$7x - 4y = 29$$

A. $x = -3, y = -2$
B. $x = 2, y = 3$
C. $x = 3, y = -2$
D. $x = -2, y = -3$.

S1964

2. Mr. Brown makes deposits and writes checks as follows:

May 1, $375 deposit
May 6, $150 check
May 10, $35 check
May 11, $42 deposit
May 20, $140 check
May 26, $18 check.

Mr. Brown's bank balance on April 30 was $257. What is his balance on May 31?

A. $465
B. $331
C. $185
D. $165.

3. The above graphs show the temperatures in a certain city for 2 different dates. How many degrees higher was the lowest temperature on March 10 than the lowest temperature on January 10?

A. 35°
B. 30°
C. 25°
D. 45°.

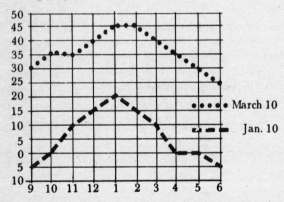

4. From the same graph estimate the temperature at 3:30 on March 10.

A. 37-1/2°
B. 42-1/2°
C. 30°
D. 5°.

5. From the same graph determine the times on January 10 when the temperature was 5°.

A. 11:30 and 3:30
B. 10:30 and 2:30
C. 10:30 and 3:30
D. 11:30 and 2:30.

**DO YOUR FIGURING HERE**

6. A student had averages of 87, 90, 80, 85, and 75 for the first 5 terms in school. What must be his average for the sixth term in order for his overall average for the six terms to be 85%?

    A. 93%
    B. 85%
    C. 87%
    D. 90%.

7. In a class of 36 students, 28 passed an examination, 4 failed and the rest were absent. What percent of the class was absent?

    A. 14-2/7%
    B. 11-1/9%
    C. 75%
    D. 33-1/3%.

8. How many digits are there to the right of the decimal point in the square root of 74859.2401?

    A. 4
    B. 2
    C. 3
    D. 1.

9. The scale of a map is 3/8"=100 miles. How far apart are 2 cities 2-1/4" apart on the map?

    A. 1200 miles
    B. 300 miles
    C. 600 miles
    D. 150 miles.

10. Tom is preparing a circle graph to show that 1/12 of the local income tax is spent in payment of public debts. How big an angle must he measure at the center of the circle to represent this fact?

    A. 30°
    B. 15°
    C. 12°
    D. 60°.

11. The diagram at the right shows the side view of a house. What is the distance from E to AB?

    A. 41'
    B. 25'
    C. 20'
    D. 39'.

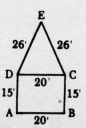

12. A weather bureau reported the following temperatures on a certain day:

1 A.M.—5°
5 A.M.—2°
9 A.M.  0°
1 P.M.  10°
5 P.M.  10°
9 P.M.  5°

What was the average temperature for the day?

A. −3°
B. 0°
C. +3°
D. +6°.

13. If you have 3 hrs. and 20 minutes to travel 150 miles, what is the average speed at which you must travel?

A. 60 mph
B. 45 mph
C. 50 mph
D. 70 mph.

14. What is the square root of .0004?

A. .0002
B. .002
C. .16
D. .02.

15. The side of a square is 18″. What is its area in square feet?

A. 324
B. 9
C. 2.25
D. 3/2.

16. Reduce to its simplest form: $\dfrac{x^2 - y^2}{(x - y)^2}$

A. $x+y$
B. $\dfrac{x - y}{x + y}$

C. $x-y$
D. $\dfrac{x + y}{x - y}$.

17. Find ∠ x, where the central angles are as shown

A. 15°
B. 70°
C. 30°
D. 35°

**DO YOUR FIGURING HERE**

18.  In the same diagram, find ∠ y.

    A.  15°
    B.  70°
    C.  30°
    D.  35°.

19.  If the sides of a parallelogram are 8″ and 10″ and the included angle is 60°, find its area.

    A.  80 square inches
    B.  40 $\sqrt{2}$ square inches
    C.  40 square inches
    D.  40 $\sqrt{3}$ square inches.

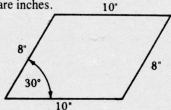

20.  If the numerical value of the circumference of a circle is equal to the numerical value of its area, find its radius.

    A.  4
    B.  1
    C.  8
    D.  2.

21.  A tower casts a shadow of 40′ at the same time that a yardstick casts a shadow of 2′. How high is the tower?

    A.  80′
    B.  40′
    C.  60′
    D.  100′.

22.  How high must a box be if its base is 5″ by 6″, and its contents must be 135 cubic inches?

    A.  9″
    B.  4″
    C.  5″
    D.  4-1/2″.

23.  What is the probability that a random selection from a box containing 6 black balls and 4 white balls will be a white ball?

    A.  4:6
    B.  6:10
    C.  4:10
    D.  6:4.

24.  What common fraction is the equivalent of .625?

    A.  3/5
    B.  5/8
    C.  4/5
    D.  2/3.

25. What is the value of the following expression when reduced to its simplest form?

$$\left(\frac{x}{y} - \frac{y}{x}\right) \div \left(\frac{x - y}{xy}\right)$$

A. 1
B. x−y
C. y−x
D. x+y.

26. A rectangular tabletop is 30″ by 48″. How many square feet of glass will it take to cover it?

A. 20 square feet
B. 5 square feet
C. 15 square feet
D. 10 square feet.

27. What will $2000 amount to after 2 years if invested at 5% interest, compounded annually?

A. $2100
B. $2205
C. $2500
D. $2700.

28. A is 20 miles east of B. C is 15 miles north of A. What is the shortest airline distance from B to C?

A. 35 miles
B. 25 miles
C. 30 miles
D. 20 miles.

29. Mr. A paid $90 a share for stock, the par value of which was $100. After he had the stock for a year, the company paid him a $9 dividend. What rate of interest did he make on his investment?

A. 9%
B. 10%
C. 18%
D. 20%.

30. If $V = 1/3\pi r^2 h$, express h in terms of $\pi$, V and r.

A. $h = \dfrac{3\pi r}{V}$

B. $h = \dfrac{\pi r}{3V}$

C. $h = \dfrac{3V}{\pi r^2}$

D. $h = \dfrac{3r^2}{\pi V}$.

31. If $S = 1/2 \, gt^2$ , express t in terms of S and g.

    A. $t = \dfrac{2S}{g}$

    B. $t = \dfrac{g}{2S}$

    C. $t = \sqrt{\dfrac{2S}{g}}$

    D. $t = \sqrt{\dfrac{g}{2S}}$.

DO YOUR FIGURING HERE

32. An auto supply company has 7 stores in one city and 4 stores in another. On a certain day, the average sales for the 7 stores in the first city was $1200 per store. In the second city the average for the 4 stores was $900 per store. What was the average for that day for all 11 stores? (Give answer to nearest dollar.)

    A. $1500
    B. $1091
    C. $1200
    D. $1100.

33. A man bought a car on the installment plan for $5500. He paid $300 down. Assuming that the other charges, including interest, were $1460, and he had to pay the balance in one year in equal monthly installments, what was the amount of each payment?

    A. $380
    B. $620
    C. $515
    D. $555.

34. The formula for the area of a circle is $A = \pi r^2$. The largest possible circle is cut from a square 42″ on a side. What is the area of the remainder of the square?

    A. 478 square inches
    B. 378 square inches
    C. 587 square inches
    D. 243 square inches.

35. The expression $2x^2 - x - 6$ when divided by $x - 2$ is

    A. $2x + 3$
    B. $2x - 3$
    C. $2x + 6$
    D. $2x - 6$.

36. Six boys agreed to buy an old car together, but one boy changed his mind at the last moment, and each had to pay $12 more for his share. What was the cost of the car?

   A. $240
   B. $300
   C. $420
   D. $360.

37. A plumber and his helper together earn $150. The plumber's hourly wage is twice the helper's. If the plumber worked 6 hours and the helper worked 8 hours, how much does the helper earn per hour?

   A. $5.00
   B. $11.50
   C. $7.50
   D. $9.00.

38. Mr. Brown invested $7500 in 2 enterprises. On one he made a 5% profit. On the other he lost 2%. His net profit for the year was $130. How much did he invest at 5%?

   A. $3000
   B. $4000
   C. $6000
   D. $5000.

39. The formula for the volume of a sphere is $V = 4/3\ \pi r^3$. Find the volume of a sphere whose radius is 21, if $\pi = 3\text{-}1/7$.

   A. 36,000
   B. 39,808
   C. 38,808
   D. 40,008.

40. If the length of a rectangle is increased by 2″, the area equals 36 square inches. If the width is increased by 3″, the area is 49 square inches. What is the original width of the rectangle?

   A. 4″
   B. 8″
   C. 6″
   D. 10″.

**DO YOUR FIGURING HERE**

# TEST VII. PERCEPTUAL MOTOR ABILITY

### TIME: 20 Minutes

*The following are representative examination type questions. They should be carefully studied and completely understood. The actual test questions will probably not be quite as difficult as these.*

DIRECTIONS: *Each question in this test consists of a numbered picture showing a box that is to be unfolded. If the box were unfolded it would look like one of the four cardboard patterns, lettered A, B, C, or D, in the other frames in the row. Choose the cardboard pattern which is unfolded from the lettered picture, and blacken your answer sheet accordingly.*

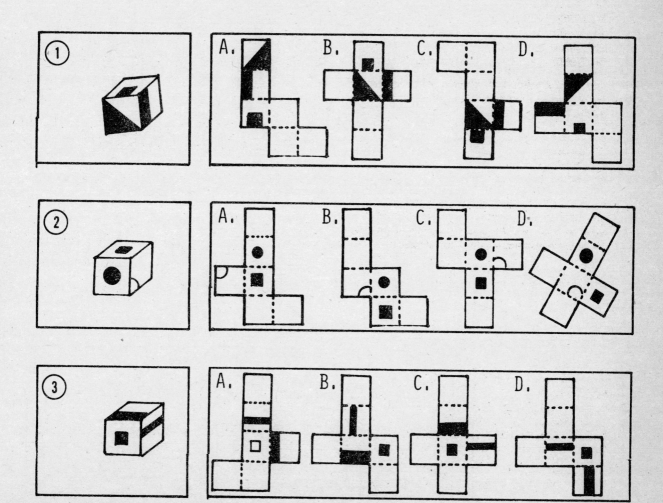

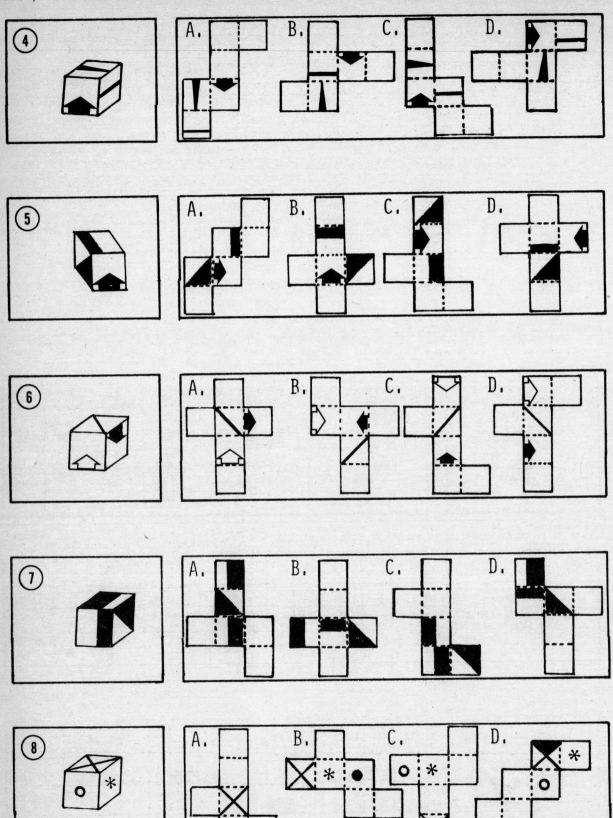

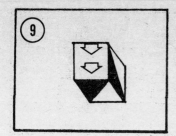
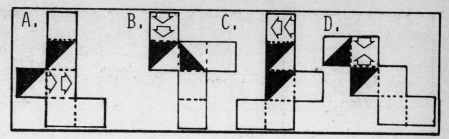

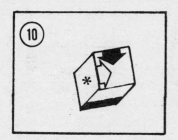
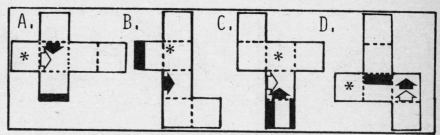

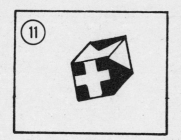
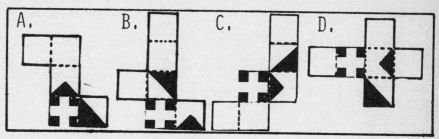

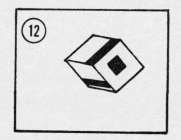
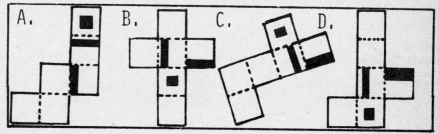

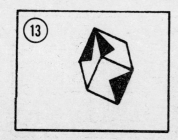
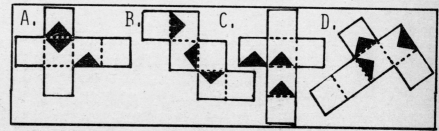

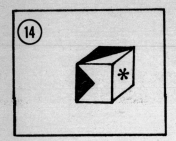

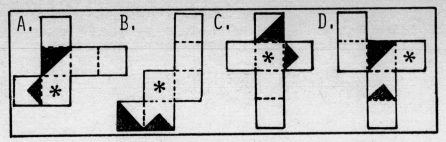

# AFTER TAKING EXAMINATION IV.

*STEP ONE — Check all your answers with the Correct Answers that follow. Then compare your total score with the Unofficial Percentile Ranking Table below. This Table will give you a reasonably good idea of how you stand with others taking the Exam. For example, if your percentile ranking is 61, according to your score, you are superior to 60% and inferior to 39% of those who have taken the Exam. Your percentile ranking on the Examination is a major factor in determining your eligibility.*

## PERCENTILE RANKING TABLE
### (unofficial)

| Approximate Percentile Ranking | Score On Test | Approximate Percentile Ranking | Score On Test |
|:---:|:---:|:---:|:---:|
| 99 | 183–185 | 69 | 120–121 |
| 98 | 181–182 | 68 | 118–119 |
| 97 | 178–180 | 67 | 116–117 |
| 96 | 175–177 | 66 | 114–115 |
| 95 | 172–174 | 65 | 112–113 |
| 94 | 170–171 | 64 | 110–111 |
| 93 | 168–169 | 63 | 108–109 |
| 92 | 166–167 | 62 | 106–107 |
| 91 | 164–165 | 61 | 104–105 |
| 90 | 162–163 | 60 | 102–103 |
| 89 | 160–161 | 59 | 100–101 |
| 88 | 158–159 | 58 | 98–99 |
| 87 | 156–157 | 57 | 96–97 |
| 86 | 154–155 | 56 | 94–95 |
| 85 | 152–153 | 55 | 92–93 |
| 84 | 150–151 | 54 | 90–91 |
| 83 | 148–149 | 53 | 88–89 |
| 82 | 146–147 | 52 | 86–87 |
| 81 | 144–145 | 51 | 84–85 |
| 80 | 142–143 | 50 | 82–83 |
| 79 | 140–141 | 49 | 80–81 |
| 78 | 138–139 | 48 | 78–79 |
| 77 | 136–137 | 47 | 76–77 |
| 76 | 134–135 | 46 | 74–75 |
| 75 | 132–133 | 45 | 72–73 |
| 74 | 130–131 | 44 | 70–71 |
| 73 | 128–129 | 43 | 68–69 |
| 72 | 126–127 | 42 | 66–67 |
| 71 | 124–125 | 41 | 64–65 |
| 70 | 122–123 | 0–40 | 0–63 |

*STEP TWO* — *Use the results of the Examination you have just taken to diagnose yourself. Pinpoint the areas in which you show the greatest weakness. Fill in the Diagnostic Table to spotlight the subjects in which you need the most practice.*

## DIAGNOSTIC TABLE FOR EXAMINATION IV.

| SUBJECT TESTED | QUESTIONS ANSWERED CORRECTLY ON EXAM | | |
|---|---|---|---|
| | Strong | Average | Weak |
| TEST I. BIOMEDICAL SCIENCE | 41–50 | 26–40 | 20–25 |
| TEST II. INTERPRETATION OF SCIENCE READINGS | 9–11 | 7–8 | 5–6 |
| TEST III. VOCABULARY | 21–30 | 16–20 | 10–15 |
| TEST IV. VERBAL ANALOGIES | 16–20 | 11–15 | 5–10 |
| TEST V. SENTENCE COMPLETIONS | 16–20 | 11–15 | 5–10 |
| TEST VI. QUANTITATIVE ABILITY | 31–40 | 21–30 | 10–20 |
| TEST VII. PERCEPTUAL MOTOR ABILITY | 10–14 | 8–9 | 4–7 |

*STEP THREE—Use the following Check List to establish areas that require the greatest application on your part. One check (√) after the item means* moderately weak; *two checks (√ √) means* seriously weak.

| Area of Weakness | Check Below | Area of Weakness | Check Below |
|---|---|---|---|
| BIOLOGY | | VERBAL ANALOGIES | |
| CHEMISTRY | | SENTENCE COMPLETIONS | |
| SCIENCE READINGS | | MATHEMATICS | |
| SYNONYMS | | SPATIAL PROBLEM SOLVING | |
| OPPOSITES | | | |

*STEP FOUR — The Pinpoint Practice chapters which follow provide all the drill material you need for every phase of the Examination. Plan your attack systematically. Concentrate on your weaknesses. Answer the practice questions in these areas. As you will discover, the material is presented so that the areas tested in the actual exam are individually treated in this book.*

# CORRECT ANSWERS FOR PREDICTIVE EXAMINATION IV.

*(Please make every effort to answer the questions on your own before looking at these answers. You'll make faster progress by following this rule.)*

## TEST I. BIOMEDICAL SCIENCE

| | | | | | | | |
|---|---|---|---|---|---|---|---|
| 1. 1 | 8. 4 | 15. 1 | 21. 3 | 27. 4 | 33. 3 | 39. 3 | 45. 3 |
| 2. 3 | 9. 2 | 16. 1 | 22. 3 | 28. 2 | 34. 2 | 40. 1 | 46. 4 |
| 3. 2 | 10. 1 | 17. 2 | 23. 4 | 29. 3 | 35. 3 | 41. 1 | 47. 3 |
| 4. 3 | 11. 4 | 18. 2 | 24. 3 | 30. 2 | 36. 3 | 42. 3 | 48. 2 |
| 5. 2 | 12. 2 | 19. 2 | 25. 4 | 31. 4 | 37. 4 | 43. 2 | 49. 3 |
| 6. 3 | 13. 1 | 20. 1 | 26. 3 | 32. 4 | 38. 1 | 44. 2 | 50. 3 |
| 7. 3 | 14. 3 | | | | | | |

## TEST II. INTERPRETATION OF SCIENCE READINGS

| | | | | | | | |
|---|---|---|---|---|---|---|---|
| 1. A | 3. B | 5. D | 7. A | 8. D | 9. C | 10. C | 11. D |
| 2. A | 4. A | 6. B | | | | | |

## TEST III. VOCABULARY

| | | | | | | | |
|---|---|---|---|---|---|---|---|
| 1. C | 5. B | 9. D | 13. B | 17. D | 21. A | 25. C | 28. A |
| 2. D | 6. C | 10. C | 14. D | 18. A | 22. D | 26. A | 29. A |
| 3. A | 7. D | 11. D | 15. C | 19. D | 23. B | 27. B | 30. D |
| 4. B | 8. D | 12. B | 16. A | 20. A | 24. D | | |

## TEST IV. VERBAL ANALOGIES

| | | | | | | | |
|---|---|---|---|---|---|---|---|
| 1. E | 4. B | 7. D | 10. A | 13. A | 15. C | 17. D | 19. C |
| 2. C | 5. A | 8. E | 11. C | 14. E | 16. D | 18. E | 20. E |
| 3. C | 6. B | 9. B | 12. B | | | | |

## TEST IV. EXPLANATORY ANSWERS

*Elucidation, clarification, explication and a little help with the fundamental facts covered in the Previous Test.*

1. **(E)** An argument has considerable emotional implication—a debate has little such implication; a fight has considerable emotional implication—a contest has little such implication.

2. **(C)** Grass and lettuce are green; snow and milk are white.

3. **(C)** Sodium is one of the elements that make up salt; oxygen is one of the elements that make up water.

4. **(B)** A dam obstructs the flow of water; an embargo obstructs the flow of trade.

5. **(A)** One allays (reduces) pain; one damps (reduces) noise.

6. **(B)** Latent means potential; late means tardy.

7. **(D)** Caliber is a standard of measurement for guns; gauge is a standard of measurement for rails.

8. **(E)** To mince is more extreme than to chop; to beat is more extreme than to stir.

9. **(B)** A peccadillo is a small offense—a crime is a large one; the biblical story of David and his slaying of the giant Goliath is well known.

10. **(A)** Wood is used to make paper; iron is used to make steel.

11. **(C)** A person with a limp is likely to use a cane; a person with a cold is likely to use a tissue.

12. **(B)** Concrete is a modern building material —adobe is little used today; paper, as a writing material, has replaced papyrus.

13. **(A)** We speak of being in the arms (antonym = legs) of Morpheus and in the hands (antonym = feet) of Destiny.

14. **(E)** Libel is written defamation; slander is oral defamation.

15. **(C)** A canal cuts right through the country of Panama; a diameter cuts right through a circle.

16. **(D)** Alleviate and aggravate are antonyms —so are plastic and rigorous.

17. **(D)** A derogatory form of behavior is an impropriety; an incorrect use of a word is a malapropism.

18. **(E)** An elm is a type of tree; a dollar is a type of money.

19. **(C)** A doctor seeks to eliminate disease; a sheriff seeks to eliminate crime.

20. **(E)** To cheat on an examination is against regulations; to graft in politics is against the law.

## TEST V. SENTENCE COMPLETIONS

| | | | | | | | |
|---|---|---|---|---|---|---|---|
| 1. D | 4. E | 7. D | 10. E | 13. E | 15. E | 17. A | 19. C |
| 2. A | 5. C | 8. B | 11. D | 14. B | 16. A | 18. E | 20. D |
| 3. B | 6. E | 9. A | 12. B | | | | |

## TEST VI. QUANTITATIVE ABILITY

| | | | | | | | |
|---|---|---|---|---|---|---|---|
| 1. C | 6. A | 11. D | 16. D | 21. C | 26. D | 31. C | 36. D |
| 2. B | 7. B | 12. C | 17. A | 22. D | 27. B | 32. B | 37. C |
| 3. B | 8. B | 13. B | 18. D | 23. C | 28. B | 33. D | 38. B |
| 4. A | 9. C | 14. D | 19. D | 24. B | 29. B | 34. B | 39. C |
| 5. C | 10. A | 15. C | 20. D | 25. D | 30. C | 35. A | 40. A |

## TEST VII. PERCEPTUAL MOTOR ABILITY

| | | | | | | | |
|---|---|---|---|---|---|---|---|
| 1. B | 3. C | 5. D | 7. C | 9. B | 11. D | 13. D | 14. B |
| 2. A | 4. C | 6. A | 8. A | 10. A | 12. B | | |

# Practice Using Answer Sheets

**Alter numbers to match the practice and drill questions in each part of the book.**
**Make only ONE mark for each answer. Additional and stray marks may be counted as mistakes.**
**In making corrections, erase errors COMPLETELY. Make glossy black marks.**

| | | | | |
|---|---|---|---|---|
| 1 A B C D E | 1 A B C D E | 1 A B C D E | 1 A B C D E | 1 A B C D E |
| 2 A B C D E | 2 A B C D E | 2 A B C D E | 2 A B C D E | 2 A B C D E |
| 3 A B C D E | 3 A B C D E | 3 A B C D E | 3 A B C D E | 3 A B C D E |
| 4 A B C D E | 4 A B C D E | 4 A B C D E | 4 A B C D E | 4 A B C D E |
| 5 A B C D E | 5 A B C D E | 5 A B C D E | 5 A B C D E | 5 A B C D E |
| 6 A B C D E | 6 A B C D E | 6 A B C D E | 6 A B C D E | 6 A B C D E |
| 7 A B C D E | 7 A B C D E | 7 A B C D E | 7 A B C D E | 7 A B C D E |
| 8 A B C D E | 8 A B C D E | 8 A B C D E | 8 A B C D E | 8 A B C D E |
| 9 A B C D E | 9 A B C D E | 9 A B C D E | 9 A B C D E | 9 A B C D E |
| 0 A B C D E | 0 A B C D E | 0 A B C D E | 0 A B C D E | 0 A B C D E |

| | | | | |
|---|---|---|---|---|
| 1 A B C D E | 1 A B C D E | 1 A B C D E | 1 A B C D E | 1 A B C D E |
| 2 A B C D E | 2 A B C D E | 2 A B C D E | 2 A B C D E | 2 A B C D E |
| 3 A B C D E | 3 A B C D E | 3 A B C D E | 3 A B C D E | 3 A B C D E |
| 4 A B C D E | 4 A B C D E | 4 A B C D E | 4 A B C D E | 4 A B C D E |
| 5 A B C D E | 5 A B C D E | 5 A B C D E | 5 A B C D E | 5 A B C D E |
| 6 A B C D E | 6 A B C D E | 6 A B C D E | 6 A B C D E | 6 A B C D E |
| 7 A B C D E | 7 A B C D E | 7 A B C D E | 7 A B C D E | 7 A B C D E |
| 8 A B C D E | 8 A B C D E | 8 A B C D E | 8 A B C D E | 8 A B C D E |
| 9 A B C D E | 9 A B C D E | 9 A B C D E | 9 A B C D E | 9 A B C D E |
| 0 A B C D E | 0 A B C D E | 0 A B C D E | 0 A B C D E | 0 A B C D E |

| | | | | |
|---|---|---|---|---|
| 1 A B C D E | 7 A B C D E | 13 A B C D E | 19 A B C D E | 25 A B C D E |
| 2 A B C D E | 8 A B C D E | 14 A B C D E | 20 A B C D E | 26 A B C D E |
| 3 A B C D E | 9 A B C D E | 15 A B C D E | 21 A B C D E | 27 A B C D E |
| 4 A B C D E | 10 A B C D E | 16 A B C D E | 22 A B C D E | 28 A B C D E |
| 5 A B C D E | 11 A B C D E | 17 A B C D E | 23 A B C D E | 29 A B C D E |
| 6 A B C D E | 12 A B C D E | 18 A B C D E | 24 A B C D E | 30 A B C D E |

TEAR OUT ALONG THIS LINE AND MARK YOUR ANSWERS AS INSTRUCTED IN THE TEXT

# TEST – TAKING MADE SIMPLE

*Having gotten this far, you're almost an expert test-taker because you have now mastered the subject matter of the test. Proper preparation is the real secret. The pointers on the next few pages will take you the rest of the way by giving you the strategy employed on tests by those who are most successful in this not-so-mysterious art.*

## BEFORE THE TEST

### T-DAY MINUS SEVEN

You're going to pass this examination because you have received the best possible preparation for it. But, unlike many others, you're going to give the best possible account of yourself by acquiring the rare skill of effectively using your knowledge to answer the examination questions.

First off, get rid of any negative attitudes toward the test. You have a negative attitude when you view the test as a device to "trip you up" rather than an opportunity to show how effectively you have learned.

APPROACH THE TEST WITH SELF-CONFIDENCE. Plugging through this book was no mean job, and now that you've done it you're probably better prepared than 90% of the others. Self-confidence is one of the biggest strategic assets you can bring to the testing room.

Nobody likes tests, but some poor souls permit themselves to get upset or angry when they see what they think is an unfair test. The expert doesn't. He keeps calm and moves right ahead, knowing that everyone is taking the same test. Anger, resentment, fear . . . they all slow you down. "Grin and bear it!"

Besides, every test you take, including this one, is a valuable experience which improves your skill. Since you will undoubtedly be taking other tests in the years to come, it may help you to regard this one as training to perfect your skill.

Keep calm; there's no point in panic. If you've done your work there's no need for it; and if you haven't, a cool head is your very first requirement.

Why be the frightened kind of student who enters the examination chamber in a mental coma? A test taken under mental stress does not provide a fair measure of your ability. At the very least, this book has removed for you some of the fear and mystery that surrounds examinations. A certain amount of concern is normal and good, but excessive worry saps your strength and keenness. In other words, be prepared EMOTIONALLY.

### Pre-Test Review

If you know any others who are taking this test, you'll probably find it helpful to review the book and your notes with them. The group should be small, certainly not more than four. Team study at this stage should seek to review the material in a different way than you learned it originally; should strive for an exchange of ideas between you and the other members of the group; should be selective in sticking to important ideas; should stress the vague and the unfamiliar rather than that which you all know well; should be businesslike and devoid of any nonsense; should end as soon as you get tired.

One of the *worst* strategies in test taking is to do *all* your preparation the night before the exam. As a reader of this book, you have scheduled and spaced your study properly so as not to suffer from the fatigue and emotional disturbance that comes from cramming the night before.

Cramming is a very good way to *guarantee poor test results.*

However, you would be wise to prepare yourself factually by *reviewing your notes* in the 48 hours preceding the exam. You shouldn't have to spend more than two or three hours in this way. Stick to salient points. The others will fall into place quickly.

Don't confuse cramming with a final, calm review which helps you focus on the significant areas of this book and further strengthens your confidence in your ability to handle the test questions. In other words, prepare yourself FACTUALLY.

### Keep Fit

Mind and body work together. Poor physical condition will lower your mental efficiency. In preparing for an examination, observe the common-sense rules of health. Get sufficient sleep and rest, eat proper foods, plan recreation and exercise. In relation to health and examinations, two cautions are in order. Don't miss your meals prior to an examination in order to get extra time for study. Likewise, don't miss your regular sleep by sitting up late to "cram" for the examination. Cramming is an attempt to learn in a very short period of time what should have been learned through regular and consistent study. Not only are these two habits detrimental to health, but seldom do they pay off in terms of effective learning. It is likely that you will be *more confused* than better prepared on the day of the examination if you have broken into your daily routine by missing your meals or sleep.

On the night before the examination go to bed at your regular time and try to get a good night's sleep. Don't go to the movies. Don't date. In other words, prepare yourself PHYSICALLY.

## T-HOUR MINUS ONE

After a very light, leisurely meal, get to the examination room ahead of time, perhaps ten minutes early . . . but not so early that you have time to get into an argument with others about what's going to be asked on the exam, etc. The reason for coming early is to help you get accustomed to the room. It will help you to a better start.

### Bring all necessary equipment . . .

. . . pen, two sharpened pencils, watch, paper, eraser, ruler, and any other things you're instructed to bring.

### Get settled . . .

. . . by finding your seat and staying in it. If no special seats have been assigned, take one in the front to facilitate the seating of others coming in after you.

The test will be given by a test supervisor who reads the directions and otherwise tells you what to do. The people who walk about passing out the test papers and assisting with the examination are test proctors. If you're not able to see or hear properly notify the supervisor or a proctor. If you have any other difficulties during the examination, like a defective test booklet, scoring pencil, answer sheet; or if it's too hot or cold or dark or drafty, let them know. You're entitled to favorable test conditions, and if you don't have them you won't be able to do your best. Don't be a crank, but don't be shy either. An important function of the proctor is to see to it that you have favorable test conditions.

### Relax . . .

. . . and don't bring on unnecessary tenseness by worrying about the difficulty of the examination. If necessary wait a minute before beginning to write. If you're still tense, take a couple of deep breaths, look over your test equipment, or do something which will take your mind away from the examination for a moment.

If your collar or shoes are tight, loosen them.

Put away unnecessary materials so that you have a good, clear space on your desk to write freely.

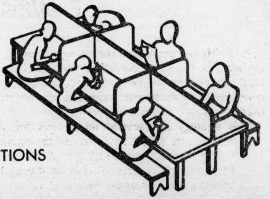

**You Must Have** TO GIVE YOUR **Best Test** PERFORMANCE

(1) A GOOD TEST ENVIRONMENT

(2) A COMPLETE UNDERSTANDING OF DIRECTIONS

(3) A DESIRE TO DO YOUR BEST

# WHEN THEY SAY "GO" — TAKE YOUR TIME!

Listen very carefully to the test supervisor. If you fail to hear something important that he says, you may not be able to read it in the written directions and may suffer accordingly.

If you don't understand the directions you have heard or read, raise your hand and inform the proctor. Read carefully the directions for *each* part of the test before beginning to work on that part. If you skip over such directions too hastily, you may miss a main idea and thus lose credit for an entire section.

## Get an Overview of the Examination

After reading the directions carefully, look over the entire examination to get an over-view of the nature and scope of the test. The purpose of this over-view is to give you some idea of the nature, scope, and difficulty of the examination.

It has another advantage. An item might be so phrased that it sets in motion a chain of thought that might be helpful in answering other items on the examination.

Still another benefit to be derived from reading all the items before you answer any is that the few minutes involved in reading the items gives you an opportunity to relax before beginning the examination. This will make for better concentration. As you read over these items the first time, check those whose answers immediately come to you. These will be the ones you will answer first. Read each item carefully before answering. It is a good practice to read each item at least twice to be sure that you understand it.

## Plan Ahead

In other words, you should know precisely where you are going before you start. You should know:

1. whether you have to answer all the questions or whether you can choose those that are easiest for you;
2. whether all the questions are easy; (there may be a pattern of difficult, easy, etc.)
3. The length of the test; the number of questions;
4. The kind of scoring method used;
5. Which questions, if any, carry extra weight;
6. What types of questions are on the test;
7. What directions apply to each part of the test;
8. Whether you must answer the questions consecutively.

## Budget Your Time Strategically!

Quickly figure out how much of the allotted time you can give to each section and still finish ahead of time. Don't forget to figure on the time you're investing in the overview. Then alter your schedule so that you can spend more time on those parts that count most. Then, if you can, plan to spend less time on the easier questions, so that you can devote the time saved to the harder questions. Figuring roughly, you should finish half the questions when half the allotted time has gone by. If there are 100 questions and you have three hours, you should have finished 50 questions after one and one half hours. So bring along a watch whether the instructions call for one or not. Jot down your "exam budget" and stick to it INTELLIGENTLY.

# EXAMINATION STRATEGY

Probably the most important single strategy you can learn is to do the easy questions first. The very hard questions should be read and temporarily postponed. Identify them with a dot and return to them later.

This strategy has several advantages for you:
1. You're sure to get credit for all the questions you're sure of. If time runs out, you'll have all the sure shots, losing out only on those which you might have missed anyway.

2. By reading and laying away the tough ones you give your subconscious a chance to work on them. You may be pleasantly surprised to find the answers to the puzzlers popping up for you as you deal with related questions.

3. You won't risk getting caught by the time limit just as you reach a question you know really well.

### A Tested Tactic

It's inadvisable on some examinations to answer each question in the order presented. The reason for this is that some examiners design tests so as to extract as much mental energy from you as possible. They put the most difficult questions at the beginning, the easier questions last. Or they may vary difficult with easy questions in a fairly regular pattern right through the test. Your survey of the test should reveal the pattern and your strategy for dealing with it.

If difficult questions appear at the beginning, answer them until you feel yourself slowing down or getting tired. Then switch to an easier part of the examination. You will return to the difficult portion after you have rebuilt your confidence by answering a batch of easy questions. Knowing that you have a certain number of points "under your belt" will help you when you return to the more difficult questions. You'll answer them with a much clearer mind; and you'll be refreshed by the change of pace.

### Time

Use your time wisely. It's an important element in your test and you must use every minute effectively, working as rapidly as you can without sacrificing accuracy. Your exam survey and budget will guide you in dispensing your time. Wherever you can, pick up seconds on the easy ones. Devote your savings to the hard ones. If possible, pick up time on the lower value questions and devote it to those which give you the most points.

### Relax Occasionally and Avoid Fatigue

If the exam is long (two or more hours) give yourself short rest periods as you feel you need them. If you're not permitted to leave the room, relax in your seat, look up from your paper, rest your eyes, stretch your legs, shift your body. Break physical and mental tension. Take several deep breaths and get back to the job, refreshed. If you

don't do this you run the risk of getting nervous and tightening up. Your thinking may be hampered and you may make a few unnecessary mistakes.

Do not become worried or discouraged if the examination seems difficult to you. The questions in the various fields are purposely made difficult and searching so that the examination will discriminate effectively even among superior students. No one is expected to get a perfect or near-perfect score.

Remember that if the examination seems difficult to you, it may be even more difficult for your neighbor.

### Think!

This is not a joke because you're not an IBM machine. Nobody is able to write all the time and also to read and think through each question. You must plan each answer. Don't give hurried answers in an atmosphere of panic. Even though you see a lot of questions, remember that they are objective and not very time-consuming. Don't rush headlong through questions that must be thought through.

### Edit, Check, Proofread . . .

. . . after completing all the questions. Invariably, you will find some foolish errors which you needn't have made, and which you can easily correct. Don't just sit back or leave the room ahead of time. Read over your answers and make sure you wrote exactly what you meant to write. And that you wrote the answers in the right place. You might even find that you have omitted some answers inadvertently. You have budgeted time for this job of proofreading. PROOFREAD and pick up points.

One caution, though. Don't count on making major changes. And don't go in for wholesale changing of answers. To arrive at your answers in the first place you have read carefully and thought correctly. Second-guessing at this stage is more likely to result in wrong answers. So don't make changes unless you are quite certain you were wrong in the first place.

## FOLLOW DIRECTIONS CAREFULLY

In answering questions on the objective or short-form examination, it is most important to follow all instructions carefully. Unless you have marked the answers properly, you will not receive credit for them. In addition, even in the same examination, the instructions will not be consistent. In one section you may be urged to guess if you are not certain;

in another you may be cautioned against guessing. Some questions will call for the best choice among four or five alternatives; others may ask you to select the one incorrect or the least probable answer.

On some tests you will be provided with worked out fore-exercises, complete with correct answers. However, avoid the temptation to skip the directions and begin working just from reading the model questions and answers. Even though you may be familiar with that particular type of question, the directions may be different from those which you had followed previously. If the type of question should be new to you, work through the model until you understand it perfectly. This may save you time, and earn you a higher rating on the examination.

If the directions for the examination are written, read them carefully, at least twice. If the directions are given orally, listen attentively and then follow them precisely. For example, if you are directed to use plus (+) and minus (−) to mark true—false items, then don't use "T" and "F". If you are instructed to "blacken" a space on machine-scored tests, do not use a check (✔) or an "X". Make all symbols legible, and be sure that they have been placed in the proper answer space. It is easy, for example, to place the answer for item 5 in the space reserved for item 6. If this is done, then all of your following answers may be wrong. It is also very important that you understand the method they will use in scoring the examination. Sometimes they tell you in the directions. The method of scoring may affect the amount of time you spend on an item, especially if some items count more than others. Likewise, the directions may indicate whether or not you should guess in case you are not sure of the answer. Some methods of scoring penalize you for guessing.

*Cue Words*. Pay special attention to qualifying words or phrases in the directions. Such words as *one, best reason, surest, means most nearly the same as, preferable, least correct*, etc., all indicate that *one* response is called for, and that you must select the response which best fits the qualifications in the question.

*Time*. Sometimes a time limit is set for each section of the examination. If that is the case, follow the time instructions carefully. Your *exam budget* and your watch can help you here. Even if you haven't finished a section when the time limit is up, pass on to the next section. The examination has been planned according to the time schedule.

If the examination paper bears the instruction "Do not turn over page until signal is given," or "Do not start until signal is given," follow the instruction. Otherwise, you may be disqualified.

*Pay Close Attention*. Be sure you understand what you're doing at all times. Especially in dealing with true-false or multiple-choice questions it's vital that you understand the meaning of every question. It is normal to be working under stress when taking an examination, and it is easy to skip a word or jump to a false conclusion, which may cost you points on the examination. In many multiple-choice

and matching questions, the examiners deliberately insert plausible-appearing false answers in order to catch the candidate who is not alert.

*Answer clearly*. If the examiner who marks your paper cannot understand what you mean, you will not receive credit for your correct answer. On a True-False examination you will not receive any credit for a question which is marked both true and false. If you are asked to underline, be certain that your lines are under and not through the words and that they do not extend beyond them. When using the separate answer sheet it is important *when you decide to change an answer*, you erase the first answer completely. If you leave any graphite from the pencil on the wrong space it will cause the scoring machine to cancel the right answer for that question.

*Watch Your "Weights."* If the examination is "weighted" it means that some parts of the examination are considered more important than others and rated more highly. For instance, you may find that the instructions will indicate "Part I, Weight 50; Part II, Weight 25, Part III, Weight 25." In such a case, you would devote half of your time to the first part, and divide the second half of your time among Parts II and III.

## A Funny Thing . . .

. . . happened to you on your way to the bottom of the totem pole. You *thought* the right answer but you marked the *wrong* one.

1. You *mixed answer symbols!* You decided (rightly) that Baltimore (Choice D) was correct. Then you marked *B* (for Baltimore) instead of *D*.

2. You *misread* a simple instruction! Asked to give the *latest* word in a scrambled sentence, you correctly arranged the sentence, and then marked the letter corresponding to the *earliest* word in that miserable sentence.

3. You *inverted digits!* Instead of the correct number, 96, you wrote (or read) 69.
Funny? Tragic! Stay away from accidents.

Record your answers on the answer sheet one by one as you answer the questions. Care should be taken that these answers are recorded next to the appropriate numbers on your answer sheet. It is poor practice to write your answers first on the test booklet and then to transfer them all at one time to the answer sheet. This procedure causes many errors. And then, how would you feel if you ran out of time before you had a chance to transfer all the answers.

### When and How To Guess

Read the directions carefully to determine the scoring method that will be used. In some tests, the directions will indicate that guessing is advisable if you do not know the answer to a question. In such tests, only the right answers are counted in determining your score. If such is the case, don't omit any items. If you do not know the answer, or if you are not sure of your answer, then *guess*.

On the other hand, if the directions state that a scoring formula *will* be used in determining your score or that you are *not to guess,* then *omit* the question if you do not know the answer, or if you are not sure of the answer. When the scoring formu-

la is used, a percentage of the *wrong* answers will be subtracted from the number of *right* answers as a correction for haphazard guessing. It is improbable, therefore, that mere guessing will improve your score significantly. *It may even lower your score.* Another disadvantage in guessing under such circumstances is that it consumes valuable time that you might profitably use in answering the questions you know.

If, however, you are uncertain of the correct answer but have *some* knowledge of the question and are able to eliminate one or more of the answer choices as wrong, your chance of getting the right answer is improved, and it will be to your advantage to *answer* such a question rather than *omit* it.

## BEAT THE ANSWER SHEET

Even though you've had plenty of practice with the answer sheet used on machine-scored examinations, we must give you a few more, last-minute pointers.

The present popularity of tests requires the use of electrical test scoring machines. With these machines, scoring which would require the labor of several men for hours can be handled by one man in a fraction of the time.

The scoring machine is an amazingly intricate and helpful device, but the machine is not human. The machine cannot, for example, tell the difference between an intended answer and a stray pencil mark, and will count both indiscriminately. The machine cannot count a pencil mark, if the pencil mark is not brought in contact with the electrodes. For these reasons, specially printed answer sheets with response spaces properly located and properly filled

in must be employed. Since not all pencil leads contain the necessary ingredients, a special pencil must be used and a heavy solid mark must be made to indicate answers.

(a) Each pencil mark must be heavy and black. Light marks should be retraced with the special pencil.

(b) Each mark must be in the space between the pair of dotted lines and entirely fill this space.

(c) All stray pencil marks on the paper, clearly not intended as answers, must be completely erased.

(d) Each question must have only one answer indicated. If multiple answers occur, all extraneous marks should be thoroughly erased. Otherwise, the machine will give you *no* credit for your correct answer.

Be sure to use the special electrographic pencil!

HERE'S HOW TO MARK YOUR ANSWERS ON MACHINE-SCORED ANSWER SHEETS:

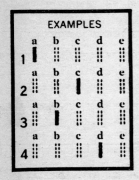

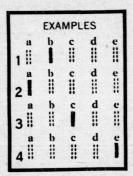

**Make only ONE mark for each answer. Additional and stray marks may be counted as mistakes. In making corrections, erase errors COMPLETELY. Make glossy black marks.**

Your answer sheet is the only one that reaches the office where papers are scored. For this reason it is important that the blanks at the top be filled in completely and correctly. The proctors will check

this, but just in case they slip up, make certain yourself that your paper is complete.

Many exams caution competitors against making any marks on the test booklet itself. Obey that caution even though it goes against your grain to work neatly. If you work neatly and obediently with the test booklet you'll probably do the same with the answer sheet. And that pays off in high scores.

# THE GIST OF TEST STRATEGY

● APPROACH THE TEST CONFIDENTLY. TAKE IT CALMLY.

● REMEMBER TO REVIEW, THE WEEK BEFORE THE TEST.

● DON'T "CRAM." BE CAREFUL OF YOUR DIET AND SLEEP ... ESPECIALLY AS THE TEST DRAWS NIGH.

● ARRIVE ON TIME ... AND READY.

● BRING THE COMPLETE KIT OF "TOOLS" YOU'LL NEED.

● CHOOSE A GOOD SEAT. GET COMFORTABLE AND RELAX.

● LISTEN CAREFULLY TO ALL DIRECTIONS.

● APPORTION YOUR TIME INTELLIGENTLY WITH AN "EXAM BUDGET."

● READ ALL DIRECTIONS CAREFULLY. TWICE IF NECESSARY. PAY PARTICULAR ATTENTION TO THE SCORING PLAN.

● LOOK OVER THE WHOLE TEST BEFORE ANSWERING ANY QUESTIONS.

● START RIGHT IN, IF POSSIBLE. STAY WITH IT. USE EVERY SECOND EFFECTIVELY.

● DO THE EASY QUESTIONS FIRST; POSTPONE HARDER QUESTIONS UNTIL LATER.

● DETERMINE THE PATTERN OF THE TEST QUESTIONS. IF IT'S HARD-EASY ETC., ANSWER ACCORDINGLY.

● READ EACH QUESTION CAREFULLY. MAKE SURE YOU UNDERSTAND EACH ONE BEFORE YOU ANSWER. RE-READ, IF NECESSARY.

● THINK! AVOID HURRIED ANSWERS. GUESS INTELLIGENTLY.

● WATCH YOUR WATCH AND "EXAM BUDGET," BUT DO A LITTLE BALANCING OF THE TIME YOU DEVOTE TO EACH QUESTION.

● GET ALL THE HELP YOU CAN FROM "CUE" WORDS.

● REPHRASE DIFFICULT QUESTIONS FOR YOURSELF. WATCH OUT FOR "SPOILERS."

● REFRESH YOURSELF WITH A FEW, WELL-CHOSEN REST PAUSES DURING THE TEST.

● USE CONTROLLED ASSOCIATION TO SEE THE RELATION OF ONE QUESTION TO ANOTHER AND WITH AS MANY IMPORTANT IDEAS AS YOU CAN DEVELOP.

● NOW THAT YOU'RE A "COOL" TEST-TAKER, STAY CALM AND CONFIDENT THROUGHOUT THE TEST. DON'T LET ANYTHING THROW YOU.

● EDIT, CHECK, PROOFREAD YOUR ANSWERS. BE A "BITTER ENDER." STAY WORKING UNTIL THEY MAKE YOU GO.

# ARCO BOOKS FOR MORE HELP

*Now what? You've read and studied the whole book, and there's still time before you take the test. You're probably better prepared than most of your competitors, but you may feel insecure about one or more of the probable test subjects. If so, you can still do something about it. Glance over this comprehensive list of books written with a view to solving your problems. One of them may be just what you need at this time . . . for the extra help that will assure your success.*

## ARCO BOOKS FOR TESTS OF ALL TYPES

Countless attractive careers are open to test takers, as you will see from this selective listing of Arco Books. One or more of them can assure success in the test you are now taking. Perhaps you've discovered that you are weak in language, verbal ability or mathematics. You can brush up in the privacy of your own home with a specialized Arco Book. Why flounder and fail when help is so easily available? Perhaps even more important than doing your best on your present test is to consider other opportunities that are open to you. Look over the lists and make plans for your future. You might get a few ideas for other tests you can start to study for *now*. By taking job tests now you place yourself in the enviable position of picking and choosing the *ideal* job. You'll be able to select from several positions. You won't have to settle for the one (or none).

Each of the following books was created under the same expert editorial supervision that produced the excellent book you are now using.

So even though we only list titles and prices, you can be sure that each book performs a real service . . . saves floundering and failure.

Every Arco Book is guaranteed. Return it for full refund in 10 days if not completely satisfied.

Whatever your goal . . . CIVIL SERVICE . . . TRADE LICENSE . . . TEACHING . . . PROFESSIONAL LICENSE . . . SCHOLARSHIP . . . ENTRANCE TO THE SCHOOL OF *YOUR* CHOICE . . . you can achieve it through the PROVEN QUESTION AND ANSWER METHOD.

## START YOUR CAREER BY MAILING THIS COUPON TODAY

**ORDER NOW** from your bookseller or direct from:

**ARCO PUBLISHING COMPANY, INC. 219 Park Avenue South, New York, N.Y. 10003**

*Please Rush The Following Arco Books*
*(Order by Number or Title)*

............................................................

............................................................

............................................................

............................................................

............................................................

☐ I enclose check, cash or money order for $_____(price of books, plus 50 ¢ for first book and 10¢ for each additional book, packing and mailing charge). No C.O.D.'s accepted.

☐ Please tell me if you have an ARCO COURSE for the position of . . . . . . . . . . . .
(Write in name of position)

☐ Please send me your free COMPLETE CATALOG

NAME_____

STREET_____

CITY_____STATE_____ZIP #_____

S3210

# CIVIL SERVICE AND TEST PREPARATION—GENERAL

| | | |
|---|---|---|
| Able Seaman, Deckhand, Scowman | 01376-1 | 5.00 |
| Accountant—Auditor | 00001-5 | 6.00 |
| Addiction Specialist, Senior, Supervising, Principal, Turner | 03351-7 | 8.00 |
| Administrative Assistant | 00148-8 | 6.00 |
| Air Traffic Controller, Turner | 02088-1 | 5.00 |
| American Foreign Service Officer | 00081-3 | 5.00 |
| Apprentice, Mechanical Trades | 00571-8 | 5.00 |
| Assistant Accountant—Junior Accountant—Account Clerk | 00056-2 | 6.00 |
| Assistant Station Supervisor, Turner | 03736-9 | 6.00 |
| Attorney, Assistant—Trainee | 01084-3 | 8.00 |
| Auto Machinist | 00513-0 | 6.00 |
| Auto Mechanic, Autoserviceman | 00514-9 | 6.00 |
| Bank Examiner—Trainee and Assistant | 01642-6 | 5.00 |
| Battalion and Deputy Chief, F.D. | 00515-7 | 6.00 |
| Beginning Office Worker | 00173-9 | 5.00 |
| Beverage Control Investigator | 00150-X | 4.00 |
| Bookkeeper—Account Clerk, Turner | 00035-X | 6.00 |
| Bridge and Tunnel Officer—Special Officer | 00780-X | 5.00 |
| Bus Maintainer—Bus Mechanic | 00111-9 | 5.00 |
| Bus Operator Conductor | 01553-5 | 5.00 |
| Buyer (Purchase Inspector) | 01366-4 | 4.00 |
| Captain, Fire Department | 00121-6 | 8.00 |
| Captain, Police Department | 00184-4 | 8.00 |
| Carpenter | 00135-6 | 6.00 |
| Cashier, Housing Teller | 00703-6 | 4.00 |
| Cement Mason—Mason's Helper, Turner | 03745-8 | 6.00 |
| Chemist—Assistant Chemist | 00116-X | 5.00 |
| City Planner | 01364-8 | 6.00 |
| Civil Engineer, Senior and Supervising, Turner | 00146-1 | 8.00 |
| Civil Service Arithmetic and Vocabulary | 00003-1 | 4.00 |
| Civil Service Handbook | 00040-6 | 1.50 |
| Claim Examiner—Law Investigator | 00149-6 | 5.00 |
| Clerk New York City—Clerk Income Maintenance | 00045-7 | 4.00 |
| Clerk—Steno Transcriber | 00838-5 | 5.00 |
| College Office Assistant | 00181-X | 5.00 |
| Complete Guide to U.S. Civil Service Jobs | 00537-8 | 2.00 |
| Construction Foreman—Supervisor—Inspector | 01085-1 | 5.00 |
| Correction Captain—Deputy Warden | 01358-3 | 8.00 |
| Correction Officer | 00186-0 | 5.00 |
| Court Officer | 00519-X | 6.00 |
| Criminal Law Quizzer, Salottolo | 02399-6 | 10.00 |
| Criminal Science Quizzer, Salottolo | 02407-0 | 5.00 |
| Detective Investigator, Turner | 03738-5 | 6.00 |
| Dietitian | 00083-X | 5.00 |
| Draftsman, Civil and Mechanical Engineering (All Grades) | 01225-0 | 6.00 |
| Electrical Engineer | 00137-2 | 5.00 |
| Electrical Inspector | 03350-9 | 8.00 |
| Electrician | 00084-8 | 6.00 |
| Electronic Equipment Maintainer, Turner | 01836-4 | 6.00 |
| Elevator Operator | 00051-1 | 3.00 |
| Employment Interviewer | 00008-2 | 6.00 |
| Employment Security Clerk | 00700-1 | 5.00 |
| Engineering Technician (All Grades), Turner | 01226-9 | 4.00 |
| Exterminator Foreman—Foreman of Housing Exterminators | 03740-7 | 6.00 |
| Federal Service Entrance Examinations | 00528-9 | 5.00 |
| File Clerk | 00962-4 | 5.00 |
| Fire Administration and Technology | 00604-8 | 6.00 |
| Firefighting Hydraulics, Bonadio | 00572-6 | 7.50 |
| Fireman, F.D. | 00010-4 | 5.00 |
| Food Service Supervisor—School Lunch Manager | 01378-8 | 6.00 |
| Foreman of Auto Mechanics | 01360-5 | 4.00 |
| Foreman | 00191-7 | 5.00 |
| Foreman (Tracks) T.A., Turner | 03739-3 | 6.00 |
| Gardener, Assistant Gardener | 01340-0 | 4.00 |
| General Entrance Series, Arco Editorial Board | 01961-1 | 4.00 |
| General Test Practice for 92 U.S. Jobs | 00011-2 | 5.00 |
| Guard—Patrolman | 00122-4 | 5.00 |
| Heavy Equipment Operator (Portable Engine) | 01372-9 | 5.00 |
| High School Civil Service Course | 00702-8 | 4.00 |
| Homestudy Course for Civil Service Jobs, Turner | 01587-X | 5.00 |
| Hospital Attendant | 00012-0 | 4.00 |
| Hospital Care Investigator Trainee (Social Case Worker I) | 01674-4 | 5.00 |
| Hospital Clerk | 01718-X | 3.00 |
| Housing Assistant | 00054-6 | 5.00 |
| Housing Caretaker | 00504-1 | 4.00 |
| Housing Inspector | 00055-4 | 5.00 |
| Housing Manager—Assistant Housing Manager | 00813-X | 5.00 |
| Housing Patrolman | 00192-5 | 5.00 |
| How to Pass Employment Tests, Liebers | 00715-X | 5.00 |
| Internal Revenue Agent | 00093-7 | 5.00 |
| Investigator—Inspector | 01670-1 | 5.00 |
| Janitor—Custodian | 00013-9 | 6.00 |
| Junior Administrator Development Examination (JADE) | 01643-4 | 5.00 |
| Junior and Assistant Civil Engineer | 01228-5 | 5.00 |
| Junior Federal Assistant | 01729-5 | 5.00 |
| Laboratory Aide, Arco Editorial Board | 01121-1 | 5.00 |
| Laborer—Federal, State and City Jobs | 00566-1 | 4.00 |
| Landscape Architect | 01368-0 | 5.00 |
| Laundry Worker | 01834-8 | 4.00 |
| Law and Court Stenographer | 00783-4 | 6.00 |
| Law Enforcement Positions | 00500-9 | 6.00 |
| Librarian | 00060-0 | 4.00 |
| Lieutenant, F.D. | 00123-2 | 8.00 |
| Lieutenant, P.D. | 00190-9 | 8.00 |
| Machinist—Machinist's Helper | 01123-8 | 6.00 |
| Mail Handler—U.S. Postal Service | 00126-7 | 5.00 |
| Maintainer's Helper, Group A and C—Transit Electrical Helper | 00175-5 | 5.00 |
| Maintenance Man | 00113-5 | 5.00 |
| Management and Administration Quizzer | 01537-3 | 6.00 |
| Mathematics, Simplified and Self-Taught | 00567-X | 4.00 |
| Mechanical Apprentice (Maintainer's Helper B) | 00176-3 | 5.00 |
| Mechanical Aptitude and Spatial Relations Tests | 00539-4 | 5.00 |
| Mechanical Engineer—Junior, Assistant & Senior Grades | 03314-2 | 8.00 |
| Messenger | 00017-1 | 3.00 |
| Mortuary Caretaker | 01354-0 | 4.00 |
| Motor Vehicle License Examiner | 00018-X | 5.00 |
| Motor Vehicle Operator | 00576-9 | 4.00 |
| Motorman (Subways) | 00061-9 | 6.00 |
| Nurse | 00143-7 | 6.00 |
| Office Assistant GS 1-4 Office Aide | 00043-0 | 5.00 |
| Office Machines Operator | 00728-1 | 4.00 |
| 1540 Questions and Answers for Electricians | 00754-0 | 5.00 |
| 1340 Questions and Answers for Firefighters, McGannon | 00857-1 | 4.00 |
| Operations and Maintenance Trainee | 01241-2 | 4.00 |
| Painter | 01772-4 | 5.00 |
| Parking Enforcement Agent | 00701-X | 4.00 |
| Patrol Inspector | 00101-1 | 4.00 |
| Peace Corps Placement Exams, Turner | 01641-8 | 4.00 |
| Personnel Examiner, Junior Personnel Examiner | 00648-X | 6.00 |
| Plumber—Plumber's Helper | 00517-3 | 6.00 |
| Police Administration and Criminal Investigation | 00565-3 | 6.00 |
| Police Administrative Aide, Turner | 02345-7 | 5.00 |
| Police Officer—Trainee P.D., Murray | 00019-8 | 5.00 |
| Police Science Advancement—Police Promotion Course | 02636-7 | 10.00 |
| Policewoman | 00062-7 | 5.00 |
| Post Office Clerk-Carrier | 00021-X | 4.00 |
| Post Office Motor Vehicle Operator | 01162-9 | 4.00 |
| Postal Inspector | 00194-1 | 5.00 |
| Postal Promotion Foreman—Supervisor | 00538-6 | 6.00 |
| Postal Service Officer | 01658-2 | 5.00 |
| Postmaster | 01522-5 | 5.00 |
| Practice for Civil Service Promotion | 00023-6 | 6.00 |
| Practice for Clerical, Typing and Stenographic Tests | 00005-8 | 5.00 |
| Principal Clerk—Stenographer | 01523-3 | 5.00 |

## MILITARY EXAMINATION SERIES

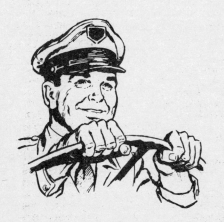
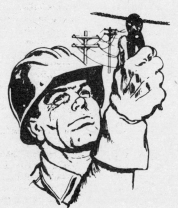
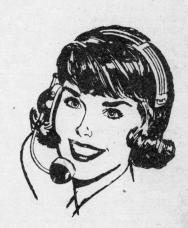

# EDUCATIONAL BOOKS

## HIGH SCHOOL AND COLLEGE PREPARATION

| | | |
|---|---|---|
| American College Testing Program Exams | 00694-3 | 5.00 |
| Arco Arithmetic Q & A Review, Turner | 02351-1 | 4.00 |
| The Arco Book of Biology, Mackean | 01913-1 | 4.00 |
| Better Business English, Classen | 01350-8 | 3.50 |
| Catholic High School Entrance Examination | 00987-X | 4.00 |
| The College Board's Examination, McDonough & Hansen | 02623-5 | 4.00 |
| College By Mail, Jensen | 02592-1 | 4.00 |
| College Entrance Tests, Turner | 01858-5 | 4.00 |
| College-Level Examination Program (CLEP), Turner | 02574-3 | 6.00 |
| College Scholarships | 00569-6 | 2.00 |
| Elements of Debate, Klopf & McCroskey | 01901-8 | 2.00 |
| Encyclopedia of English, Zeiger | 00655-X | 2.50 |
| English Grammar: 1,000 Steps | 02012-1 | 2.00 |
| Good English with Ease, Beckoff | 00859-8 | 2.00 |
| Guide to Financial Aids for Students in Arts and Sciences for Graduate and Professional Study, Searles & Scott | 02496-8 | 3.95 |
| High School Entrance and Scholarship Tests, Turner | 00666-8 | 4.00 |
| High School Entrance Examinations—Special Public and Private High Schools | 02143-8 | 4.00 |
| How to Prepare Your College Application, Kussin & Kussin | 01310-9 | 2.00 |
| How to Write Reports, Papers, Theses, Articles, Riebel | 02391-0 | 5.00 |
| New York State Regents Scholarship | 00400-2 | 4.00 |
| Organization and Outlining, Peirce | 02425-9 | 4.00 |
| Practice for Scholastic Aptitude Tests | 01035-5 | .95 |
| Q and A Biology—Question and Answer Course in General Biology, Hechtlinger | 00755-9 | 1.50 |
| Scholastic Aptitude Tests | 02038-5 | 4.00 |
| Scoring High on the NMSQT-PSAT, Turner | 00413-4 | 5.00 |
| Scoring High on Reading Tests | 00731-1 | 5.00 |
| Triple Your Reading Speed, Cutler | 02083-0 | 3.00 |
| Typing for Everyone, Levine | 02212-4 | 2.95 |

### GED PREPARATION

| | | |
|---|---|---|
| Comprehensive Math Review for the High School Equivalency Diploma Test, McDonough | 03420-3 | 4.00 |
| High School Equivalency Diploma Tests, Turner | 00110-0 | 5.00 |
| Learning to Use Our Language, Pulaski | 01518-7 | 2.50 |
| Preliminary Arithmetic For The High School Equivalency Diploma Test | 02165-9 | 3.00 |
| Preliminary Practice for the High School Equivalency Diploma Test | 01441-3 | 4.00 |
| Preparation for the Spanish High School Equivalency Diploma (Preparacion Para El Exam De Equivalencia De La Escuela Superior—En Espanol) | 02618-9 | 6.00 |
| Step-By-Step Guide to Correct English, Pulaski | 03402-5 | 3.95 |

### General Education Development Series

| | | |
|---|---|---|
| Correctness and Effectiveness of Expression (English HSEDT). Castellano, Guercio & Seitz | 03688-5 | 4.00 |
| General Mathematical Ability (Mathematics HSEDT). Castellano, Guercio & Seitz | 03689-3 | 4.00 |
| Reading Interpretation in Social Sciences, Natural Sciences, and Literature (Reading HSEDT). Castellano, Guercio & Seitz | 03690-4 | 4.00 |
| Teacher's Manual for the GED Series, Castellano. Guercio & Seitz | 03692-2 | 2.00 |

### COLLEGE BOARD ACHIEVEMENT TESTS

| | | |
|---|---|---|
| American History and Social Studies Achievement Test, Altman | 01722-8 | 1.45 |
| Biology Achievement Test, Miller & Weiss | 01263-3 | .95 |
| Chemistry Achievement Test, Spector & Weiss | 01264-1 | .95 |
| English Composition Achievement Test | 01247-1 | .95 |
| French Achievement Test, Biezunski & Boisrond | 01668-X | 1.45 |
| German Achievement Test, Greiner | 01698-1 | 1.45 |
| Latin Achievement Test | 01743-0 | 1.45 |
| Mathematics: Level I Achievement Test, Bramson | 01266-8 | .95 |
| Mathematics: Level II Achievement Test, Bramson | 01456-3 | .95 |
| Physics Achievement Test, Bruenn | 01265-X | 1.95 |
| Spanish Achievement Test, Jassey | 01741-4 | 1.45 |

## PROFESSIONAL CAREER EXAM SERIES

| | | |
|---|---|---|
| Action Guide for Executive Job Seekers and Employers, Uris | 01787-2 | 3.95 |
| Bar Exams | 01124-6 | 5.00 |
| The C.P.A. Exam: Accounting by the "Parallel Point" Method (Two Volumes), Lipscomb | 02020-2 | 15.00 |
| Certified General Automobile Mechanic, Turner | 02900-5 | 5.00 |
| Computer Programmer, Luftig | 01232-3 | 6.00 |
| Computers and Automation,—Revised Edition, Brown | 01745-7 | 5.00 |
| Graduate Business Admission Test | 01063-0 | 5.00 |
| Graduate Record Examination Aptitude | 00824-5 | 4.00 |
| Health Insurance Agent (Hospital, Accident, Health, Life) | 02153-5 | 5.00 |
| How A Computer System Works, Brown & Workman | 03424-6 | 5.95 |
| How to Become a Successful Model, Krem | 03625-7 | 5.00 |
| The Installation and Servicing of Domestic Oil Burners, Mitchell & Mitchell | 00437-1 | 10.00 |
| Insurance Agent and Broker | 02149-7 | 6.00 |
| Law School Admission Test, Turner | 00840-7 | 4.00 |
| Life Insurance Agents' Examination | 02343-0 | 5.00 |
| Miller Analogies Test—1400 Analogy Questions | 01114-9 | 4.00 |
| The 1974-75 Airline Guide to Stewardess and Steward Careers, Morton | 02435-6 | 4.95 |
| Notary Public | 00180-1 | 4.00 |
| Oil Burner Installer | 00096-1 | 6.00 |
| Pharmacist License Tests | 00516-5 | 4.00 |
| Playground and Recreation Director's Handbook | 01096-7 | 4.00 |
| Quizzer for Students of Education, Walton | 01447-4 | 4.00 |
| Real Estate License Examination, Gladstone | 03755-5 | 5.00 |
| Real Estate Salesman and Broker | 00098-8 | 6.00 |
| Refrigeration License Manual, Harfenist | 02726-6 | 10.00 |
| Resumes for Executive Job Hunters, Shykind | 02424-0 | 4.00 |
| Resumes That Get Jobs, Resume Service | 01076-2 | 2.00 |
| Security Representatives' Examinations, Stefano | 01934-4 | 5.00 |
| Stationary Engineer and Fireman | 00070-8 | 6.00 |
| The Test of English as a Foreign Language (TOEFL), Moreno, Babin & Scallon | 02944-7 | 6.00 |

### ADVANCED GRE SERIES

| | | |
|---|---|---|
| Biology: Advanced Test for the G.R.E., Miller | 01068-1 | 3.95 |
| Business: Advanced Test for the G.R.E., Berman, Malea & Yearwood | 01599-3 | 3.95 |
| Chemistry: Advanced Test for the G.R.E., Weiss | 01069-X | 3.95 |
| Economics: Advanced Test for the G.R.E., Zabrenski & Heydari-Darafshian | 01557-8 | 3.95 |
| Education: Advanced Test for the G.R.E., Jassey | 01223-4 | 3.95 |
| Engineering: Advanced Test for the G.R.E., Ingham & Nesbitt | 01604-3 | 3.95 |
| French: Advanced Test for the G.R.E., Dethierry | 01070-3 | 3.95 |
| Geography: Advanced Test for the G.R.E., White | 01710-4 | 3.95 |
| Geology: Advanced Test for the G.R.E., Dolgoff | 01071-1 | 3.95 |
| History: Advanced Test for the G.R.E., Smith | 01072-X | 3.95 |
| Literature: Advanced Test for the G.R.E. | 01073-8 | 3.95 |
| Mathematics: Advanced Test for the G.R.E., Bramson | 01458-X | 3.95 |
| Music: Advanced Test for the G.R.E., Murphy | 01471-7 | 3.95 |
| Philosophy: Advanced Test for the G.R.E., Steiner | 01472-5 | 3.95 |
| Physical Education: Advanced Test for the G.R.E., Rubinger | 01609-4 | 3.95 |
| Physics: Advanced Test for the G.R.E., Bruenn | 01074-6 | 3.95 |
| Political Science: Advanced Test for the G.R.E., Meador & Stewart | 01459-8 | 3.95 |
| Psychology: Advanced Test for the G.R.E., Millman & Nisbett | 01145-9 | 3.95 |
| Sociology: Advanced Test for the G.R.E., Reddan | 01444-X | 3.95 |
| Spanish: Advanced Test for the G.R.E., Jassey | 01075-4 | 3.95 |
| Speech: Advanced Test for the G.R.E., Graham | 01526-8 | 3.95 |

S3210